Innovative Smart Healthcare and Bio-Medical Systems

Innovative Smart Healthcare and Bio-Medical Systems

AI, Intelligent Computing, and Connected Technologies

Edited by
Abdel-Badeeh M. Salem

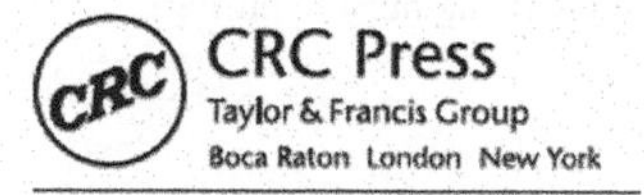

CRC Press is an imprint of the
Taylor & Francis Group, an informa business

First edition published 2021
by CRC Press
6000 Broken Sound Parkway NW, Suite 300
Boca Raton, FL 33487-2742

and by CRC Press
2 Park Square, Milton Park, Abingdon, Oxon OX14 4RN

ISBN: 9780367490614 (hbk)
ISBN: 9781003044291 (ebk)

Contents

Contributors

Tamer Abdelkader
Faculty of Computer and Information Sciences
Ain Shams University
Cairo, Egypt

Shaymaa Adnan Abdulrahman
Department of Computer Engineering
Imam Ja'afar Al-Sadiq University
Baghdad, Iraq
Ain Shams University
Cairo, Egypt

Ibrahim M. Ahmed
Department of Information Technology,
Faculty of Computer and Information Technology
Karary University
Khartoum, Sudan

Marco Alfonse
Department of Computer Science,
Faculty of Computer and Information Sciences
Ain Shams University
Cairo, Egypt

Vitalina Babenko
Full professor
International E-commerce and Hotel & Restaurant Business Department
V.N. Karazin Kharkiv National University
Kharkiv, Ukraine

Adriana Burlea-Schiopoiu
University of Craiova
Craiova, Romania

T.N. Bzhalava
Georgian Technical University (GTU)
Tbilisi, Georgia

Olena Chebanyuk
Software Engineering Department
National Aviation University
Kyiv, Ukraine

Khaled El-Bahnasy
Faculty of Computer and Information Sciences
Ain Shams University
Cairo, Egypt

El-Sayed A. El-Dahshan
Professor
Computational Physics
Ain Shams University
Cairo, Egypt

Koudoua Ferhati
University of Craiova
Craiova, Romania

Galib Hamidov
Information Technologies Department
Baku, Azerbaijan

Seyed Mojtaba Mir Hosseini
Kerman University of Medical Sciences
Kerman, Iran

Rania R. Hussein
Lecturer
Computer Science department
Higher Technological Institute
Cairo, Egypt

P.J. Kervalishvili
Georgian Technical University (GTU)
Tbilisi, Georgia

Antoanela Naaji
Vasile Goldis Western University of Arad
Arad, Romania

Nasim Nasiri
Kerman University of Medical Sciences
Kerman, Iran

Olexandr Palahin
V.M. Glushkov Institute of Cybernetics
National Academy of
Sciences of Ukraine
Kyiv, Ukraine

Marius Popescu
Western University of Arad
Arad, Romania

Amin Saberinia
Kerman University of Medical Sciences
Kerman, Iran

Abdel-Badeeh M. Salem
Full professor
Ain Shams University
Cairo, Egypt

Sarah A. Soliman
Assistant lecturer
Department of Computers and
Information, Higher Technological
Institute
10th of Ramadan, Egypt

S. Lenty Stuwart
Department of Electronics and
Communication Engineering
University College of Engineering,
Nagercoil
Tamil Nadu, India

Mohamad Yousef
Faculty of Computer and Information
Sciences
Ain Shams University
Cairo, Egypt

Yuriy Zaychenko
Institute for Applied System Analysis
Igor Sikorsky Kyiv Polytechnic Institute
Kyiv, Ukraine

Dina Ziadlou
Colorado Technical University
Colorado, USA

1 Smart Software for Real-Time Image Analysis

Marius Popescu and Antoanela Naaji

CONTENTS

1.1 INTRODUCTION

A digital image is the representation of a real image, being constituted as a two-dimensional data structure, which can be natural numbers, complex numbers, or real numbers represented on a finite number of bits. An image element is called pixel, the whole image being composed of a string of octets. The color components of pixel are red, green, and blue (RGB). The image formats are known according to their file extension, such as bitmap (BMP), the gross form of the image; Joint Photographic Expert Group (JPG), intended to compress the images taken from reality; Graphic Interchange Format (GIF), a good quality format and very strong compression; Tagged Image File Format (TIF), used for professional photos due to its versatility and nondestructive compression; Digital Imaging and Communications in Medicine (DICOM), used for medical images; and raw, which contain the entire information that was captured by the sensor at the moment of the shooting.

In real and legal practice, there are situations where fraudulent images are used. Detecting a fake ordinary image or video edits is not an easy task. Until recently, only few software could determine whether an image was original or whether someone manipulated it. Currently, the image can be cracked by using a technique called Deep Video Portraits (DVP) [1], which allows the imitation of a great variety of movements, including a three-dimensional (3D) head view, its rotation, shifting it, and even blinking. This uses artificial intelligence by which movement data are taken from the source and transmitted to the digital image that is to be integrated into the video. Through artificial intelligence, motion patterns are collected, analyzed, calculated, and predicted in order to create a more realistic video [2]. DVP is a very effective method for creating computerized animations, converting into realistic photo images, and is extremely easy to confound with a person's real image.

Some software that implement many filters that work automatically or semiautomatically are already available. Software developers have created 3D reconstruction algorithms over 50 smart filters, most of which are unique. These algorithms are part of the specialized software, and some of them are embedded into the visual video cameras. There are companies that patent at least five new technologies related to photo and video processing. Among these, there are algorithms that allow to perform 3D face and object reconstruction, measure the dimensions and distances between objects on photo and video, analyze the motion model of an object in a frame, etc. VOCORD VideoExpert is a powerful tool used for analyzing and improving digital photo and video materials [3]. The program restores indescribable objects on the original photos or videos – faces of people, license plates, or text, greatly improving the quality of the material.

Amped Authenticate is another software package used to authenticate forensic images and the incorrect detection of digital photos [4]. Current products and processes focus on one or several scientific instruments. With the help of authentication, *Amped* empowers law enforcement experts and legal medicine laboratories with an instrument capable of detecting any manipulation that has been done on an image and checking whether a digital photograph has been generated by a specific device. Previously, specialized applications have been highlighted in this domain, but there are other applications that can perform a similar analysis of the image (satellite), the best known being Peripheral Component Interconnect Geomatica [5], Environmental for Visualizing Images (ENVI), or ER Mapper [6].

Exelis and Environmental Systems Research Institute have joined to improve the interoperability between image processing and geographic information system (GIS) software through ENVI and ArcGIS. Practically, ENVI is a selection of workflows and tools that have been integrated into the ArcGIS ArcToolbox environment.

Most existing applications in this domain are professional applications that offer, in most cases, the "package" functionality at a fairly high cost. As a rule, they are marketed as a trial version, valid for a limited time, or as a simple editor or viewer that does not include any functionality. In addition to this impediment, many of them come as third parties, which require integration with other applications. An example is ENVI. If it is desired to use some of the processing or methods that it offers, another application, such as ArcGIS, which may be available at a cost, is required in order to enable the use of the ENVI functionalities.

These applications may also require a user guide or course as their complexity makes them inaccessible for some users. Few of them even require an Internet connection for certain packages and functionalities. Our software was developed in order to avoid these drawbacks of the existing applications and make it accessible to everyone.

This chapter is organized as follows: the second section presents some techniques related to image processing, the third section is about the theoretical background, the fourth section presents the application and its implementation, and the fifth section evaluates and validates it. Finally, few conclusions are presented in the conclusion section.

1.2 TURNING PICTURES AND VIDEOS TO RECORD/EVIDENCE

Image processing is a complex and dynamic domain with numerous applications in many areas. New technologies used in the image processing industry allow the application of new algorithms and methods for extracting useful information from the image: parallel algorithms, neural network-based classifiers, etc. There are also real-time systems implementations based on the image processing, systems such as those used in medicine, or the ones for the automated process control. Many improvements have also been made for the systems that process fingerprints, face, or writing recognition, etc.

The bias of the imaging can be performed by transforming the color components of each pixel.

The brightness of an image can be changed by adding a value to the color components of each pixel so that it does not come out of the 0.255 range. If a positive value is used, a lighter luminosity will be obtained, and if a negative value is used, a darker luminosity will be obtained.

The rotation of an image can be achieved by mapping an input pixel with the output position, determined by rotating with an angle, around an origin. Translating an image means moving the pixels from the original image, with a value that the user specifies, into the new positions.

The reflection or mirroring converts the original image so that the pixels are reflected from an axis specified in the new position in the target image. The reflection may be relative to a horizontal axis of order or to a vertical axis of abscissa. Mirroring may be after an axis pointing in an arbitrary direction also, which passes through the point of origin. In general, image processing involves two essential procedures: fusion of images and pseudo-coloring of images. Image fusion is a process of combining relevant information from a set of images into a single image, where the resulting image will contain more information than any of the images used before the merging [7]. Various methods have been developed to achieve the fusion of images. Some regions of the images, which are focused, have pixels of greater intensity than the rest.

Thus, the arithmetic mean algorithm is a way to get an image with all the focused regions. The algorithm consists in calculating the pixel average of the input images, and the resulting value is assigned to the pixel in the output image. The operation is repeated for each pixel in the image [8].

The algorithm of the maximal selection chooses the focus regions of each input image by electing the highest value of each pixel, resulting in an image with highly focused regions.

Discrete wavelet transform (DWT) is a process of image decomposition in low-high, high-low, and high-high space frequency bands on different scales, and the low-low band at the largest scale [9]. The low-low band contains the average of the information in the image, while the other bands contain information regarding the direction due to the spatial orientation.

Principal component analysis (PCA) is a mathematical *tool* that converts a number of correlated variables into a number of uncorrelated variables [10]. The algorithm is often used in compressing and classifying images. The uncorrelated transformed variables are called main components. The first main component is considered to be along the direction with the maximum variation. The second main component is constrained to stretch in the subspace that is perpendicular to the first one. The third main component is taken in the direction of the maximum variation in the subspace that is perpendicular to the first two and so on.

Pseudo-coloring, in the image processing [11], represents the color assignment for gray values according to a specific criterion. The term "pseudo-coloring" emphasizes the fact that these colors are artificially assigned in opposition to the true colors [12]. As in the fusion of images, pseudo-coloring can also be performed through different techniques.

Intensity slicing is a technique that can be better explained by interpreting the grayscale image as a 3D function that is cut by a plane that is parallel to the plane of the image. The intensity-color transformation is a method that involves performing three independent transformations on the intensity of any input pixel. The results are placed separately on the RGB channels, producing a composite image that has its colors modulated by the transformation functions.

In image acquisition, noise is the result of errors and is expressed by pixel values that do not reflect the intensity of the true image. Thus, if the image is a photocopy of a photo, the granulation of the film or photographic paper is a source of noise. If the image is purchased directly via satellite/digital camera, then the acquisition equipment can bring noise to the image.

Also, satellite image transmission can produce noise. Some image components or noise reduction are favored by filtering, which is a technique used for modifying or improving the image in order to favor certain components or remove other components. The noise of the image can be reduced by replacing the value of each pixel with the median of neighboring pixel values.

Median filtering is an effective image smoothing technique for noise abatement; however, it has the disadvantage of affecting the contours of the objects included in the image. Contours are critical in an image; therefore, we need to eliminate the noise. For a moderate noise level, the median is the ideal way to remove the noise, preserving the contours. Digital image filters are used to edit digital images in order to transform or improve them. They can also be used to modify or retouch photos, apply special effects, or make unique transformations using light and deformation effects. For example, the filters provided by Photoshop or ImageJ are organized by categories according to the desired result: stylistic and artistic effects, geometric distortions (creating 3D effects or other reforming effects), pixel displacements, etc.

1.3 THEORETICAL BACKGROUND OF THE APPLICATION

Analyzing a specific object within an image requires its contour to be highlighted with the help of the image segmentation procedure. Segmentation and contour extraction are important steps in image analysis. The segmentation process is considered as a process of classifying objects in an image. The purpose of segmentation is to simplify the representation of images in useful information by partitioning into areas. Although there are high complexity algorithms, image segmentation remains application dependent, with no unique solution identified. The segmentation method is used to detect certain objects or contours in an image. The contour of an object is given by the set of pixels of the object that have at least one neighbor outside the object. Segmenting images by this method involves locating pixels corresponding to contours of objects present in the image. After the acquisition of the image (e.g., through satellite telecommunications networks), it follows the analysis of the characteristics of a particular area/object in the image, which is a complex process having the following general processing stream: preprocessing, improvement and highlighting, and result processing.

The filters are used within each layer of the application flow, where algorithms and drivers are implemented, such as the salt and pepper filter, the low-pass filter, the high-pass filter, *contrast stretching*, *grayscale* processing, fusion, and pseudo-coloring of images.

The *salt and pepper filter/noise* is generally caused by the flaws of the photo/video sensor, memory location faults, or sync errors in the digitization process [13]. The *salt and pepper* is represented in an analytical form as follows:

$$\text{Histogram}_{\text{Salt\&Paper}} = \begin{cases} A & g = a(\text{paper}) \\ B & g = b(\text{salt}) \end{cases} \tag{1.1}$$

In the noise model type of salt and pepper, there are only two possible values. The likelihood of occurrence of each of them is generally less than 0.1. At higher values than these, the noise will dominate the image. For an 8-bit image, the typical intensity value for the pepper noise is approximately zero, and for the salt noise it is around 255.

The *low-pass filter* attenuates or blocks the passage of high frequencies, and allows only the unattenuated passage of the space low frequencies. They are usually used to reduce noise from images. The ideal low-pass filter [14] blocks all frequencies that are higher than the cut-off frequency ω_0,

$$H(k,1)=\begin{cases} 1 & \left(k^2+1^2\right) \le \omega_0^2 \\ 0 & \text{else} \end{cases} \tag{1.2}$$

and the Gaussian low-pass filter brings to the attenuation of the high frequencies without completely removing them as the ideal filter.

$$H(k,1)=e^{\left(-\frac{\omega}{\omega_0}\right)^2}, \omega^2 = k^2+1^2 \tag{1.3}$$

The effects that result from this filter are capable of smoothing the image and without effects of ringing wave. It usually applies before segmentation (based on regions or edges) to eliminate noise. Other filters are the *butterworth*

$$H(k,1) = \frac{1}{1+\left(\frac{\omega}{\omega_0}\right)^n} \tag{1.4}$$

and *trapezoidal filters* (which introduce a circular wave effect stronger than the Gaussian or butterworth, but weaker than the ideal one).

$$H(k,1) = \begin{cases} 1 & \text{for } \omega<\omega_0 \\ \frac{\omega-\omega_1}{\omega_0-\omega_1} & \text{for } \omega_0 \le \omega \le \omega_1 \\ 0 & \text{for } \omega>\omega_1 \end{cases} \tag{1.5}$$

The *high-pass filter* attenuates or blocks the passage of low frequencies, allowing only the unattenuated passage of space high frequencies. The ideal filter passes high blocks all frequencies smaller than a cut-off frequency. The resulting image after applying this filter has a circular wave pattern. The Gaussian high-pass filter performs a gradual reduction of the low frequencies so that the high frequencies could pass unaltered through the filter.

$$H(k,1)=1-e^{\left(-\frac{\omega}{\omega_0}\right)^2}, \omega^2 = k^2+1^2 \tag{1.6}$$

In practice, this filter is combined with a Gaussian low-pass filter, and thus results in the *Gaussian difference*. Another filter is the *butterworth* high-pass filter.

$$H(k,1) = 1-\frac{1}{1+\left(\frac{\omega}{\omega_0}\right)^n} \tag{1.7}$$

Contrast stretching is a simple technique for image improvement that improves the contrast of the image by "stretching" the range of pixel intensities so that it covers a range of desired values, for example, the entire range of values supported by the image to which it applies. This type of improvement is more sophisticated than the histogram equalization, where only a linear scaling function applies to the pixel intensities [15]. Before "stretching" can be performed, it is necessary to set the upper limit and lower limit of pixel value over which the image is normalized. Often, these limits are the minimum and maximum pixel values that the image supports. For example, for 8-bit *gray level* images, the lower and upper limits are 0 and 255, respectively.

Grayscale processing [16] is a very simple technique and consists in equalizing the three color components of each pixel. A commonly used method is the mediation of the three components.

Image fusion is a process of combining relevant information from a set of images belonging to the same scene into a single image [17]. This process has some requirements, namely: the merged image must contain all the input image information and the fusion of images must not introduce other artifacts which may lead to wrong analysis.

Image fusion methods can be divided into two groups: spatial domain-based fusion, which directly works on the pixels from the input image (in this group, we have algorithms such as minimum selection, maximum selection, arithmetic mean, or the analysis of the main component), and domain transformation-based fusion, which relies primarily on the image transfer in a frequency domain (in this group, we have algorithms such as DWT). In the case of the minimum selection, the result of the fusion is obtained by selecting the pixel with the minimum intensity in the fused images.

$$F(i,j) = \sum_{i=0}^{m} \sum_{j=0}^{n} \min\left(A(i,j), B(i,j), \ldots\right) \tag{1.8}$$

where $A(i,j)$, $B(i,j)$ are input images and $F(i,j)$ is the resulting image.

In the case of the arithmetic mean, the result of the fusion is obtained by calculating the arithmetic mean of the pixel intensity from the input images.

$$F(i,j) = \frac{A(i,j), B(i,j) + \ldots}{n} \tag{1.9}$$

The main component analysis is a subspace method that reduces multidimensional sets of data into smaller dimensions for analysis. This method determines the balance/ponderosity of each source image using its own proper vector at the matrix's own covariance value, for each source image.

DWT is a multi-resolution image decomposition technique that offers a variety of channels that represent the image characteristics in different frequency sub-bands. When the decomposition is accomplished, the approximation and detail components can be separated. DWT converts the image from the spatial domain to the frequency domain. The image is divided by both vertical and horizontal lines, representing the first DWT order. Let $s(n_1,n_2)$ be the input image of size $N_1 \times N_2$, then the wavelet and scaling functions are:

$$\begin{aligned} \omega_{\Phi}\left(j_0, k_1, k_2\right) &= \frac{1}{\sqrt{N_1 N_2}} \sum_{n_1=0}^{N_1-1} \sum_{n_2=0}^{N_2-1} s\left(n_1, n_2\right) \Phi_{j_0,k_1,k_2}\left(n_1, n_2\right) \\ \omega_{\in}\left(j_0, k_1, k_2\right) &= \frac{1}{\sqrt{N_1 N_2}} \sum_{n_1=0}^{N_1-1} \sum_{n_2=0}^{N_2-1} s\left(n_1, n_2\right) \in_{j_0,k_1,k_2}\left(n_1, n_2\right) \end{aligned} \tag{1.10}$$

1.4 DESCRIPTION OF THE APPLICATION

The operating principle behind the application consists in taking a stream of image-type data and processing them along a series of modules and filters to get the final result that highlights some features. Each module represents a general step in the processing line and plays a well-defined role in the processing of information, with various algorithms, data structures, and implementation technologies. These modules are:

- The image acquisition module, which takes over high-resolution TIFF format images from an external source and transforms them into a data structure and stores them externally into easily accessible (JPEG) formats.
- The preprocessing module, which is an optional one but often very necessary. If the images on which the actual processing is desired require some "adjustments," this module provides a number of filters that may prove to be useful.
- The module of image enhancement and highlighting the features of the images, which is considered to be the "heart" of the entire application, having the role of improving the features of the image by image fusion methods, and highlighting or mapping the regions of the image using pseudo-coloring techniques.
- The result processing module, which is the last in the execution thread and deals with the analysis of the data obtained in the previous step, comparing the resulting image and the areas highlighted with a legend that will determine the characteristics of interest.

1.4.1 Application Architecture and Module Description

The organization of the application under the "pipes and filters" pattern [18] is an ideal structure for the systems that process a data stream, each step being encapsulated into a filter that represents a *pipeline* processing unit.

The advantages of organizing the application under this pattern include flexibility in changing filters (changing between filters and the interface and functionality is easy), flexibility by recombination (ease of reconfiguring a *pipeline* for including new filters, or using the existing filters in another sequence), reuse of filters (small filters are easy to reuse if the environment allows them to be connected in a simple way), and efficiency through parallel processing (filters run on different threads, and from this point of view, pipes-and-filters systems can benefit from the advantage of a multiprocessor).

The disadvantages include expensive or inflexible information exchange (the information must be encoded, transmitted, and then decoded), gaining efficiency by paralleling processes is just an illusion (the cost of data and synchronization can be high), and error handling (the disadvantage of the structure lies in the dependence of the current module on the previous one and the fact that the occurrence of a possible data processing error in one of the modules from the first steps may propagate an error along the entire process line). Despite these disadvantages, this architectural pattern fits the application developed by us and presented in this chapter. The implementation of the application by using the "pipes and filters" pattern was done in the Java programming language. The image pickup module has the role of uploading the image from an external source to the application (hard disk, CD/DVD), for processing. The application allows the processing of a single image as well as the simultaneous processing of two images. Thus, the user interface will have dedicated areas for uploading these images. Once the external files are taken in, they are intermediary saved in an easily accessible (JPEG) file format. This will be done after each processing, each step being seen as a filter that represents a processing unit.

Preprocessing prepares the information for the next stage, the processing step, by applying filtration operations. This step in the execution flow can be optional, depending on the user's requirements. From the previous module, data ready for processing reach this module in which it is decided to preprocess them. The steps that run here are similar to those of the image acquisition. The user can dynamically add the filter(s) and the order in which the image(s) passes. This is done with the ease of a JPanel where each process is represented by a *drop-down* menu called JComboBox, which contains the entire list of processes available in the application.

Improving and highlighting the image features is the main application module, including processing, such as fusion of images and pseudo-coloring. On the fusion of images, algorithms for minimum and maximal selection, fusion by calculating the arithmetic mean, and DWT were implemented, as well as an intensity slicing algorithm for pseudo-coloring, which uses seven coloring levels. The algorithms were implemented without using any external bookstore, or the Application Programming Interface (API). The image is read by using its location and then transformed into a BufferedImage-type object. The transformation into this object will allow an easy extraction of the image pixel matrix.

Thus, the following steps will represent the pure processing for accomplishing the above-mentioned methods. Image fusion requires two or more images. The application will only fuse for two images. Typically, of the two images, one will be a panchromatic image and the other one will be a different frequency band image (Table 1.1 [19]).

Once the two images are available as BufferedImage objects, the actual processing may start. The fusion technique consists in selecting the minimum pixel value from the same position in both images and creating a new image with them. This theory

TABLE 1.1
Wave Length Bands

Band	Name	Band width(λ, μm)	Space resolution
1.	Blue	0.45–0.515	30 m
2.	Green	0.525–0.605	30 m
3.	Red	0.63–0.69	30 m
4.	Near infrared	0.75–0.90	30 m
5.	Shortwave IR-1	1.55–1.75	30 m
6.	Thermal IR	10.4–12.5	60 m/120 m
7.	Shortwave IR-2	2.09–2.35	30 m
8.	Panchromatic	0.52–0.9	15 m

applied in our situation undergoes some changes. As shown in Table 1.1, the eight-band image has a much higher resolution than the others, in which case the pixels in the same position will no longer match. However, whatever the second image will be, excluding the one of the eight bands, the following relationship will occur:

```
panchromatic.dimension() = α*secondImage.dimension();
```

where α represents how many times the eight-band image is larger than any of the other images. If the value of α is set, then the selection can begin. A first step will be to find out which of the two images is larger. Thus, the dimensions of the two images will be calculated and will be compared in order to determine which one is the eight-band image. Once the dimensions are calculated, it is known which of the two images has the higher resolution, but the value of α is still unknown. In the present case, α will consist of two components: αW, which represents how many times the eight-band image is larger in width than any other image, and αH, which means the same thing, but in height. Finally, it will be determined how many pixels in the panchromatic image correspond to a pixel from any other image. Finding this, we can begin to scroll through the two images and select the minimum. The browsing is performed using two repetitive type *for*. structures, one in width and the other one in height. The pixels are extracted from the BufferedImage object as follows:

```
intpixelValue = bufferedImage.getRGB(x,y);
intredPixelValue = (pixelValue&0x00ff0000)>>16;
intgreenPixelValue = (pixelValue&0x0000ff00)>>8;
intbluePixelValue = pixelValue&0x000000ff;
```

where x and y are the coordinates from which we wish to extract the pixel, and redPixelValue, greenPixelValue, and bluePixelValueare are, respectively, the intensity values for the red, green, and blue colors of that pixel.

In this case, the image will be gray scale, and all three values for red, green, and blue are equal; therefore, we only need one of them. Extracting the pixels in the above case is only valid for the lower resolution image, and for the panchromatic image we will have to extract the corresponding αW × αH pixels. Having all the pixel values in the eight-band image and of the pixel in the other image, one can unanimously calculate these values, and that minimum will be the pixel from the current position of the final image. The maximum selection method consists in selecting the maximum pixel value from the same position in both images and creating a new image with them. This method is almost identical to the fusion method by selecting the minimum, the only thing that changes being the one from the final step.

Thus, instead of calculating the minimum value between all the pixels in the panchromatic image and the pixel in the different band image, the maximum will be calculated, and this will be a result in the final image. The fusion by calculating the arithmetic mean uses the same principle, instead, at the final step, for the pixels extracted from both images, the arithmetic mean is calculated. The value resulting from this calculation is the pixel value in the result image.

The DWT method is slightly different from the one presented above, due to the fact that it may contain them, plus high-pass and low-pass filters in the preprocessing module. Implementation of this method involves the following three steps:

- Decomposing the image by a coefficient, using high-pass and low-pass filters
- The fusion of the decomposed images using a simple method previously described
- Composing the resulting images until reaching one image, namely, the final image. Both loaded images will undergo the same decomposition transformations. The initial images will be applied by a high-pass and a low-pass filter, resulting in two images. The two resulting images will also be submitted to the same methods and filters. This transformation will be repeated by a number of times equal to the decomposition coefficient. The decomposition coefficient can be entered by the user from the keyboard. Finally, after decomposing, there will be $2n$ (where n is the decomposition coefficient) for the panchromatic band and the other band of choice. Following each decomposition process, the result will be saved in the project directory. The images resulting from applying the high-pass and low-pass filters on the first image will fuse, using a simple fusion method, with the images resulting from applying the filters to the second image. As in the decomposition coefficient, the fusion modality can be selected by the user. Having the $2n$ merged images, their composition may begin. This composition is also called *inverse discrete wavelet transform* and consists in adding the pixels from these images until a single image is reached, which is the final image. All the states of this process are presented in Figure 1.1 [19].

The last step of this module is the pseudo-coloring function. Once we have the enhanced image, we can apply the transformation in order to map the areas of the image in color. For pseudo-coloring, we will use the intensity slicing procedure with seven ramps for coloring. Thus, the image will be browsed pixel by pixel, and for each pixel a gray value will be drawn; according to this value, it will fit in a certain color as shown in Table 1.2 [19].

After this processing, the final image, which will be transmitted to the resulting processing module, will be analyzed. In order to better highlight the relationships between all these functionalities, a class diagram was added for the improvement and highlighting of the features belonging to the preprocessing module presented (see Figure 1.2)[19].

The resulted processing module is the part where the processed image, ready to be analyzed, is shown to the user. The actual displaying is done in a JFrame object type that will contain a panel with the final image. In addition to this panel containing the final image, there will be a panel with a legend in which the meaning of each color, and therefore each region, plus a set of rules or combinations of results will be presented (because the classification of the images based on the information extracted from one channel is quite inconclusive) to help with this analysis process. In order to get as much information as possible, needed for classification, combinations of bands

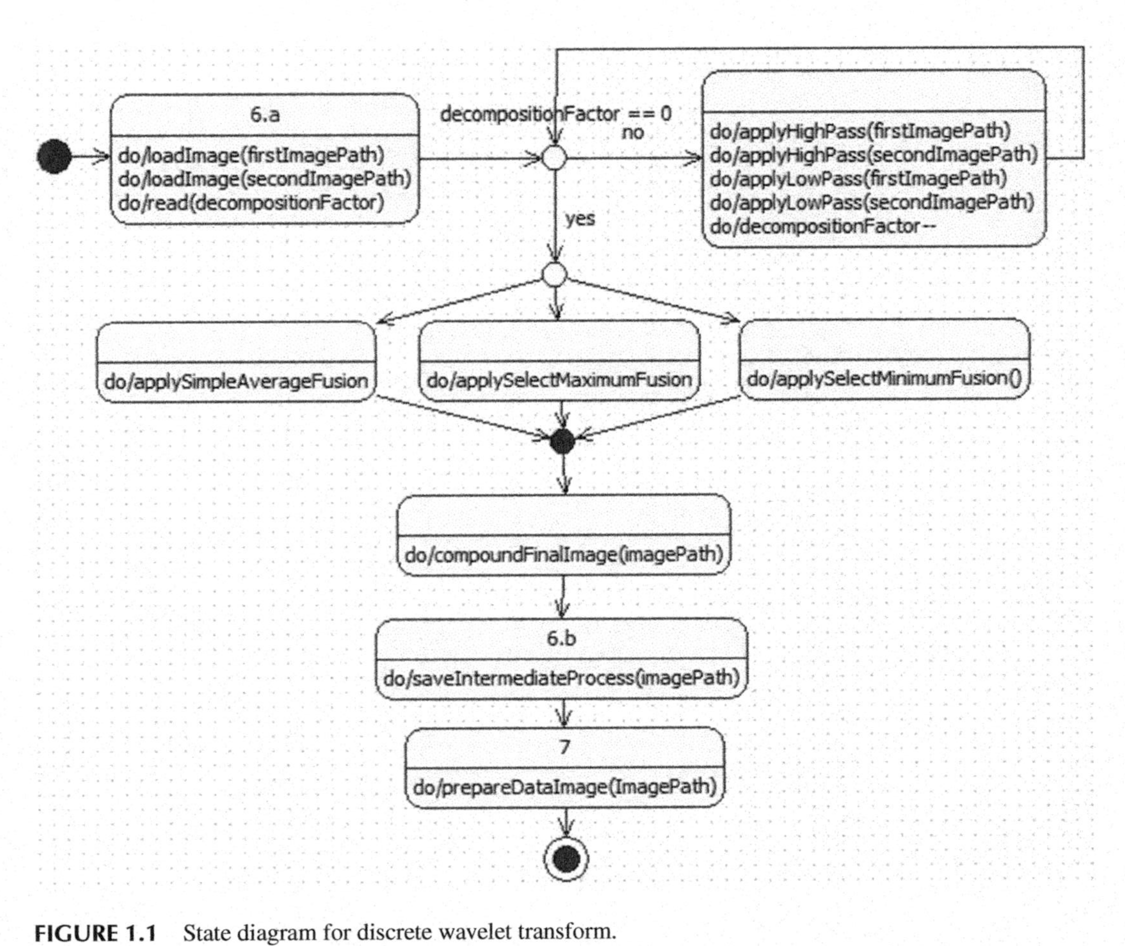

FIGURE 1.1 State diagram for discrete wavelet transform.

TABLE 1.2
Pseudo-Coloring – Calculation of the Color Ramps

Grey Intervals	Color Transition	Calculation of the Color Intensity
0–72	Red ->yellow	Color(255, (grayintensity*3), 0)
73–108	Yellow->green	Color(255 – ((grayintensity – 72)*7, 255, 0)
109–144	Green->bleu ciel	Color(0, 255 – ((grayintensity – 108)*7))
145–180	Bleu ciel->blue	Color(0, 255 – ((grayintensity – 144)*7),255)
181–216	Blue->pink	Color(((grayintensity – 108)*7),0,255)
217 – 255	Pink->red	Color(255,0, 255 – ((grayintensity – 216)*7))

are used or various indexes are calculated. Depending on the module in which it is assisted or not, in case of the classification made by a human specialist, the supervised and unsupervised classifications are distinguished.

The supervised classification is achieved when all existing knowledge concerning the studied area is taken into account, and the classification is assisted by a human expert in the field. Unsupervised classification is based only on the results obtained from pixel-based calculations without any supervision by the expert. This way of classification is useful when studying hard-to-reach areas or areas not yet explored. Practically, the classification consists in determining the attributes that can be mapped on the areas that were identified after processing an image.

The proposed modalities of classification for these types of images are:

- The Anderson classification, which is a hierarchical one, where the information is clearly structured into classes and subclasses. This classification system is mainly used to identify different entities at national level.
- The decision trees-based classification. This algorithm uses certain rules learned to classify the pixels of an image [20].

1.4.2 Functionalities and Scenario/Photoplay

The user has total access, benefits from all the functionality offered by the application, and can control a large part of them with the help of the user interface available.

The functionalities and settings to which the user has access are the following:

- Selecting the number of images, when the entire execution thread can be made on a single input image, or on two such images. If the transition through the image enhancement module is considered, then two images are required, but the application does not constrain the user to do so. Thus, the user can choose the number of images that he or she wishes to load, provided that the image fusion process is used or not. Another flexibility provided in the scenario where two images are loaded is the order of their loading, which does not matter.

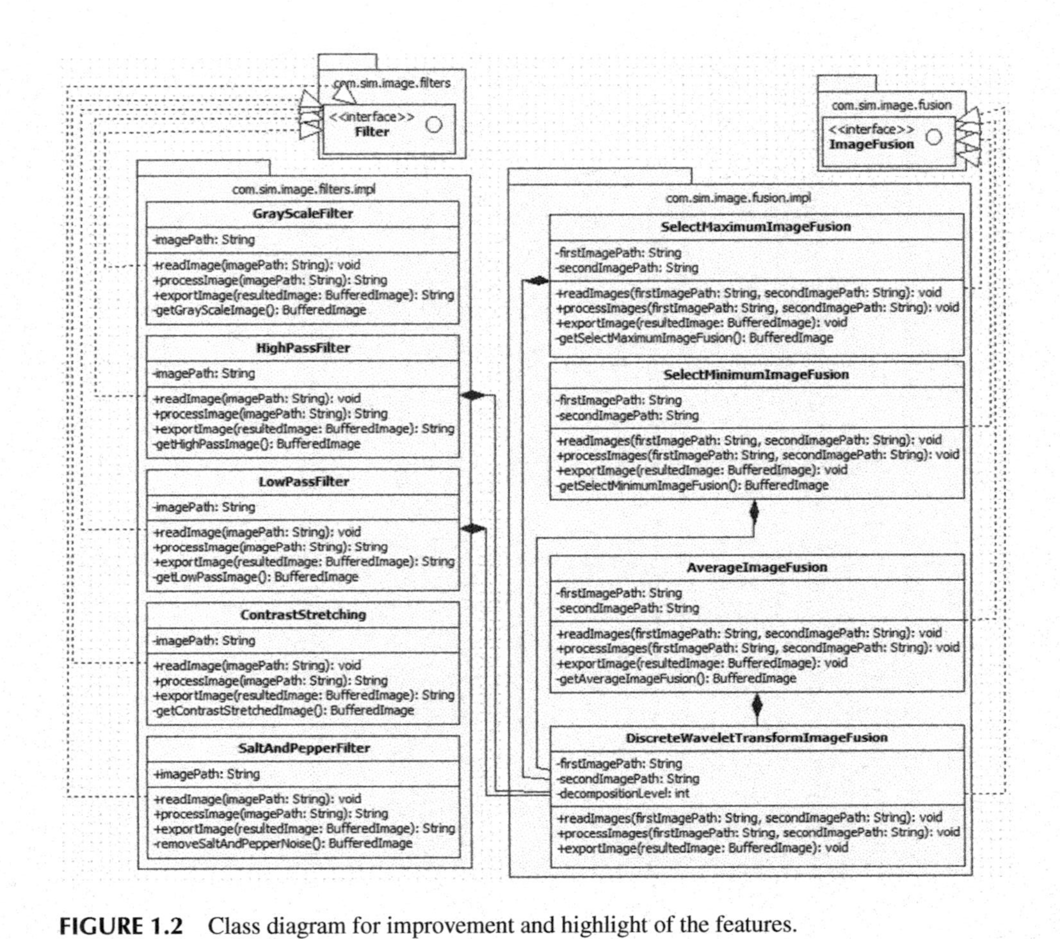

FIGURE 1.2 Class diagram for improvement and highlight of the features.

- Selecting the number of times it was processed, when the user has two buttons that allow him to add or remove a step from the execution thread. The number of these steps is not a default one but a choice of the user.
- Selecting the order of processing, when the same can be said also about the order in which the processes are to be executed. When the user adds a process, he or she basically adds a step containing a list of processes that he or she can choose from. That list of processes represents all the processing methods that the application has at its disposal. In this way, the order and the number of processes are not imposed but determined by the one using the application.
- Selecting the degree of decomposition, if the image fusion method called DWT is chosen as a step in the execution thread, the user will be allowed to choose the degree of decomposition. This degree of decomposition represents the number of times the high-pass and low-pass filters are applied to the image. This number should be between 1 and 5 inclusive. Choosing a higher degree of decomposition is not allowed, as it would result in cumbersome processing that would decrease from the performance of the application.
- Selecting the fusion method, when choosing the method of merging decomposed images will be allowed (in the case of the DWT merger). One of the three methods (minimum selection, maximum selection, or arithmetic mean calculation) can be selected by the user as a method of fusing between decomposed images. Two cases will be analyzed.
- For single image processing (considered as a scenario: image upload, application of the *grayscale* filter, also of the *contrast stretching* one, and pseudo-coloring), the order of the steps will be as shown in Figure 1.3.
- Creating the project directory, when the application is launched, named after the current date and time.
- Loading the image, the user using one of the two reserved spaces to load the desired image; this will need to have the .tif extension.
- Saving the intermediate image that is saved in the project directory.
- Applying the *grayscale* filter, which applies to the image saved in previous step.
- Saving the intermediate image; this is saved in the project directory.
- Applying the *contrast stretching* filter; this applies to the image saved in previous step.
- Saving an intermediate image that is saved in the project directory.
- Pseudo-coloring, which is applied to the image saved in previous the step.
- Saving the intermediate image; this is saved in the project directory.
- Showing the final image in an application frame.

For processing on two images (considering as a scenario: loading images, applying DWT fusion to the degree of decomposition 2 and arithmetic mean fusion, pseudo-coloring application), in which case the order of the steps will be:

- Creating the project folder, named after the current date and time, when the application starts.
- The user will use the two reserved spaces to upload the desired images, which will need to be in the TIFF format, meaning the .tif extension.

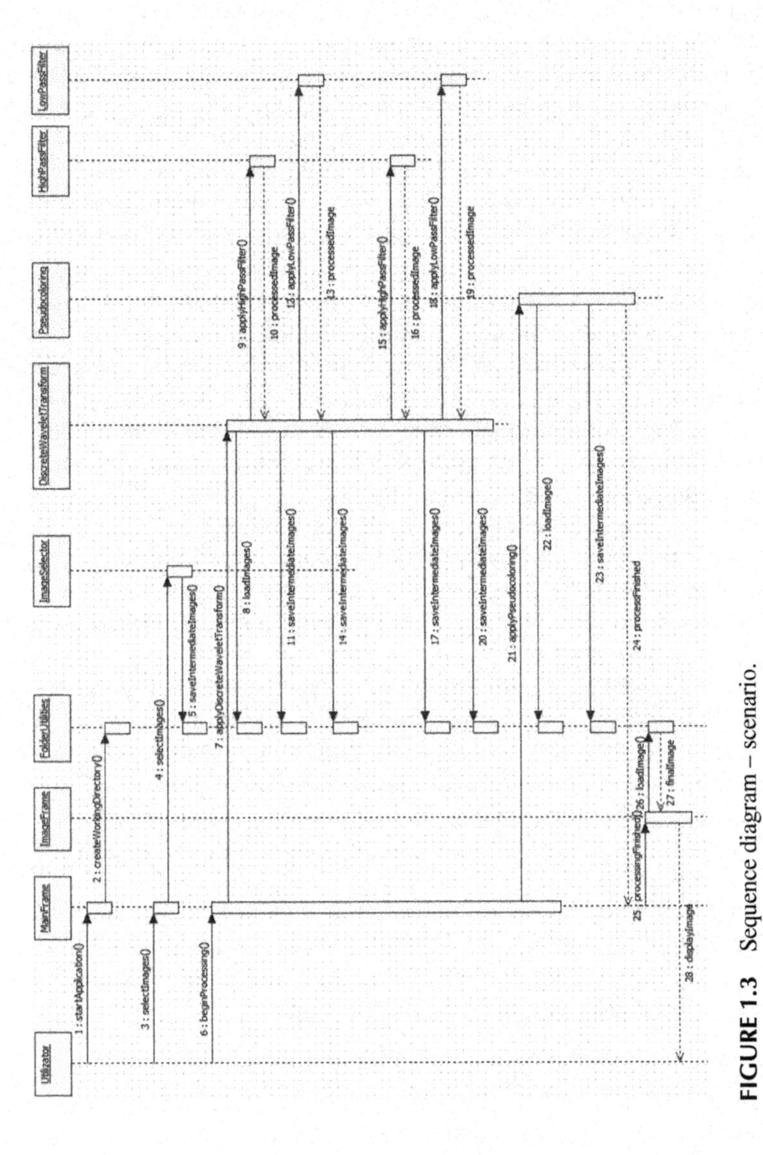

FIGURE 1.3 Sequence diagram – scenario.

- Saving the loaded images in the project directory.
- Applying to both images that were saved at the previous step, the low-pass and high-pass filters, for the decomposition degree 1.
- Saving the images resulting from the application of the filters in the project directory.
- Applying to the images saved in the previous step, the low-pass and high-pass filters, for the decomposition degree 2.
- Saving the images resulting from the application of the filters in the project directory.
- The fusion of images by calculating the arithmetic mean of two-by-two images, from those saved in the previous step, is performed.
- Saving the images resulting from the merger in the project directory.
- Composing the saved images for shifting from the decomposition degree 2 to decomposition degree 1.
- Saving the images resulting from the composition in the project directory.
- Composing the saved images for the transition from the decomposition degree 1 to the decomposition degree 0 is achieved (thus, a single image is obtained, i.e., the final image).
- Saving the image resulting from the composition (intermediate image saving) in the project directory.
- pseudo-coloring is applied on the image saved in previous step;
- Saving the image resulting from the pseudo-coloring in the project directory.
- Displaying the final image into an application frame.

1.4.3 Testing, Installing, and Using the Application

The testing of the application will consider the analysis of the application's features from different points of view. To highlight these features, a series of tests will be performed that address certain aspects such as performance, precision, or external factors.

The first test will be the performance one, which highlights the time the application manages to process an input image to a final result ready for analysis. In the present case, this would be hard to show, and even if it were done, it would not indicate any precise timing.

Determining accurate values to indicate the performance of the application depends largely on two factors: input images and processes in the execution thread.

The images on the bands may vary in size, variation that is not a small one, or one that can be neglected; there may be cases with differences of the fourth degree in the sizes of two images.

The flexibility of the program allows the user to choose the execution thread as desired. Thus, there may be processes in which only a simple fusion and a pseudo-coloring are used, resulting in relatively little processing time, or there may be processes that include 2–3 filters in the preprocessing module, a fusion of images using DWT with a decomposition factor equal to 5, and a pseudo-coloring, in which case the execution time would be totally different from the first situation. Considering this situation, performance tests will be applied on each algorithm in part on two different hardware configurations presented in Vele [19]. The algorithms implemented in the application were tested under the same conditions on both systems. The second test will be the precision one, which refers to the evaluation of the result so that it is optimal. The precision in this case, as well as the performance, is based on the way of analyzing a single result and the combined analysis of several results. The used algorithms are precise algorithms, which will always make exactly the same processing regardless of the loaded scenes. When it comes to precision, the problem comes in the analysis part. The application proposes analysis using both Anderson classification and decision trees-based classification. Prior to launching the application, the user must ensure that all software and hardware requirements are met.

The software requirements are as follows: Windows 7 operating system (recommended), or lately, Java Development Kit-JDK (recommended 1.7 or newer), Java IDE (recommended Eclipse), Apache Maven (recommended version 3.0.4, or newer). The minimum hardware requirements are as follows: 4 GB RAM, 80 GB 5400 rpm HDD, Dual Core 2.0 GHz processor. Optimal hardware requirements are as follows: 8 GB RAM, 160 GB 7200 rpm HDD, Quad Core 3.0 GHz processor. Having fulfilled the requirements, the work environment can be set in order to be able to launch the application.

For workspace configuration, the Java Development Kit, Apache Maven, and Eclipse IDE (an archive containing the preinstalled development software) will be installed. Then the application is imported using the File->Import menu. From the import section, we select Maven->Existing Maven Projects, and in the Maven Projects section we select the project using the *Browse* button. After the Eclipse is started, a series of modifications will be required to allocate more memory space for the Java Virtual Machine (VM). This is done by accessing the Run Configurations submenu from the Eclipse Run menu. In the new window, we select the application on the left side of the Java Application expandable menu. In the VMs arguments section, we pass the following command: -Xmx1024m, and click Run. The application is ready for use at this time. Once all of the settings listed above have been completed, the application can be run by performing the following steps:

- We select the project, and from the menu Project of the Eclipse, we select the submenu Clean.....
- We select from the Maven section the subsection Update Project.....
- We select from the Run As section the Maven Clean subsection –this process will be logged in Console tab of the Eclipse.
- We select from the Run As section the Maven Install subsection – the previous steps and this step make the building of the application.
- We select from the Run As section the Java Application subsection and the application is on.

On the launch, the main application interface, which is divided into quadrants (Figure 1.4), appears.

In the upper left corner there are two spaces reserved for uploading images. Once the Browse button is pressed, a window will appear allowing you to navigate through

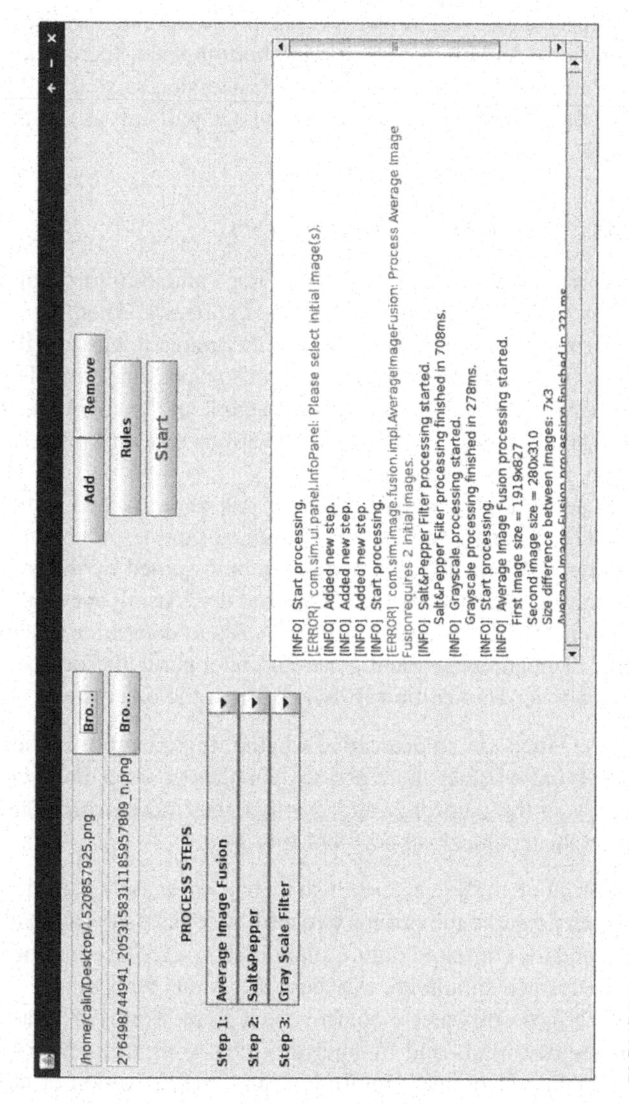

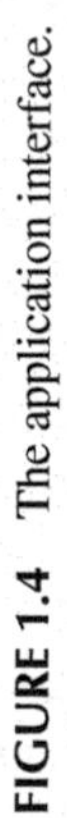
FIGURE 1.4 The application interface.

the local space for uploading the images. After the images have been uploaded, the next step is to create the runtime thread by adding processes. The two Add and Remove buttons on the top right allow adding or deleting processes. These processes will be illustrated on the bottom left through the selection menus.

If one of the processes chosen is DWT, in the top right, the mode of selection of the decomposition factor and of the fusion type for this transformation will appear (Figure 1.5). Once the execution thread is created, you can run it by pressing the Start button at the top right. As you can see, on the bottom right, there is an information panel that will contain information about each processing as well as their execution times. At the end of the process, the processed image will appear in a frame separate from the main one.

1.5 VALIDATION OF THE APPLICATION

Practical aspects are presented in this section. For validating the application, some images will be processed by using the described software. Then, they will be converted from color images to grayscale images, the image intensity will be adjusted, the image will be filtered (to reduce noise as much as possible), etc. The application is an image-processing and analysis program, capable of displaying 8, 16, and 32 bit images and performing analysis (it allows for various standard processing: smooth, contour detection, filtering, etc.).

The *bitstream* access and cloning/duplication can be performed with the following methods [21, 22, 23, 24]: non-destructive (analytical samples not being materially or digitally contaminated), repetitive (analysis can be resumed by the same user), and reproducible (analysis can be reproduced by other users using appropriate facilities). The authentication offers a variety of different tools to determine whether an image is an unmodified original, an original generated by a particular device, or the result of manipulation with a photo editing software. Then, the objective is:

> [T]to verify the video and to determine whether this record is authentic in the sense of specifying whether there are any changes or other interventions that alter the reality of the recording and whether that record corresponds to the registration on the technical support that was used.

For a complete set of analysis to establish that an ordinary registration is authentic or compatible with an authentic ordinary record, it is necessary to analyze the technical equipment and the contested digital support. Through the equipment, the digital recording was performed simultaneously with the events it contains.

Using the described software, a controversial framework [25] was analyzed by using the implemented filters and by analyzing the resulting ordinary images. The software allows the application of multiple filters, the activation or deactivation of the effect of a filter, the resetting of the filter options, the modification of the application order of the filters, etc. To reveal the photo assemblage, the inserted images and other manipulation signs, the algorithms analyze a number of parameters, such as metadata, source and direction of light in the image, general file structure, and so on. As a result, the user can understand whether the material is genuine or modified. The effects of the filters are applied in the order they are selected. Filters can be

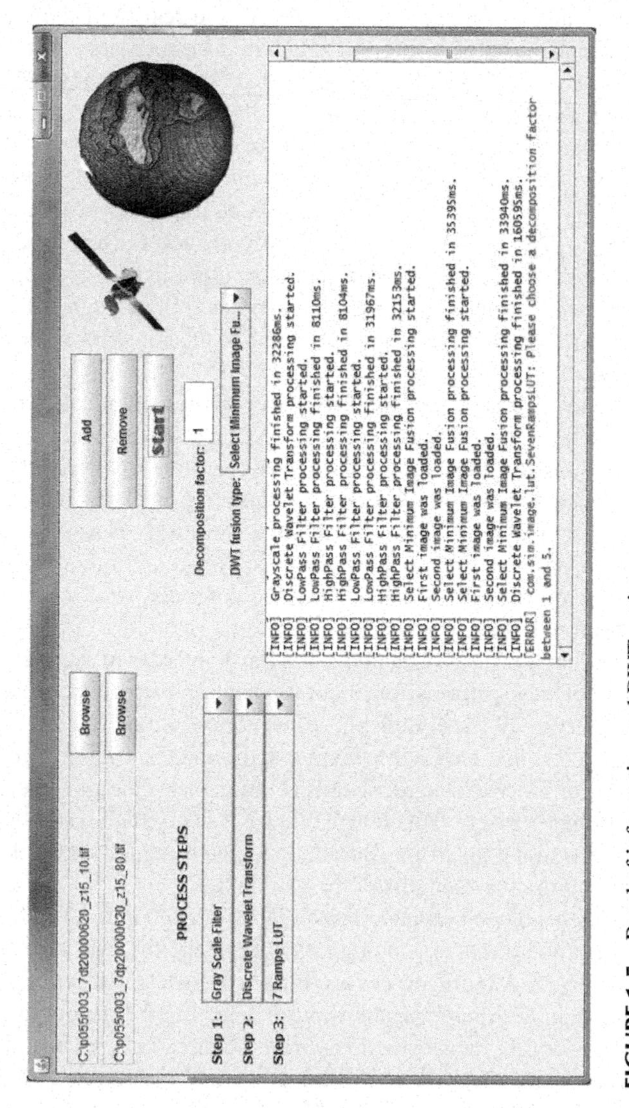

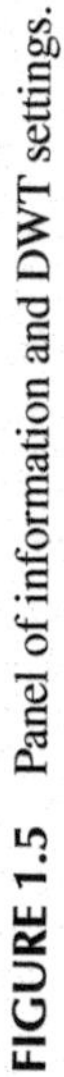

FIGURE 1.5 Panel of information and DWT settings.

rearranged after they are applied by selecting a filter name from the applied filter list. Rearranging filters can greatly change the way the ordinary image looks.

Figure 1.6 presents in detail the tested frame analysis, taken from a DVD and transposed in TIFF format, using one scenario (Figure 1.6a, b, c) or two scenarios (Figure 1.6d), and one filter (Figure 1.6a) or several filters (Figure 1.6b, c, d).

In conclusion, the content of the video on the external memory is genuine, meaning that there are no changes or interventions that alter the reality of the recording, as shown in the image analysis by using the software described above. In the case of medical imagery, the acquisition process is laborious. There are many optical sensors (ranging from hundreds to millions) that convert light into electricity and then into bits. All of these processes, in addition to the sensor features and errors that do not depend on the actual acquisition, such as equipment optics, lead to image deformation and noise addition. The changes we make on an image cover these drawbacks as much as possible, the resulting image being ready for further processing. The application allows us to switch to a grayscale image (simplifying both image coding and access to a wide spectrum of processing techniques) in cases in which the color is an irrelevant information (e.g., in order to determine the contours of the image). An example is presented in Figure 1.7.

Although segmented images are used in many medical applications (diagnosis, pathological lesion localization, structure analysis, etc.), image segmentation is difficult due to variations in the shape of the objects and the quality of the acquired images. Most medical images are taken with sampling artifacts, noise that leads to errors when strict image-processing techniques are used. Several segmentation methods have been proposed for medical images. Noise and other image artifacts can cause the occurrence of incorrect regions and contours, or discontinuity of the objects obtained through these methods.

Since long ago, humans have risen above the Earth in order to remotely observe it so that they could get more information about its shape and structure, generally about the surface characters in all the complexity of its composition. The analysis that the satellite is doing on a single area will generate eight images, each image being specific to an interval of the wavelength (band) (Figure 1.8). One of the eight images will be the panchromatic image. This image will have a very high resolution, and will be the most generous in details. A panchromatic image is actually a black-and-white image sensitive to all the wavelengths of the visible light.

After the images have been uploaded into the software application, the next step is to create the execution thread by adding processes using the Add and Remove buttons that allow adding or deleting processes. If one of the selected processes is DWT, in the upper right side, it will appear the way for selecting the decomposition factor and the fusion type for this transformation. Once the thread is created, we can run it by pressing the Start button. At the end of the process, the processed image will appear in a frame separate from the main one (Figure 1.9).

1.6 CONCLUSIONS

The application scientifically determines the origin of a photo/image from a video, not just a comparison of the different patterns contained in a database. The software

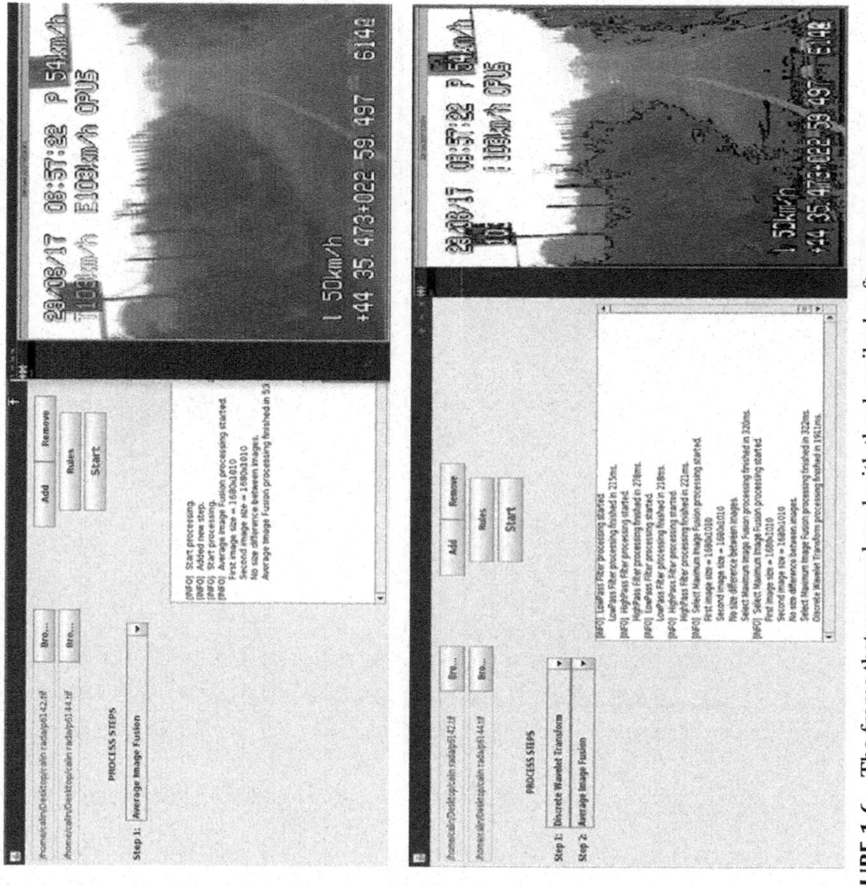

FIGURE 1.6 The frame that was analyzed with the described software.

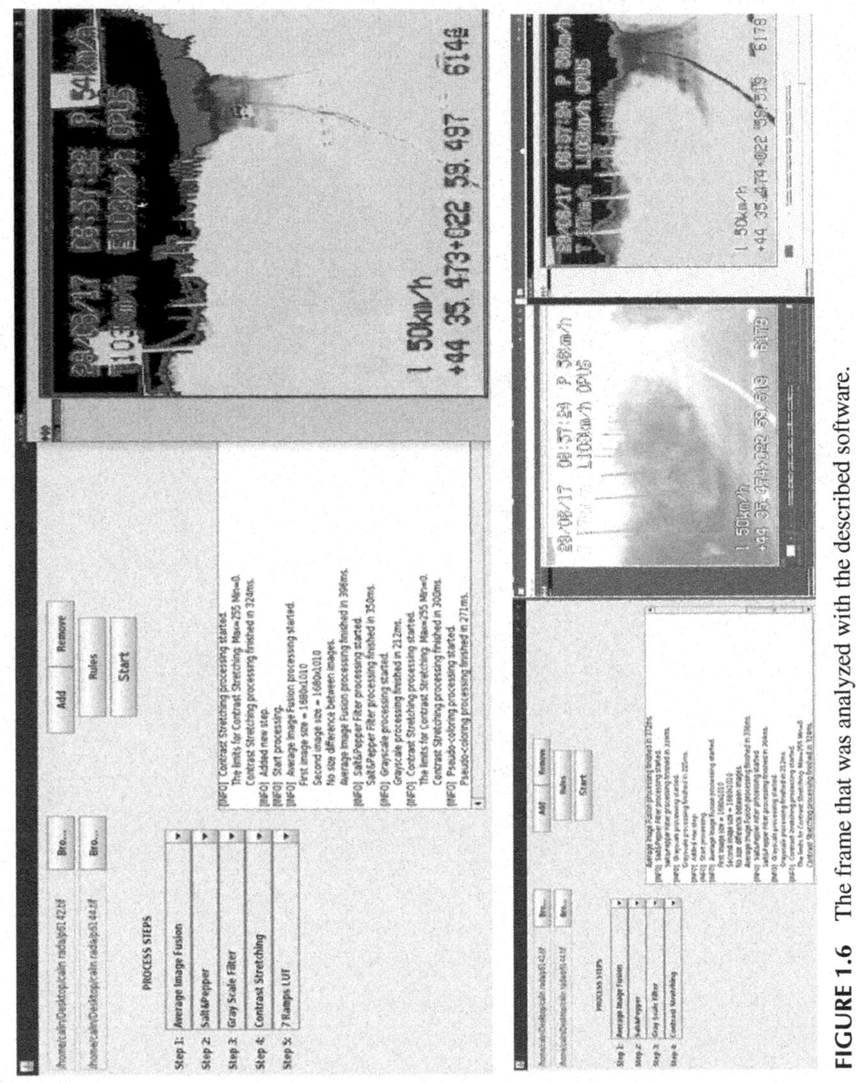

FIGURE 1.6 The frame that was analyzed with the described software.

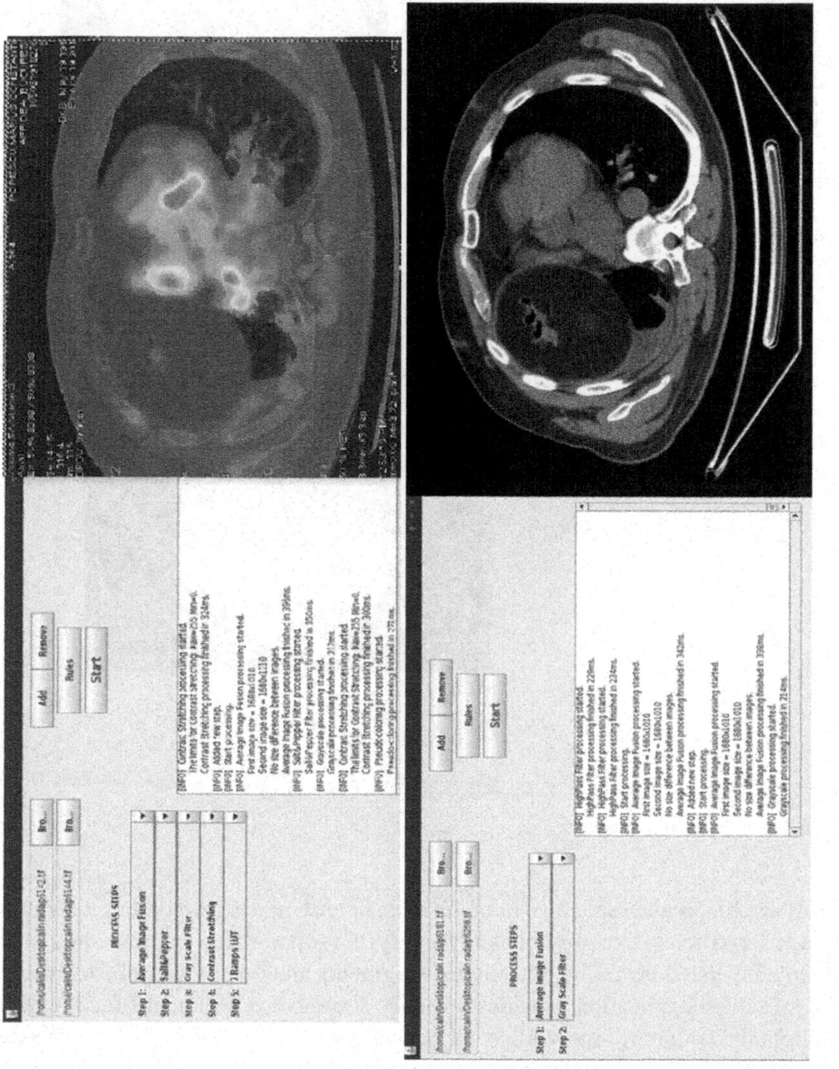

FIGURE 1.7 Medical image analyzed with the described software.

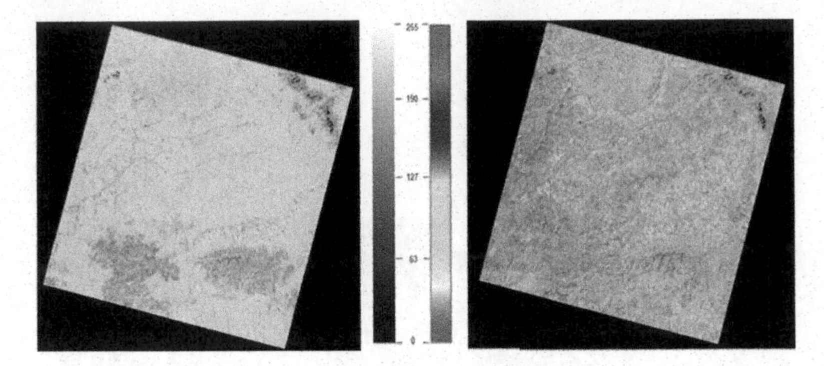

FIGURE 1.8 Image in red band (a) and middle infrared (b).

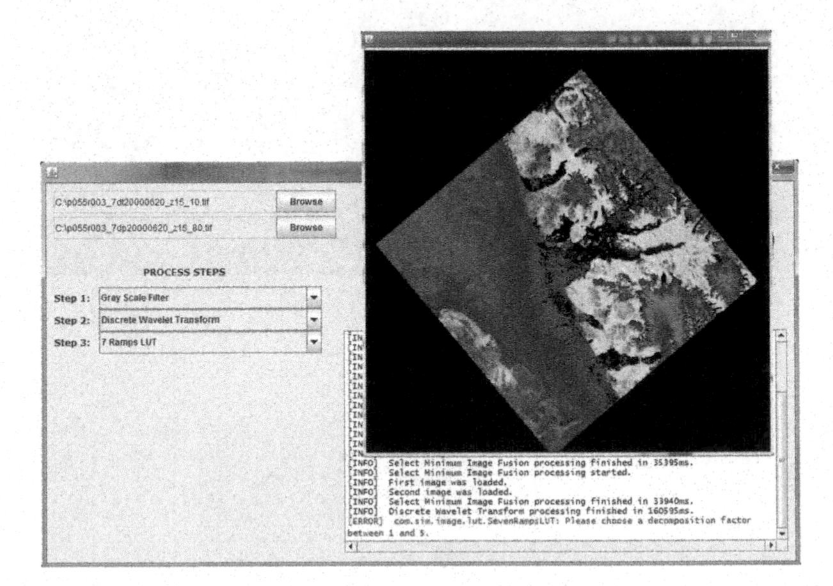

FIGURE 1.9 Finalized image.

can analyze objects and recognize human faces, license plates, and other relevant objects. In order to detect the assembly and forgery, the software has implemented filters for video conversion detection, introduced fragments and other types of forgeries.

The presented application provides not only a number of efficient functionalities to highlight the features of the studied surfaces/objects, but also the flexibility needed for reaching the best and easier method to interpret the result. Although the implemented algorithms are quite expensive in terms of execution times, the application provides quite good accuracy in highlighting the features we are interested in. The application is intuitive and allows the reuse of modules, or the choice of the processing order without an additional intervention of the user. To improve the quality of photos and images taken from videos and for identifying the relevant details in the images, the software contains ten filters.

The software integrates in a single, simple, and easy-to-use package the accepted legal, medical, and telecommunication techniques that were previously available only with personalized tools for top researchers. Unlike the professional applications, presented at the beginning of the chapter, this one does not require a beforehand qualification in order to be used.

A number of improvements can be made to the application for the satellite image analysis, such as processing images on grids into separate threads, georeferencing of the resulting images, implementing algorithms that are able to automate the analysis process using decision trees or Anderson classification.

In case of medical images, we will improve the software by developing some algorithms for detecting the contour of the investigated organ, or for recognizing its shape, in order to extract them from the original image. Also, we can connect the application to an online database for taking images directly from the hospital without a local saving process.

REFERENCES

1. H Kim, P Garrido, A Tewari, W Xu, J Thies, M Nießner, P Pérez, C Richardt, M Zollhöfer, C Theobalt (2018). Deep Video Portraits. *ACM Transactions on Graphics.*, Vol. 37, No. 4, Article 163, p. 1–14.
2. S Ylirisku, J Buur (2017). *Designing with video*, Springer.
3. VOCORD (2018). Vocord Videoexpert User's guide. An Image Processing Application, Version 1.8, p. 136. www.vocord.com/directions/authenticity_of_the_photo_video/, Accessed June 2018.
4. Amped Software. https://ampedsoftware.com/authenticate-samples, Accessed January 2018.
5. ***http://www.pcigeomatics.com/pdf/Geomatica_Prime.pdf, Accessed June 2018.
6. ERDAS. https://erdas-er-mapper.software.informer.com/, Accessed June 2018.
7. DK Sahu, MP Parsai (2012). Different Image Fusion Techniques – A Critical Review. *International Journal of Modern Engineering Research* (IJMER), Vol. 2, No. 5, September–October, p. 4298–4301.
8. G Gupta (2011). Algorithm for Image Processing Using Improved Median Filter and Comparison of Mean, Median and Improved Median Filter. *International Journal of Soft Computing and Engineering* (IJSCE), Vol. 1, No. 5, November, p. 304–311.
9. N Kashyap, GR Sinha (2012). Image Watermarking Using 3-Level Discrete Wavelet Transform. *I.J. Modern Education and Computer Science*, Vol. 4, No. 3, April, p. 50–56.
10. JE Candes, X Li, Y Ma, J Wright (2011). Robust Principal Component Analysis. *Journal of the ACM*, Vol. 58, No. 3, May, p. 1–39.
11. S Rahmani, M Strait, D Merkurjev, M Moeller, T Wittman (2010). An Adaptive IHS PanSharpening. *IEEE Geoscience and Remote Sensing Letters*, Vol. 7, No. 4, October, p. 746–750.
12. MC Popescu, N Mastorakis (2009). Applications of the Four Color Problem. *International Journal of Applied Mathematics and Informatics*, Vol. 3, No. 1, p. 17–26.
13. K Murugan, VP Arunachalam, S Karthik (2018). A Combined Filtering Approach for Image Denoising. *IEEE International Conference on Soft-Computing and Network Security*, February 14–16, 2018, Coimbatore, India.
14. MC Popescu (2008). *Telecommunications* (in Romanian). Universitaria Publishing House, Craiova.

15. M Pandey, RK Bharti, AK Bhatt (2017). A Study of Color Enhancement Techniques for Input Images. *IEEE 2nd International Conference on Computational Systems and Information Technology for Sustainable Solution*, December.
16. Y-J Shen, J-J Zhang, S Tian, K Zhu, Y-W Feng (2018). Research of Algorithm for Single Gray-Scale Image Haze Removal. *Proceedings, Optical Sensing and Imaging Technologies and Applications*, Vol. 10846, December.
17. M Saleha, S Muhammad, Y Mussarat, SM Alyas, A Rehman (2017). Image Fusion Methods: A Survey. *Journal of Engineering Science & Technology Review*, Vol. 10, No. 6, p. 186–194.
18. H-W Sehring, M Garcia (2006). Software Architectures. Chapter 5, Hamburg University of Technology, Germany, p. 1–17.
19. S Vele (2017). Highlighting Ground Surface Characteristics Based on Satellite Image Processing. Graduation Thesis (in Romanian), Vasile Goldis Western University of Arad, Romania. United States Government Printing Office, Washington, p. 1–28
20. JR Anderson, EE Hardy, JT Roach, RE Witmer (2001). A Land Use and Land Cover Classification System for Use with Remote Sensor Data.
21. A Marshall (2008). *Digital Forensics – Digital Evidence in Criminal Investigation.* Wiley-Blackwell, New Jersey, USA.
22. ASTM E2916-13 Standard Terminology for Digital and Multimedia Evidence Examination, Accessed June 2018. https://www.astm.org/DATABASE.CART/WORKITEMS/WK63874.htm, Accessed June 2018
23. J. Sammons (2014). Chapter 13 – Digital Forensics in Introduction to Information Security – A Strategic Based Approach. P. 275–302. Elsevier.
24. A Grigoras, D Rappaport, J Smith (2012). Analytical Framework for Digital Audio Authentication. *AES 46th International Conference on Audio Forensics*, Denver, June 14–15.
25. MC Popescu (2018). Report of Judicial Expertise (in Romanian). Craiova.

2 A Best Practice for Establishing a Telemedicine Project

Dina Ziadlou, Seyed Mojtaba Mir Hosseini, Nasim Nasiri, and Amin Saberinia

CONTENTS

2.1 INTRODUCTION

Telemedicine refers to use the health information technology and telecommunication tools for providing digital healthcare and medical services via distance, specially, for population who live in rural areas or have limited access to providers and healthcare teams (Beck, 2016; Blanton & Balch, 1995; Sandhu, 2020). Telemedicine removes the geographical and time zone barriers and creates equity in digital healthcare services for people around the world. The goals of telemedicine are to increase patient access to clinicians and healthcare professionals to improve the quality of care by managing chronic diseases at a distance and deliver medical services to deprived rural areas (Schwamm, 2014; Schwamm et al., 2017).

Kerman province, located in central south of Iran, has vast geographical area including rural and urban areas that have encountered with a lack of specialists in different medical fields; most of the available areas are considered as deprived areas in which some of the medical facilities locate in remote areas and refer the therapeutics patients to the specialists in bigger cities that needs long-distance transportation. Most of the time, the transportation for even a simple one visit not only costs the patient but also puts them in trouble and road accidents. Therefore, one of the solutions to overcome the barrier like accessability is telemedicine service. The challenges like physician shortage, access to care, cost of care services, expansion of chronic diseases, and increasing demand of aging population for caring services can be facilitated by telemedicine technologies (AMMC, 2018; Baker et al., 2017; Beck, 2016; Waters, 2009). However, before starting to implement technology in a hospital or healthcare organization, it is essential to evaluate the needs of the organization and the readiness of employees for digital healthcare technology changes (Sandhu, 2020).

The first users of digital technologies are the physicians, nurses, and professionals of medical centres, and thus it is essential to evaluate their awareness of and opinion about implementing digital changes (AHA, 2016; Ziadlou, Islami, & Hassani, 2008). Study and analyze available status in different dimensions, such as awareness and viewpoints of employees about telemedicine technology, in order to calculate the acceptance level of this technology (Davis 1989; Hadeel & Sandhu, 2021; Venkatesh & Davis 2000) for implementing the project is the first step of success in digital transformation. Moreover, it can reduce the resistance to the change while the employees engage in decision-making and strategic makers perceive the preference and opinion of employees. This research evaluated the awareness and attitude of managers and personnel regarding this technology (telemedicine) in Kerman University of Medical Sciences.

2.2 BACKGROUND

Digital technologies have created a revolution in all industries including the healthcare industry in which digital and healthcare have merged as one and referred to as digital healthcare (Sandhu, 2020). One of the digital technologies that has changed the healthcare service deliveries and resulted in quality improvement, cost reduction, and accessibility is telemedicine (Beck, 2016; Schwamm, 2014). However, developing the digital technologies in healthcare organizations needs an in-depth understanding of the organization's situation and employees' readiness to embrace changes, while factors such as cultural, legal, political, social, and technological factors have direct and indirect impacts on achieving successful outcomes in digital technology establishment (Van Dyk, 2014; Ziadlou, 2019). Given the reports, between 35% and 75% of projects change are failed, and most of HIT (Health Information Technology) projects' failures derive from the lack of well-developed planning phase, 50% of failures are due to managerial issues, and 20% of failures come from a lack of effective communication (Scheer, 2016; Tait, 2013). To do so, one of the most essential and first step in telemedicine projects is to assess the awareness of employees and their viewpoints regarding telemedicine services.

The primary goal of this project was to evaluate the awareness and viewpoints of professionals about telemedicine. This population were directly involve in patient treatment and health services in healthcare network of Kerman University of Medical Sciences. The study was conducted in 2011–2012 in order to answer to the question, "How can primary awerness and knowledge of healthcare workers impact on success of telemedicine establishment". The survey was conducted randomly by distributing a questionnaire consisting of three sections: demographic specifications, awareness level assessment, and viewpoints evaluation.

The awareness assessment survey was consisted of evaluating the awareness of employees about telemedicine services, including online consultation, online educational services, online nursing services, and distance treatment. Moreover, the viewpoints assessment was consisted of evaluating the impact of technology in culture, decision-making, and medical diagnosis, along with their opinions about telemedicine as a technology for fair distribution of digital healthcare services in deprived areas, financial cost reduction for patients, unnecessary travel prevention, medical error reduction, and quality improvement. The data were analyzed by SPSS software.

2.3 LITERATURE REVIEW

In Ancient Greek, the term *tele* means "distance," and telemedicine refers to distance medicine. The first documented report of telehealth history was recorded in Haukeland Hospital of Norway in 1920 (Schmeida, 2005). In the United States of America (USA), the modern telemedicine began in the early 1950s by transferring neurological examination images at the University of Nebraska. Then, the National Aeronautics and Space Administration (NASA) utilized telemedicine services for monitoring the astronauts' vital signs on space missions; the Mercury flight used telecardiology to monitor the cardiac status of astronauts in the space station (Ryu, 2010; Schmeida, 2005). Nowadays, telemedicine is widely used in different forms: from simple types of video conferencing in telepsychiatry and telephycology to remote patient monitoring and tele-home care, Moreover, in complex services – namely, telesurgery, teleradiology, teledermatology, and telepathology – telemedicine has an effective role in transferring electronic patient records from one site to another for consultation, decision sharing, education, and treatment.

Telemedicine refers to the clinical side of telehealth services that provide digital healthcare deliveries, prevention, diagnosis, treatment, prescription, and follow-up for patients. From the nonclinical side of telehealth, it provides educational services to promote the knowledge of individuals (e.g., patients, physicians, nurses, and clinicians), to enhance the relationship between patients and providers, and to increase the quality of health and well-being of society. However, the American Telemedicine Association has described telehealth and telemedicine as synonyms for technologies and telecommunication tools delivering healthcare via online digital services to patients with no geographical limitation and time dependency (Richard, 2012; Ziadlou, 2013). Telemedicine and telehealth services are cost-effective technologies to deliver patient care equitably, improve quality care, manage chronic diseases, improve patient satisfaction, and develop digital healthcare outcomes (Adler-Milstein, Kvedar & Bates, 2014; AHA, 2016; Center for Information Technology Leadership Partners HealthCare, 2015; Chen, 2017; Phillips, 2012).

In 1968, Boston Logan Airport and Massachusetts Hospital were connected to visit patients in the airport via video camera (Blanton & Balch, 1995). In 1989, the US Public Health connected physicians to 37 rural areas via telemedicine, and it could save 22% of the cost of healthcare service delivery (Blanton & Balch, 1995). Similarly, Blanton and Balch (1995) reported North Carolina's Central Prison linked to North Carolina University of Medicine via telemedicine to treat dangerous prisoners; this telemedicine service was a monitoring console to display skin rash of prisoners to the dermatologist. It was a valuable achievement in the medical world to improve access to medical services at distance. However, Schooley (1998) stated that reimbursement, malpractice liability, physicians licensing, and patients' privacy were the challenges of telemedicine.

Ashley (2002) and Stanberry (2006) indicated that licensing, credentialing, malpractice liability and patients' information confidentiality were the significant barriers to telemedicine development. Moreover, the study of Medeiros De Bustos, Moulin, and Audebert (2009) found that these barriers remain in the healthcare system. In 2010, the Agency for Healthcare Research and Quality (AHRQ) emphasized on developing a system of training and empowerment for physicians in advanced technology usage (Phillips, 2012).

According to the AHRQ law, physicians were required to learn telemedicine policies, guidelines, and regulations relevant to origin state. Brown (2006), Mazzolini (2013), and Adler-Milstein et al. (2014) argued that the most significant relevant element that has contributed to telehealth adoption (Rogers 1995) in US hospitals is reimbursement. Lewis (2015) asserted that a lack of precise definition for each type of telemedicine service and a lack of uniform policy are the critical negative factors for insurance plans not to utilize this technology widely. Consequently, Callahan (2015) and Scott (2015) argued that the lack of unique regulation and inadequate reimbursement rules/policies among states, federal, and insurance companies had created the policy barriers in telehealth development. Telemedicine critics have stated that telemedicine could not sufficiently be a reliable and trustable way for consumers (Chen, 2017). They believe that dehumanization (medical ethics issue), lack of confidentiality (privacy issue), and loss of details for evaluating patients' health (technology issues) may affect the quality, access, and cost of telemedicine (Chen, 2017).

Despite critics of telemedicine, "[i]n 2006, telehealth celebrated its 100th anniversary"(Scott, 2015, p. 11). The Center for Information Technology Leadership Partners HealthCare (CITLPH) reported that establishing telemedicine services has resulted in saving $327 million in transportation cost (indirect medical cost) between nursing homes and emergency departments, and $479 million cost-saving in transportation from nursing homes to physicians' offices (Center for Information Technology Leadership Partners HealthCare, 2015). Hermar (2016) in the article of Blue Cross and Blue Shield of Alabama, conducted that more insurers are willing to use telehealth for patients in a rural area because a $50 telehealth visit for ear infection treatment is much cheaper than $600 cost of the trip from a rural area to an emergency department. Ultimately, many studies have asserted that telehealth could (1) improve cost-effectiveness, (2) increase patient satisfaction, (3) improve quality, (4) expand networking, (5) reduce the readmission, (6) improve chronic diseases management and infection control, (7) develop medication management, (8)

improve peer-to-peer review, (10) improve mental health management, (11) reduce transportation cost, (12) reduce the lengthy time for a visit, (13) improve post-op follow-up, and (14) improve primary care management without geographical limitation and time zone dependency (American College of Medical Practice Executives, 2014; Augsburger, 2017; Dinesen et al., 2016; LeRouge & Garfield, 2013; Moran, Juan, & Roudsari, 2015; Scott, 2015; Ziadlou, 2013).

In recent years, considerable advancement in telehealth barriers, including technological, financial, strategical, and legal challenges, has happened. Following are the example of advancement in telemedicine to remove the barriers: (1) technical barriers: considerable advancement has been established in HIPAA (Health Insurance Portability and Accountability Act) and standardization of security and network integration (Pinkney, 2013); (2) legal barriers: advancement in Medicare's and Medicaid's new policies happens (CMS, 2018); (3) financial barriers: sustainable ROI and reimbursement have been improved during recent years, and the Centers for Medicare & Medicaid has developed the procedural terminology codes and Healthcare Common Procedure Coding System (HCPCS) (Goedert, 2017); (4) strategy barrier: shifting viewpoints from telemedicine as a luxury project to a sustainable project is a part of strategical advancement in telehealth; the Office for the Advancement of Telehealth (AOT) provides policies and strategies to facilitate this technology and promote the critical factors for suitable success (McKinnon, 2017); and (5) organizational barriers: increasing trust and engagement of patients in their healthcare and developing a willingness to utilize telemedicine among providers and nurses have been the recent achievement of telemedicine (LeRouge & Garfield, 2013).

An intervention study in Minnesota indicated that 30% of adult population in the USA has high blood pressure (BP), and the annual cost of in-person visits for monitoring BP is around $50 billion (Beck, 2016). This study involved patients with high blood pressure and compared in-person visits in doctors' office and virtual visits via telemonitoring. The result illuminated that the number of patients with controlled blood pressure via telemedicine was significantly higher and more efficient. In this study, Beck stated that the cost of remote visiting is around $45 for nonemergency problems, which save costs for patients compared with the same service in-person visit with $100 in doctor's office and $160 at an urgent-care clinic (Beck, 2016). Also, the Department of Veteran Affairs in the telemedicine program has had a significant reduction in hospitalization over 40%, 30% for heart failure and 20% for diabetes and chronic obstructive pulmonary disease (COPD). John Hopkins Medicine, in a tele-home care project for the elderly, estimated that the total cost of care in the home via telehealth is 30% less than hospital stay and also calculated the shorter length of stay in bed, 3.2 versus 4.9 (AHA, 2016; Schwamm, 2014).

The Best Practices Poll Results reported by *Modern Healthcare* in 2016 revealed that people in the USA had ranked telehealth technology 2 out of 25 for boosting patient outcomes. In contrast, providers still look at telemedicine as an inconvenient and cumbersome technology, and among 1.500 family physicians, only 15% use telemedicine in practices, and 90% of providers argue about the reimbursement issues (Beck, 2016). In 2010, the AHRQ emphasized to develop the system of training and empowerment of physicians for advanced technology usage. The physicians, in different states, require learning about each state policy, guideline, and regulation because the providers also comply with the regulations that need an appropriate licensing board in the patient's state (Phillips, 2012; TRC, 2016). Moreover, the Congressional Budget Office (CBO) estimated the cost of telemedicine for Medicare approximately $150 million in 2001, but in 2014 document of the Center for Telehealth and eHealth law showed that the average cost of telemedicine had been around $57 million (AHA, 2016; Beck, 2016; Lewis, 2015).

On the other hand, what happens in Iran and telemedicine advancement in this country? According to the report of the Iranian Space Agency (2012) to the United Nations on using technologies for online digital healthcare improvement, Iran has developed a web-based influenza surveillance system in Shahid Beheshti Medical University (SBMU), Tehran, and connected 10 district hospitals to the system, and also has created web-based Vaccination Supplies Stock Management services for 435 vaccination stores in 2004. Moreover, a successful online e-learning service (Hadeel & Sandhu, 2021) in digital healthcare was created in 2003 in Shiraz, Iran, along with telehealth system implementation between Ghadir Mother and Child Hospital in Shiraz and three other hospitals, namely, Shahid Rajaei Hospital, Gerash Hospital, and Iranian Hospital in Dubai, UAE (Iranian Space Agency, 2012). Respectively, telemedicine services establishment including teleradiology, tele-ICU (intensive care unit), and tele-spirometry in the National Research Institute of Lung Diseases and Tuberculosis (NRITLD) in 2006 have been the progressive activities in utilizing digital technologies to reduce the cost of pulmonary care services to rural areas. While according to this earlier report, one of the major causes of death in Iran is road accidents, with 25,000 fatal cases and 250,000 injuries per year, telemedicine can be a good solution to reduce the transportation rate between hospitals and homes, and it can result in a reduction in road accidents (Iranian Space Agency, 2012).

Another example of advanced telemedicine services in Iran is the Iranian Retinopathy Teleophthalmology Screening (IRTOS) service, as a community-based telemedicine screening project (Safi et al., 2019). It is an m-Health system for early detection of diabetic retinopathy (DR) through telescreen services in the regions where the population has the most report of DR issues. The telescreens are used in rural areas, such as Islamshahr, to screen the patients. The images of the retina and the information of patients are communicated to ophthalmologists and experts via smartphones and cameras, and the patients who need further investigation are referred to hospitals. According to Safi et al. (2019), 50% of patients can be distinguished for early detection of DR, and they can be treated in advance before the problem turns into the chronic condition. Likewise, Salehahmadi and Hajialiasghari (2013) reported the cost reduction and recovery rate improvement in high-risk pregnancies where patients were monitored by telemedicine. Ayatollahi, Mirani, Nazari, and Razavi (2018) in a survey among 295 physicians and nurses found that most of the participants agreed with the advantages of telemedicine in diabetics management, cost-effectiveness, transportation reduction, and patient safety improvement. However, the resistance to adopt digital technologies, lack of appropriate infrastructure in rural areas, cultural differences among patients, standard guidelines, and security considerations are still the challenges of telemedicine services in Iran (Ayatollahi et al., 2018; Salehahmadi & Hajialiasghari, 2013).

2.4 THE MAIN FOCUS OF THE CHAPTER

This quantitative study was a cross-sectional study with descriptive desing. The main focus of the study was to present the essential, first step of establishing digital healthcare technologies, such as telemedicine, in healthcare organizations, which is to evaluate the readiness of healthcare workers to accept a new digital health technology. While developing digital technologies in healthcare organizations results in challenges and changes in the organization's context – namely, changes in structure, infrastructure, culture, operation, technology, process, and strategies – it is essential to analyze the situation and employee readiness to create the actionable strategic plans for overcoming the challenges and reducing the resistance to change at first place and before implementing the technologies (Van Dyk, 2014; Ziadlou, 2019).

2.4.1 Research Methodology Design

This sectional and descriptive study collected data from 276 healthcare professional employees in 30 centers at Kerman University of Medical Sciences between 2010 and 2011. The research utilized a quantitative design. The awareness assessment survey was consisted of evaluating the awareness of employees about telemedicine services, including online consultation, online educational services, online nursing services, and distance treatment. Moreover, the viewpoints assessment was consisted of evaluating the impact of technology in culture, decision-making, and medical diagnosis along with their opinions about telemedicine as a technology for fair distribution of digital healthcare services in deprived areas, financial cost reduction for patients, unnecessary travel prevention, medical error reduction, and quality improvement. The data were analyzed by using SPSS software.

2.4.1.1 Population and Sample

The sample size was included healthcare workers who provide treatment and medical services at Kerman University of Medical Sciences, including senior managers, managers, matrons, nurses, nurse assistants, practical nurses, physicians, specialists, reception personnel, medical deeds of hospitals, employees, and experts of health centers which include Shafa Hospital, Afzali Pour, Shahid Bahonar, Shahid Beheshti, Emam Reza Sirjan, Pastor Bam, Hazrat Ghaem Bardsir, Sina Zarand, Valiasr Shahre Babak, Khatamolanbia Baft, Aliebn Abitaleb Ravar, Arzoieyeh.

These medical centers are working under the supervision of the Kerman University of Medicine. This research attempted to include all different types of employees, while digital technologies impact all departments and workflows of the cross-functional activities. At the beginning, based on a sample volume of 276 personnel working for 30 centers, cluster sampling was done in some processes, and after situating on clusters, the sample selection was done randomly. Among considered indexes in the plan, age, sex, education, service records, type of employment, and educational level were included. The information was gathered by using interview techniques and encouragement of participants for partnership with telemedicine technology performance by using data gathering in this research, which was the questionnaire.

2.4.2 Data Collection

The ascertaining instrument and questions of the questionnaire were prepared with the method of brainstorming by the executives and colleagues of the plan by using reviewed studies and using the latest scientific issues and Persian and Latin essays in three sections.

The first section included demographic features including sex-age (below 20 years old with 5-year classification and maximum up to 60 years old in 9 branches), marital status, education, place of service, type of employment, service records (less than 5 years with 5-year classification up to more than 30 years with 7-year classification). The second section is a survey section that consisted of ten closed-ended questions for determining the awareness of employees. Moreover, the third section consisted of 18 questions for determining the viewpoints of employees about the object.

For determining the awareness manner, awareness evaluation questions were used, and respondents expressed their answer through options such as true, false, and no information. Also, for obtaining the opinion of attendesss, a prospective evaluation was designed based on five-degree scales, where respondents expressed their answer through the following options: fully agree, agree, neither agree nor disagree, disagree, and fully disagree). For determining the validity of the questionnaire, books, similar articles, and polling from some clear-sighted scholars (scholars and faculty members of Kerman University of Medical Sciences) were used. The reliability of the questionnaire was determined by using the introductory study and the Cronbach's alpha coefficient using SPSS software, was 0.88, as indicated correctly in internal affiliation.

2.4.2.1 Specifications of Interviewers

Some educated persons in the field of computer software and nurses were invited to interview the study population. However, before conducting the interview, the researchers provided techniques and other required training for adhering to ethical consideration, human subject standards, and collecting the precise data through the interview and also through the observation of body language of interviewers. The interviewers submitted the questionnaire to the employees in person. The place of the interview was the place of employee service listed in the population section.

2.4.2.2 Sampling Procedure

The sample size was included the healthcare workers who involved in treatment and healthcare services at Kerman University of Medical Sciences. The researchers used Morgan's formula, as follows:

$$z = 1.96, p = q = 0.5, d = 0.06 \ (n = 276 \text{ Confidence level: } 95\%)$$

The factor z is the reliability level and normal variable volume of standard unit, p is the expected prevalence volume, d is the accuracy or authorized error volume, and n is the volume of sample. Using this formula indicated that the sample size

TABLE 2.1
Listwise Deletion Based on All Variables in the Procedure

Case Processing Summary

		N	%
Cases	Valid	10	100.0
	Excluded	0	.0
	Total	10	100.0

$$n = \frac{z^2 pq}{d^2}$$

Reliability Statistics

Cronbach's Alpha	No. of Items
0.888	30

would include 267 persons; their random selection after locating in cluster is shown in Table 2.1.

2.4.3 Data Analysis

This study attempted to measure the awareness of employees and their viewpoints in modern technologies such as telemedicine. Thus, by designing a questionnaire and analyzing information, the two factors of awareness and viewpoints of employees were evaluated. The researchers applied the SPSS software, descriptive and deductive statistics, multivariate analysis, and distributing Fisher's and K-test. Afterward, the findings were presented in graphical format in four dimensions as follows:

- Awareness concerning telemedicine technology and the efficiency of its usage.
- Awareness for performing consultation of patients with telemedicine
- Awareness for using telemedicine for providing training and information to patients
- Awareness for providing nursing services and treatment by using telemedicine.

In evaluating the knowledge of attendees the following factors were collected:

- Impact of telemedicine in decision-making
- Impact of telemedicine on the fair distribution of healthcare services
- Impact of telemedicine in reducing financial costs of patients
- Impact of telemedicine in preventing unnecessary travels
- Impact of telemedicine on reducing errors in medical affairs
- Impact of telemedicine on performance

2.4.4 Findings

In awareness factor, the findings clarified that 61.45% of participants had awareness about telemedicine technologies, 17.9% had limited knowledge about telemedicine, and 20.8% were unaware of this technology (Table 2.2). Moreover, the awareness for providing digital healthcare services through telemedicine ranked second after the

TABLE 2.2
The Results of Evaluating Telemedicine Awareness

Type of Telemedicine Service	Unaware		Poor		Good	
	Percent	Number	Percent	Number	Percent	Number
Awareness concerning telemedicine technology and the efficiency of its usage	(20.8)	58	(17.9)	49	(61.4)	169
Awareness for performing consultation of patients with telemedicine	(22.8)	63	(15.9)	44	(61.3)	169
Awareness level for using telemedicine to provide training and information to patients	(10.1)	28	(10.9)	30	(79.0)	218
Awareness level for providing nursing services and treatment by using telemedicine	(17.8)	49	(15.2)	42	(67.0)	185

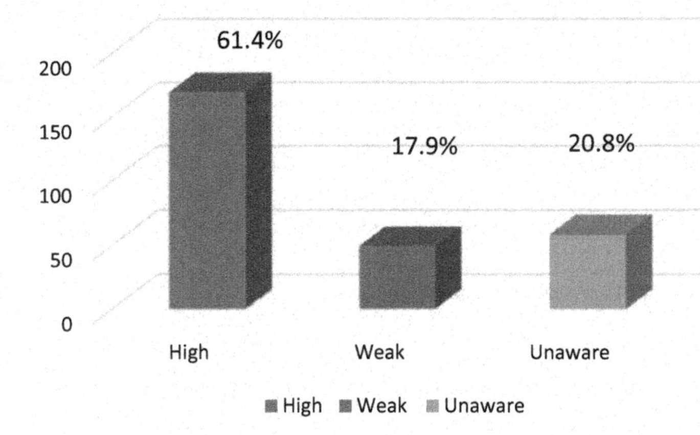

FIGURE 2.1 Awareness level about telemedicine technology and efficiency of its usage.

awareness of using telemedicine for training. Therefore, first essential factor was to train the healthcare employees in order to increase their knowledge of digital technologies and telemedicine. About 79% of participants stated that the first step of implementing telemedicine must be started with establishing an e-learning platform as well as simple model of telemedicine such as SMS (short massage system) data centre to start the adaptation phase and then start to develop multiple telemedicine services (see Figures 2.1–2.4).

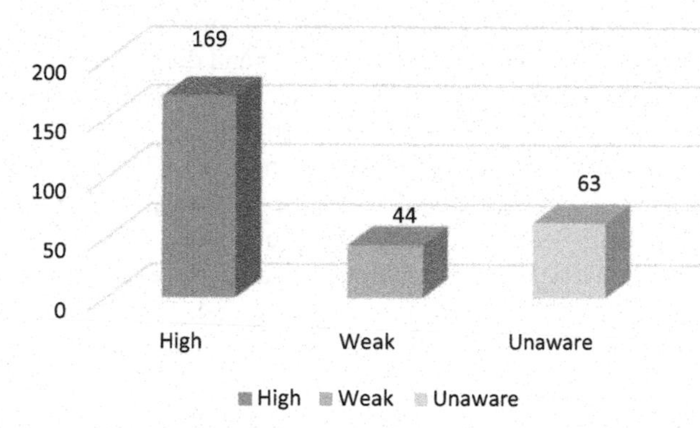

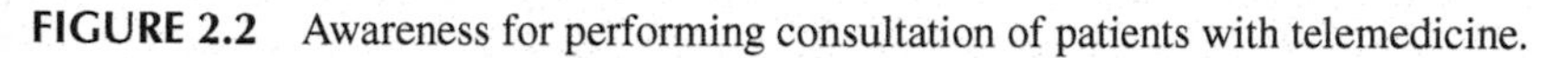
FIGURE 2.2 Awareness for performing consultation of patients with telemedicine.

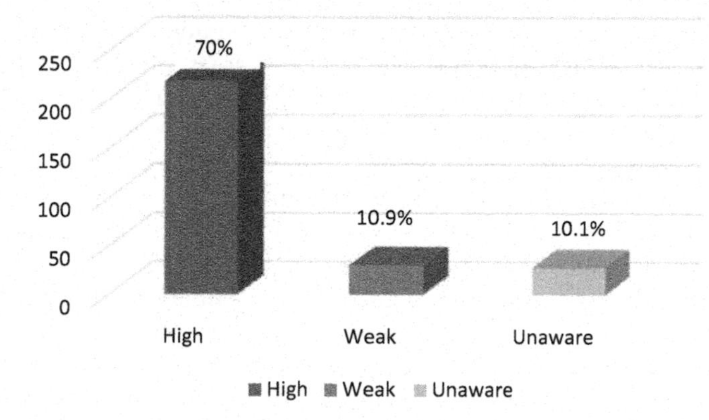

FIGURE 2.3 Awareness for using telemedicine for providing training and information to patients.

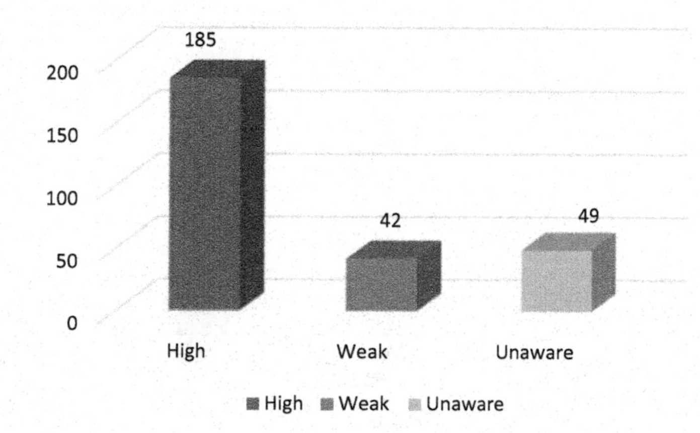

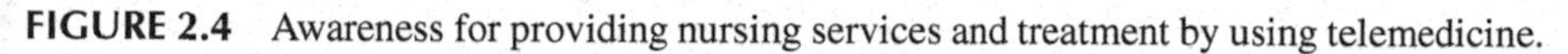
FIGURE 2.4 Awareness for providing nursing services and treatment by using telemedicine.

Data statistics indicated that employees had an agreement with regard to the impact of telemedicine on medical decision-making and diagnosis. Respectively, the culture of using modern technologies and reducing road transportation were the most significant advantages of telemedicine from the employee's viewpoints. Of the 276 participants, 141 stated that telemedicine is not improving the quality of care services, 136 participants stated that it could improve fair distribution, and 120 participants stated that telemedicine is a cost-effective technology.

In investigating the viewpoint of employees regarding the cultural impact of new digital technologies, 29.8% of participants totally agreed, 37.6% agreed, 18.3% neither agreed nor disagreed, 5.8% disagreed, and 11% totally disagreed as shown in Figure 2.5.

Figure 2.6 shows that the impact of telemedicine in treatment and prevention of different diseases obtained 52 participants (18.7%) complete agreement, 87 (40.4%) agree, 73 (26.6%) neither agree nor disagree, 53 (5.8%) disagree, and 11 (8.5%) completely disagree.

In evaluating the attitude of people toward telemedicine in the fair distribution of healthcare services in remote and deprived areas, 86 (1.2%) participants agreed completely, 136 (49.2%) agreed, 38 (13.8%) neither agreed nor disagreed,15 (6.4%) disagreed, and 1 (0.4%) participant was in complete disagreement (see Figure 2.7).

Figure 2.8 shows the attitude of people regarding the effect of telemedicine in reducing financial costs of patients for treatment and health services, where 14 (5.1%) participants agreed completely, 120 participants (43.5%) agreed, 62 (22.5%) participants neither agreed nor disagreed, 40 (14.5%) participants disagreed, and 40 (14.5%) participants completely disagreed with the statement.

Figure 2.9 shows the data concerning the attitude of people toward telemedicine in preventing required travels for treatment and health services , where 81 (29.3%)

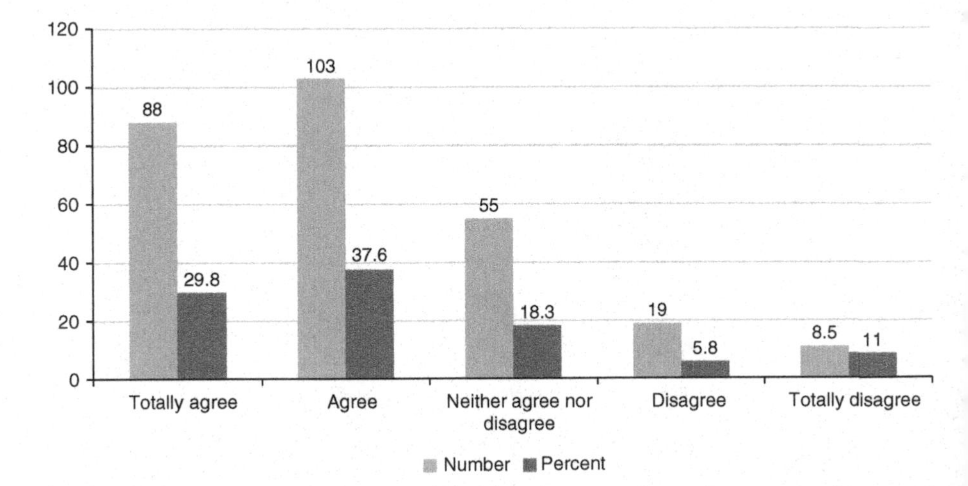

FIGURE 2.5 The viewpoint of employees in culture development by telemedicine.

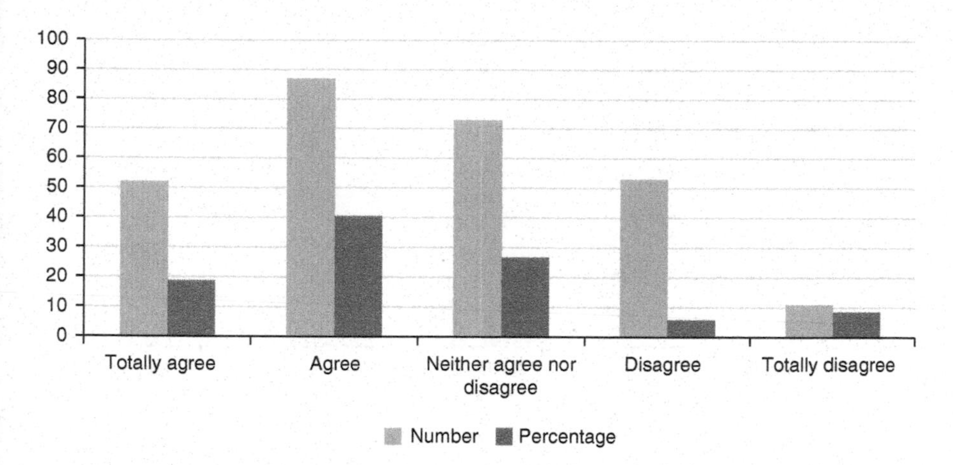

FIGURE 2.6 The viewpoint of employees in improving treatment and preventive medicine by telemedicine.

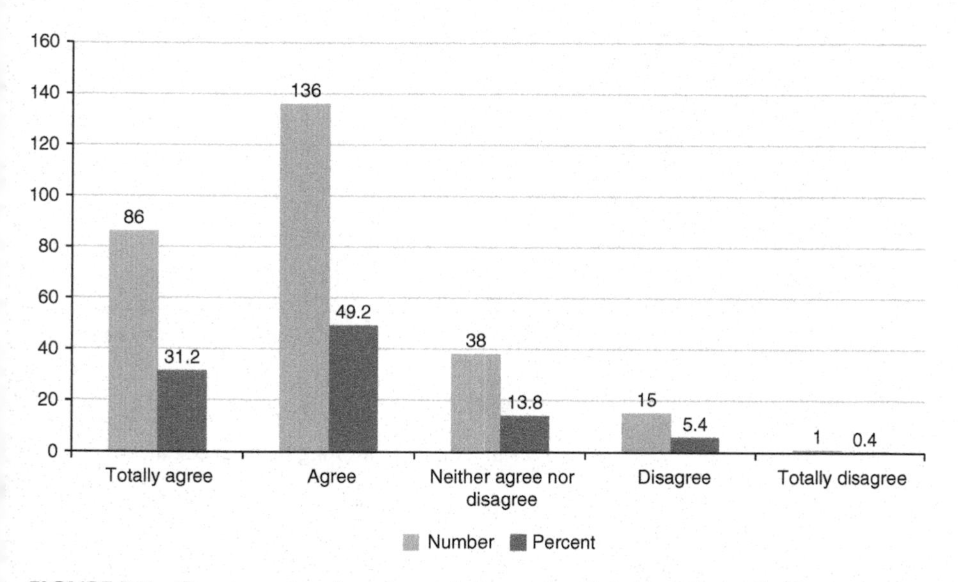

FIGURE 2.7 The viewpoint of employees in increasing digital healthcare distributive justice by telemedicine.

participants agreed completely, 138 (50%) participants agreed, 28 (0.2%) participants neither agreed nor disagreed, 20 (7.2%) participants disagreement and 9 participants (3.3%) completely disagreement.

Concerning the attitude of people regarding the impact of telemedicine in reducing errors in medical affairs, 58 (21%) participants agreed completely, 109 (39.5%) participants agreed, 103 (12.2%) participants neither agreed nor disagreed, 17 (6.2%) participants disagreed, and 3 (1.1%) participants completely disagreed, as shown in Figure 2.10.

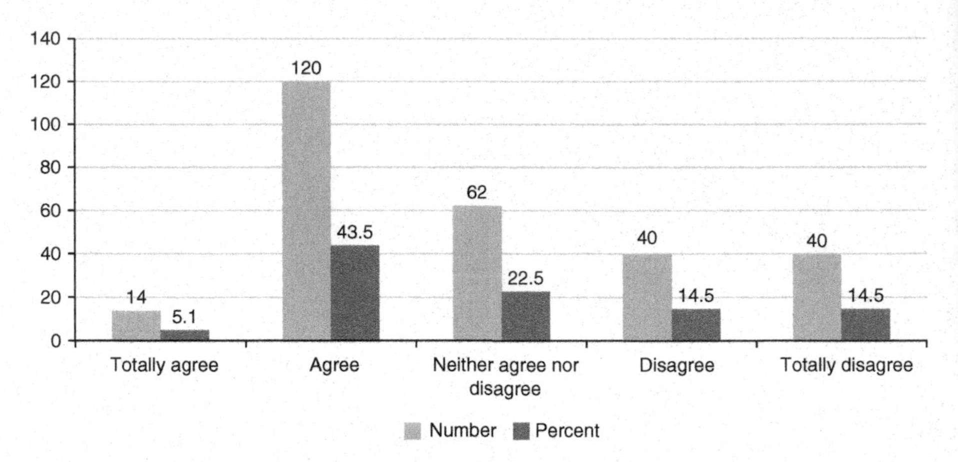

FIGURE 2.8 The viewpoint of employees in reducing cost by telemedicine.

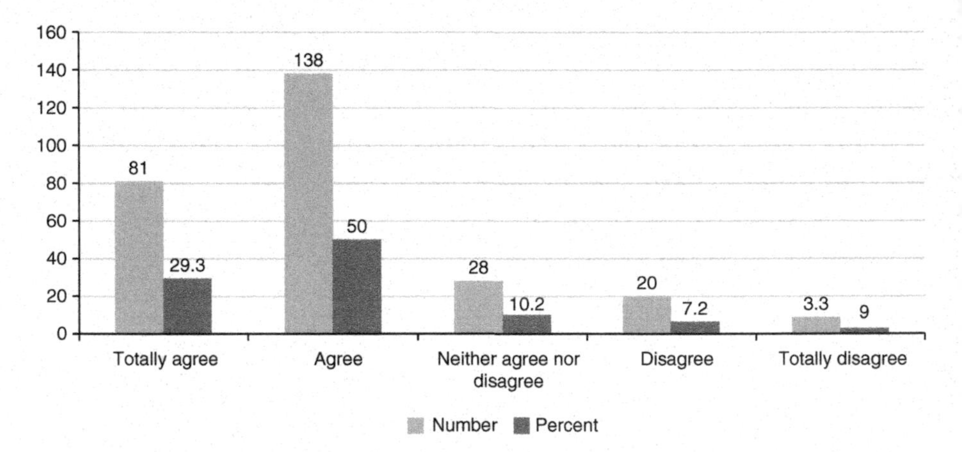

FIGURE 2.9 The viewpoint of employees in reducing travelling by telemedicine.

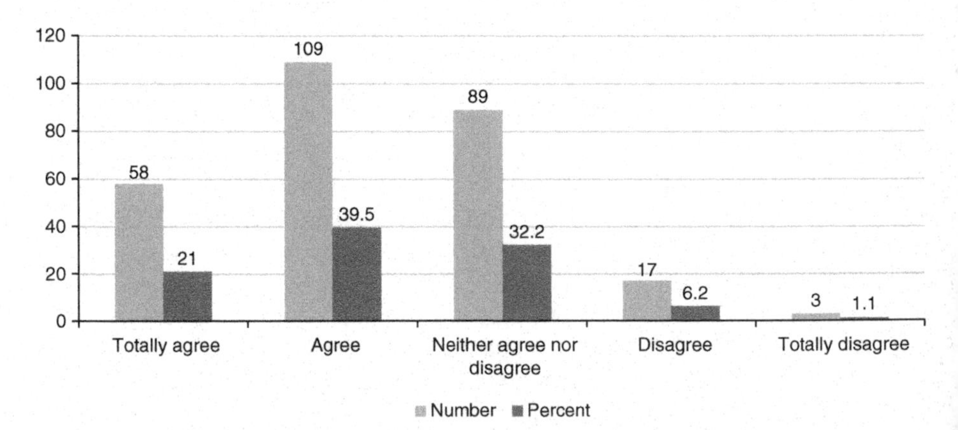

FIGURE 2.10 The viewpoint of employees in reducing medical errors by telemedicine.

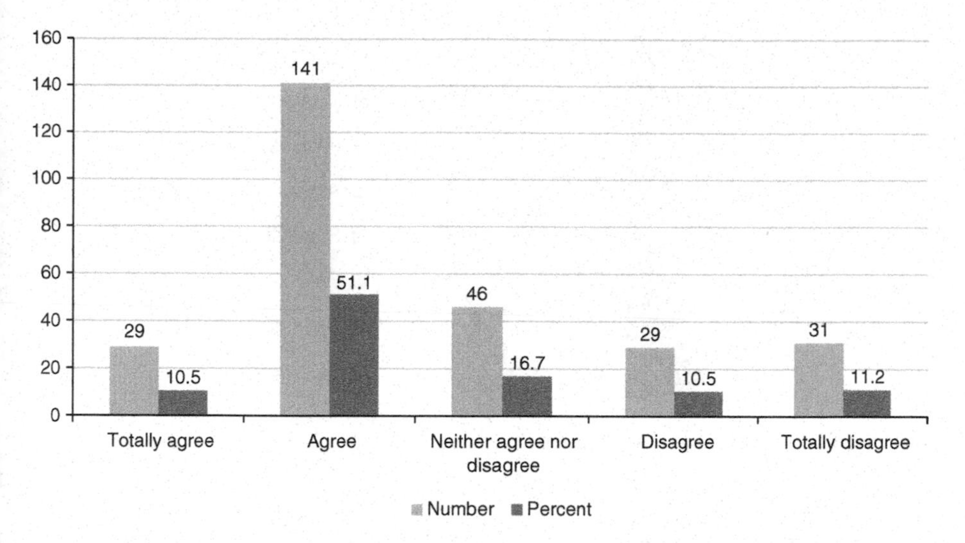

FIGURE 2.11 The viewpoint of employees in improving quality by telemedicine.

With regard to the attitude of people regarding the effects of telemedicine in improving and increasing the quality of provided services in health and treatment, 29 (10.5%) participants agreed completely, 141 (51.1%) participants agreed, 46 (16.7%) participants neither agreed nor disagreed, 29 (10.5%) participants disagreed, and 31 (11.2%) participants completely disagreed, as shown in Figure 2.11.

2.4.5 Participants' Demographics

Of the total 276 participants who filled out the questionnaire, 200 (72.5%) were females, 76 (27.5%) were males, 196 (71%) were married, and 80 (29%) were single. Most of the participants (86; 31.2%) were aged between 25 and 30 years old and only four (1.4%) participants were aged 35–40 years old. Educational status of the participants was as follows: 137 (49.6%) had a bachelor's degree, 16.3% had a professional doctorate degree, 39 (14.1%) had an associate degree, 19 (6.9%) had a master's degree, 12 (4.3%) had a specialty board (medical doctor), 10 (3.6%) had PhD, 9 (3.3%) had a high school diploma, and 5 (1.8%) had a Fellowship degree. Most of the service records were relegated to 5–10 years range, with 78 participants (28.3%), and only 2 (7%) participants had more than 30 years of service record. There were 29 contractual participants, 122 contractual staff, 16 faculty members, 89 tenured employees, and 20 persons were on a performance basis. All the participants were from 30 centers affiliated to Kerman University of Medical Science. The demographics of attendees is shown in Figures 2.12 and 2.13.

2.5 SOLUTION AND RECOMMENDATION

According to the study conducted, the results of the questionnaire confirmed that for implementing telemedicine project in the Kerman province requires

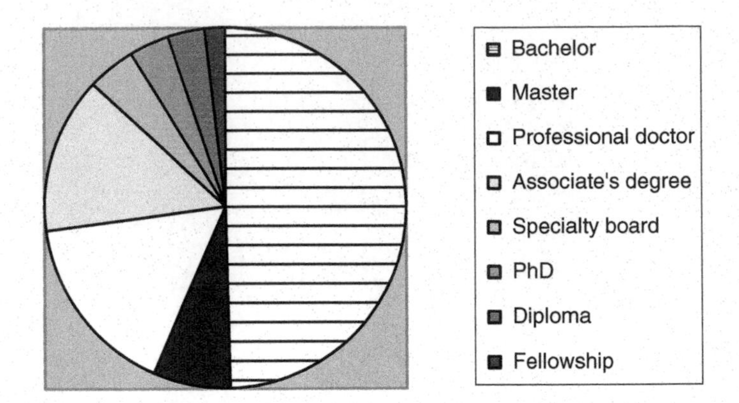

FIGURE 2.12 Education of participants.

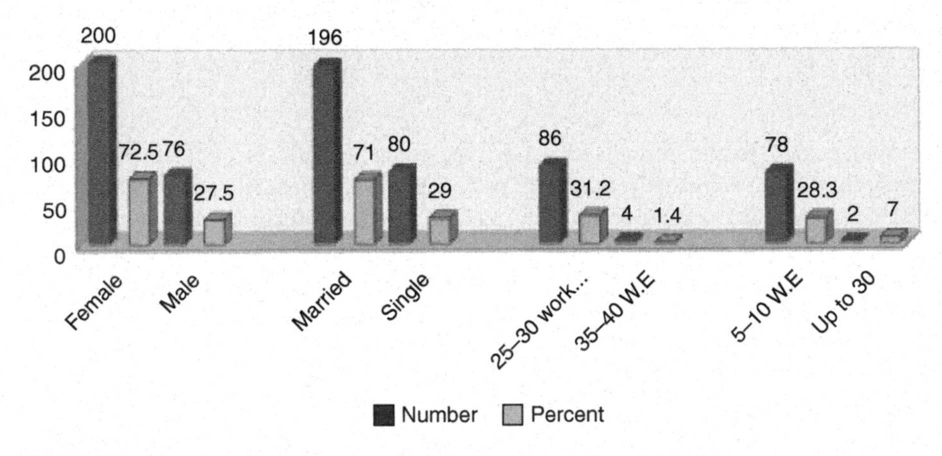

FIGURE 2.13 Sex, marital state, and work experience of participants.

performing necessary training for readiness and awerness development about telemedicine services. There were also high statistics of positive attitude to use e-learning services and positive attitude to use telemedicine in medical diagnosis. The e-learning can be implemented in this province between Kerman University of Medical Sciences and deprived cities for holding educational classes for healthcare providers and nurses.

Since there were many disagreed responses for treatment and prevention of diseases by telemedicine, it is necessary to provide best practice samples to illuminate the positive role of telemedicine. To obtain approval for telemedicine projects, it is essential to build a comprehensive proof of telemedicine cost-effectivness and its return on investement for decision makers and senior managers. Understanding financial benefit can be displayed through tangible, intangible, and hidden cost evaluation.

2.6 FUTURE RESEARCH DIRECTIONS

The lesson learned from this study indicated that before starting the telemedicine implementation, understanding the needs of the population, their readiness, and their awerness and knowledge about digitalization are essential. Likewise, the study of the best practices helps healthcare organizations to grasp more insights. For instance, in the USA, Hermar (2016) found that more insurers are willing to use telehealth for patients in rural areas because a $50 telehealth visit for an ear infection is much cheaper than the $600 cost of the trip from a rural area to an emergency department. Moreover, self-insured employers and some larger insurance companies, such as Athena, United Healthcare, and Anthem, are covering the telehealth services, and copay and deductible may apply for these services (Hermar, 2016). In Europe, according to the Health Technology Assessment Organization, analysis of the cost of technologies, such as telemedicine, is based on quality-adjusted life years (QALYs), healthy years equivalent (HYE), and disability-adjusted life years (DALYs) (CCHP, 2018; Dinesen et al., 2016). In Australia, the emphasis on telemedicine deployment is on supporting champions, and engaging clinicians and digital healthcare professionals is an important factor (Wade, 2013). The waiting time reduction and patient empowerment in their health have been the achievement of telemedicine usage in cities such as Adelaide; however, the lack of health literacy, the potential for dehumanization, and privacy of patient information are the biggest challenges for Australia to embrace telemedicine (Wade, 2013). Therefore, the next phase of establishing telemedicine after evaluating the awareness of individuals must be an in-depth study of payment services, patient privacy consideration, patient safety consideration, and infrastructure and connectivity improvement, as well as integrated context to create a cohesive patient health information database.

2.7 CONCLUSION

According to the findings obtained from this research, it is revealed that technology acceptance is high in this population, and telemedicine can be a useful digital technology to be established in Kerman Province. Evaluating the participants' awareness about telemedicine indicated that 61.4% believed that telemedicine is an efficient technology for teleconsultation, 79% stated that telemedicine is a useful tool for nurses and providers training, and 67% found telemedicine as a helpful technology for the treatment of patients at distance. Moreover, the majority of participants agreed with the advantages of telemedicine, and they viewed telemedicine as a digital technology that can improve cost-effectiveness, develop the digital culture of healthcare, reduce travelling cost, increase healthcare distributive justice, and improve treatment and preventive medicine services.

ACKNOWLEDGEMENTS

The authors gratefully acknowledge Dr. Nakhaei, Dr. Aflatoonian, Dr. Sepehri, Dr. Rohani, Dr. Pendar, Dr. Larizadeh, Dr. Montazer Ghaem, Dr. Bahadini, Dr. Khajavi,

Dr. Malek Pour, Dr. Mosadeg, Dr. Doost Mohamadi, Dr. Azarnoosh, and Dr. Khademi for collaborating in the process of validation of the questionnaire used in this study.

REFERENCES

Adler-Milstein, J., Kvedar, J., & Bates, D. W. (2014). Telehealth among US hospitals: Several factors, including state reimbursement and licensure policies, influence adoption. *Health Affairs, 33*(2), 207–215.

American Hospital Association. (2016). Telehealth: Helping hospitals deliver cost-effective care. *American Hospital Association.* Retrieved from www.aha.org/telehealth.

American College of Medical Practice Executives. (2014). The role of telemedicine in health care reform in 2014 and forward. *American College of Medical Practice Executives.*

AMMC. (April 2018). New research shows increasing physician shortages in both primary and specialty care. *Association of American Medical Colleges.* Retrieved from https://news.aamc.org/press-releases/article/workforce_report_shortage_04112018/.

Ashley, R. C. (2002). Telemedicine: Legal, ethical, and liability considerations. *Journal of the American Dietetic Association, 102*(2), 267.

Augsburger, M. L. (2017). Telemedicine and telehealth benefit, revenue opportunities, challenges, recent developments. *Reimbursement Advisor, 33*(4), 1–12.

Ayatollahi, H., Mirani, N., Nazari, F., & Razavi, N. (2018). Iranian healthcare professionals' perspectives about factors influencing the use of telemedicine in diabetes management. *World Journal of Diabetes, 9*(6), 92–98. doi:10.4239/wjd.v9.i6.92

Baker, T. A., Clay, O. J., Johnson-Lawrence, V., Minahan, J. A., Mingo, C. A., Thorpe, R. J., … Crowe, M. (2017). Association of multiple chronic conditions and pain among older black and white adults with diabetes mellitus. *BMC Geriatrics, 17*(1), 255–255. doi:10.1186/s12877-017-0652-8

Beck, M. (2016). How telemedicine is transforming health care. The revolution is finally here raising a host of questions for regulators, providers, insurers, and patients. *Wall Street Journal* (Online). Retrieved from www.wsj.com/articles/how-telemedicine-is-transforming-health-care-1466993402

Blanton, T., & Balch, D. C. (1995). Telemedicine. *Futurist, 29*(5), 14.

Callahan, E. (2015). Telemedicine reimbursement improving, but is it right for you? *Managed Care Contracting & Reimbursement Advisor, 12*(2), 1–3.

Center for Information Technology Leadership Partners HealthCare. (2015). *Senate appropriations subcommittee on labor, health and human services, education and related agencies hearing*. Washington: Center for Information Technology Leadership Partners HealthCare.

Chen, E. T. (2017). Considerations of telemedicine in the delivery of modern healthcare. *American Journal of Management, 17*(3), 20–28.

CCHP. (2018). Telehealth Advancement Act. *Public Health Institute Center for Connected Health Polic.* Retrieved from https://www.cchpca.org/telehealth-policy/telehealth-advancement-act

CMS. (July 2018). CMS proposes historic changes to modernize Medicare and restore the doctor-patient relationship. *The Centers for Medicare & Medicaid Services*. Retrieved from www.cms.gov/Medicare/Medicare-Fee-for-Service-Payment/SustainableGRatesConFact/Downloads/sgr2015p.pdf

Davis, F. D. (1989). Perceived usefulness, perceived ease of use, and user acceptance of information technology. *MIS Quarterly*, 13 (10) 319–340. Doi: 10.2307/249008

Dinesen, B., Nonnecke, B., Lindeman, D., Toft, E., Kidholm, K., Jethwani, K., … Nesbitt, T. (2016). Personalized telehealth in the future: A global research agenda. *Journal of Medical Internet Research, 18*(3), e53. doi:10.2196/jmir.5257

Goedert, J. (2017). Most states now have laws supporting telehealth reimbursement. *Health Data Management, 25*(4), 9.

Hadeel, A., & Sandhu, K. (2021). PLS model performance for factors influencing students acceptance of elearning analytics recommender. *International Journal of Virtual and Personal Learning Environments.* 10 (2). Doi: 10.4018/IJVPLE.2020070101

Hermar, B. (2016). Virtual reality: More insurers are embracing telehealth. *Modern Healthcare, 46*(8), 16-19.

Iranian Space Agency. (2012). *Report on the United Nations/Islamic Republic of Iran regional workshop on the use of space technology for human health improvement.* (A/AC.105/2012/CRP.13). Vienna: United Nations. Retrieved from www.unoosa.org/pdf/limited/l/AC105_2012_CRP13E.pdf

LeRouge, C., & Garfield, M. (2013). Crossing the telemedicine chasm: Have the U.S. barriers to widespread adoption of telemedicine been significantly reduced? *International Journal of Environmental Research and Public Health, 10*(12), 6472.

Lewis, C. B. (2015). Private payer parity in telemedicine reimbursement: How state mandated coverage can be the catalyst for telemedicine expansion. *The University of Memphis Law Review, 46*(2), 471–502.

McKinnon, K. J. (2017). *Telemedicine: An augmentation strategy to mitigate primary care shortage.* (10685086 D.B.A.), Walden University, Ann Arbor. ProQuest Dissertations & Theses Global database.

Medeiros De Bustos, E., Moulin, T., & Audebert, H. J. (2009). Barriers, legal issues, limitations and ongoing questions in telemedicine applied to stroke. *Cerebrovascular Diseases, 27*, 36–39.

Moran, A., Juan, J., & Roudsari, A. (2015). The importance of telehealth for directors and other decision makers. *Studies in Health Technology and Informatics, 208*, 7–11. Doi: 10.3233/978-1-67499-488-6-7

Phillips, A. B. (2012). *An integrative review of the literature on technology transformation in healthcare.* (3543483 Ph.D.), Columbia University, Ann Arbor. ProQuest Central; ProQuest Dissertations & Theses Global database.

Pinkney, L. M. (2013). *Healthcare reform: Innovative and other proven strategies for successfully managing and implementing organizational change.* (3608771 D.Mgt.), University of Maryland University College, Ann Arbor. ProQuest Central; ProQuest Dissertations & Theses Global database.

Richard, W. (2012). Twenty years of telemedicine in chronic disease management – An evidence synthesis. *Journal of Telemedicine and Telecare, 18*(4), 211–220. doi:10.1258/jtt.2012.120219

Rogers, E. (1995). *Diffusion of Innovations* (4th edn.). New York: The Free Press.

Ryu, S. (2010). History of telemedicine: Evolution, context, and transformation. *Healthcare Informatics Research, 16*(1), 65–66. doi: 10.4258/hir.2010.16.1.65

Safi, S., Ahmadieh, H., Katibeh, M., Yaseri, M., Nikkhah, H., Karimi, S., … Kheiri, B. (2019). Modeling a telemedicine screening program for diabetic retinopathy in Iran and implementing a pilot project in Tehran suburb. *Journal of Ophthalmology, 2019.* doi:10.1155/2019/2073679

Salehahmadi, Z., & Hajialiasghari, F. (2013). Telemedicine in Iran: Chances and challenges. *World Journal of Plastic Surgery, 2*(1), 18–25.

Sandhu, K. (2020). Digital systems innovation for health data analytics. In N.Wickramasinghe (Ed.), *Handbook of Research on Optimizing Healthcare Management Techniques*. Hershey, PA: IGI Global. Doi: 10.4018/978-1-7998-1371-2.ch019

Schwamm, L. H. (2014). Telehealth: Seven strategies to successfully implement disruptive technology and transform health care. *Health Affairs, 33*(2), 200–206.

Scheer, V. (2016). *Process improvement for implementing and sustaining change in healthcare* (10125146 M.S.). The College of St. Scholastica, Ann Arbor. ProQuest Dissertations & Theses Global database.

Schmeida, M. (2005). *Telehealth innovation in the American states* (3180725 Ph.D.). Kent State University, Ann Arbor. ProQuest Central; ProQuest Dissertations & Theses Global database.

Schooley, A. K. (1998). Allowing FDA regulation of communications software used in telemedicine: A potentially fatal misdiagnosis? *Federal Communications Law Journal, 50*(3), 731–751.

Schwamm, L. H. (2014). Telehealth: Seven strategies to successfully implement disruptive technology and transform health care. *Health Affairs, 33*(2), 200–206.

Schwamm, L. H., Chumbler, N., Brown, E., Fonarow, G. C., Nystrom, K., Suter, R., … Tiner, C. (2017). Recommendations for the implementation of telehealth in cardiovascular and stroke Care. *American Heart Association*, 24–44. doi: 10.1161/CIR.0000000000000475

Scott, J. A. (2015). *US telehealth state policies: A forecast of Texas telehealth trends to Medicaid beneficiaries* (3742878 Ph.D.). The University of Texas at Dallas, Ann Arbor. ProQuest Dissertations & Theses Global database.

Stanberry, B. (2006). Legal and ethical aspects of telemedicine. *Journal of Telemedicine and Telecare, 12*(4), 166–175.

Tait, I. E. (2013). *Comparison of project management software tool use in healthcare and other industries* (3607024 Ph.D.). Capella University, Ann Arbor. ProQuest Central; ProQuest Dissertations & Theses Global database.

TRC. (2016). Telehealth policy barriers. *National Organization of State Offices of Rural Health, Center for Connected Health Policy, Telehealth Resource Center*.

Van Dyk, L. (2014). A review of telehealth service implementation frameworks. *International Journal of Environmental Research and Public Health, 11*(2), 1279–1298.

Venkatesh, V., & Davis, F. D. (2000). A theoretical extension of the technology acceptance model: Four longitudinal field studies. *Management Science, 46*(2), 186–204.

Wade, V. A. (2013). *What is needed for telehealth to deliver sustainable value to the routine operation of healthcare in Australia*, Thesis (Ph.D.), University of Adelaide, School of Population Health

Waters, R. J. (2009). Ensuring success: Telemedicine boosts access to needed care. *Roll Call*. ProQuest Central. Proquest ID 324394303

Ziadlou, D. (2013). Evaluation of using telemedicine in unexpected disaster in city of Tehran. *Telemedicine and e-Health Journal, 19*(5), 79. doi: 10.1089/tmj.2013.9994-A

Ziadlou, D. (September 2019). *Digital health leadership in healthcare organizations[YouTube]*. Switzerland International Society for Telemedicine and e-Health (ISfTeH).

Ziadlou, D., Islami, A., & Hassani, H. R. (2008). Telecommunication method for implementing the telemedicine systems in crisis management. *IEEE*, 268–273. DOI: 10.1109/BROADCOM.2008.31

APPENDIX

Kerman Province Map

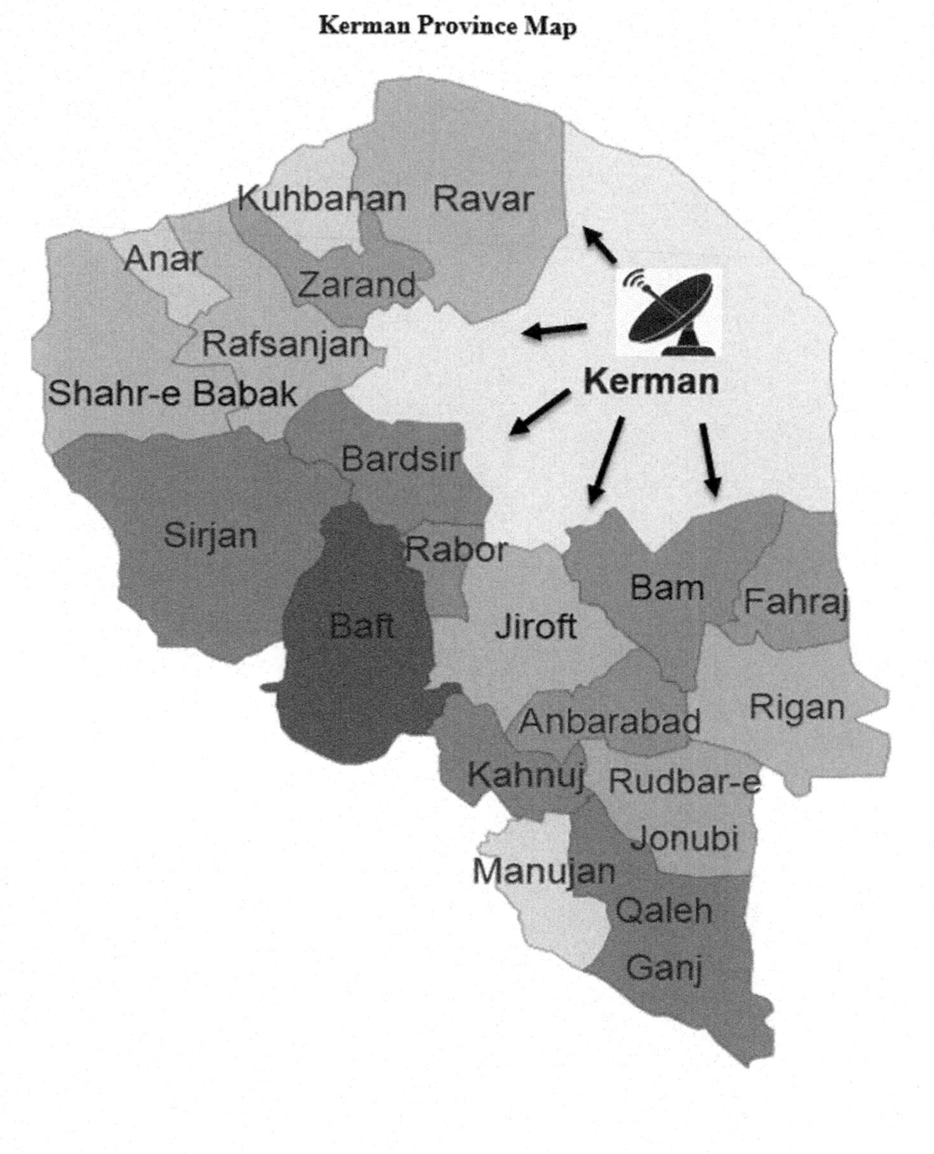

3 Intelligent Algorithms for the Diagnosis of Alzheimer's Disease

Sarah A. Soliman, Rania R. Hussein, El-Sayed A. El-Dahshan, and Abdel-Badeeh M. Salem

CONTENTS

3.1 INTRODUCTION

The most common form of dementia, Alzheimer's disease (AD), is characterized by unresolved etiology and pathophysiology. The progressive degenerative aspect of the disease is indicated by neurofibrillary tangle, plaque buildup, and tissue loss in brain parenchyma [1, 2]. In terms of patient management, early detection of AD at the pre-clinical stage is of great importance. Since the earliest symptoms of AD, such as short-term memory loss and irrational paranoia, are often mistaken for aging and anxiety, or are confused with symptoms arising from other brain disorders, it remains difficult to assess the progression of disease and AD dynamics in the dementia scenario until it demonstrates severe cognitive deterioration with typical signs of neuroimaging.

Patient history and cognitive impairment testing are usually helpful in the diagnosis of AD clinically [3]. Neuropsychological-scale diagnosis requires a variety of specialist clinical experience to be subjective and less repeatable. In addition, it is more difficult to classify patients with AD at a prodromal level, called mild cognitive impairment (MCI), as these patients have cognitive impairments beyond what is required for their age and education, but do not track AD neuropathological changes. Neuroimaging, especially high-resolution magnetic resonance imaging (MRI), was recommended for prediction of AD in more precise research criteria. The structural MR images provide additional information on pathological tissue atrophy or other unusual biomarkers that can be sensitively identified at an early stage of the disease, and therefore automated imaging methods are needed to help diagnose the disease until permanent neuronal failure has occurred or to help detect brain changes [5].

To this end, many algorithms have been proposed to distinguish AD or MCI, ranging from conceptually simple volume measurement or mathematically complex description of shape difference in a priori regions of interest (ROI) [6–7] to voxel-wise modeling of changes in tissue density across the entire brain region, for example, voxel-wise morphometry [8]–9]. Medical imaging machine learning and computer-aided diagnostics have gained more attentions in the field of medical diagnostic, where a machine learning algorithm is trained to produce a desired output from a set of input training data, such as voxel intensity, tissue density, and shape descriptor features.

Diagnostics of machine learning can also be divided into methods based on ROI and whole brain. Algorithms based on ROI also concentrate on the brain's medial temporal structures, including the hippocampus and entorhinal cortex. Support vector machine (SVM) was used in the work of Achterberg et al. [10], Gerardin et al. [11], and Sørensen et al. [12] to classify AD or MCI subjects with hippocampal volume or shape as characteristics. Another study has compared the linear discriminant analysis (LDA) and SVM for MCI classification and prediction based on hippocampal volume [11]. The entorhinal cortical thickness and modified tissue in amygdala, hippocampus gyrus have also been used as features in AD and MCI discrimination [13–14]. It is still unclear whether hippocampus, medial temporal lobe, or other ROIs would be a better choice for AD prediction. Klöppel et al. [15] developed a supervised method for grouping the gray matter segment of T1-weighted MR images into a high-dimensional space using linear SVM, treating voxels as coordinates and intensity values at each voxel location.

Aguilar et al. [16] investigated the classification performance of orthogonal projections on latent structures (OPLS), decision trees, artificial neural networks (ANNs), and SVM based on 10 features selected from 23 volumetric and 34 cortical thickness variables. Beheshti et al. [17] combined voxel-based morphometric with Fisher's criterion to pick and minimize features across the entire brain, followed by SVM for classification.

This work is aimed to analyze and study the existing algorithms for detecting AD using MRI technique. The rest of the chapter is organized as follows: Section 3.2 discusses brain imaging techniques and especially spots the light on MRI scans. Section 3.3 presents the methodology of pattern recognition for AD using MRI and discusses the most popular algorithms in detail used to build architecture system for detecting AD. Section 3.4 focuses on pattern recognition techniques and finally Section 3.5 concludes the chapter.

3.2 BRAIN IMAGING TECHNIQUES

Brain imaging techniques allow doctors and researchers, without invasive neurosurgery, to see behavior or issues within the human brain. Recent research has found that a range of approved, secure imaging techniques are in use today. There are many imaging modalities [18] that allow physicians and researchers to study the brain in a noninvasive manner. Computed tomography (CT), positron emission tomography (PET) and MRI [18–19] can provide brain tissues information from a variety of sequences of excitation. MRI provides superior contrast to various brain regions compared to all other imaging modalities. MRI is effective in the application of brain tumor detection and identification [20] due to high soft tissue contrast, high spatial resolution, and no harmful radiation, and is a non-invasive procedure.

For soft tissue delineation, MRI is often the superior medical imaging. It is used by radiologists to visualize the body's internal structure. MRI offers a wealth of human soft tissue anatomy data. It helps in AD assessment [20–21]. MRI scans are used to examine and study the brain behavior. The strength of the MRI signal depends mainly on three molecules. Other two parameters are relaxation T1 and T2 [22], representing different characteristics of individual protons' local environment. The pathological T2 test is useful to identify the area of brain damage. Usually the anatomical T1 scans have the best scan resolution and are useful for anatomical structure localization. MRI can provide high-resolution spatial images, and its rich data material can be properly used to build automated diagnostic tools that can help the medical community to draw inferences about the state of the brain being examined faster and easier.

3.3 PATTERN RECOGNITION METHODOLOGY

Recognition of patterns is a collection of processes aimed at extracting meaningful information or patterns from a data set [23]. The organizational chart in Figure 3.1 uses classification techniques that predict categorical labels to show the supervised pattern recognition steps. The first step in pattern recognition is the problem statement that gathers the data and context knowledge behind the application domain, creates assumptions, and decides what type of information is required to derive from

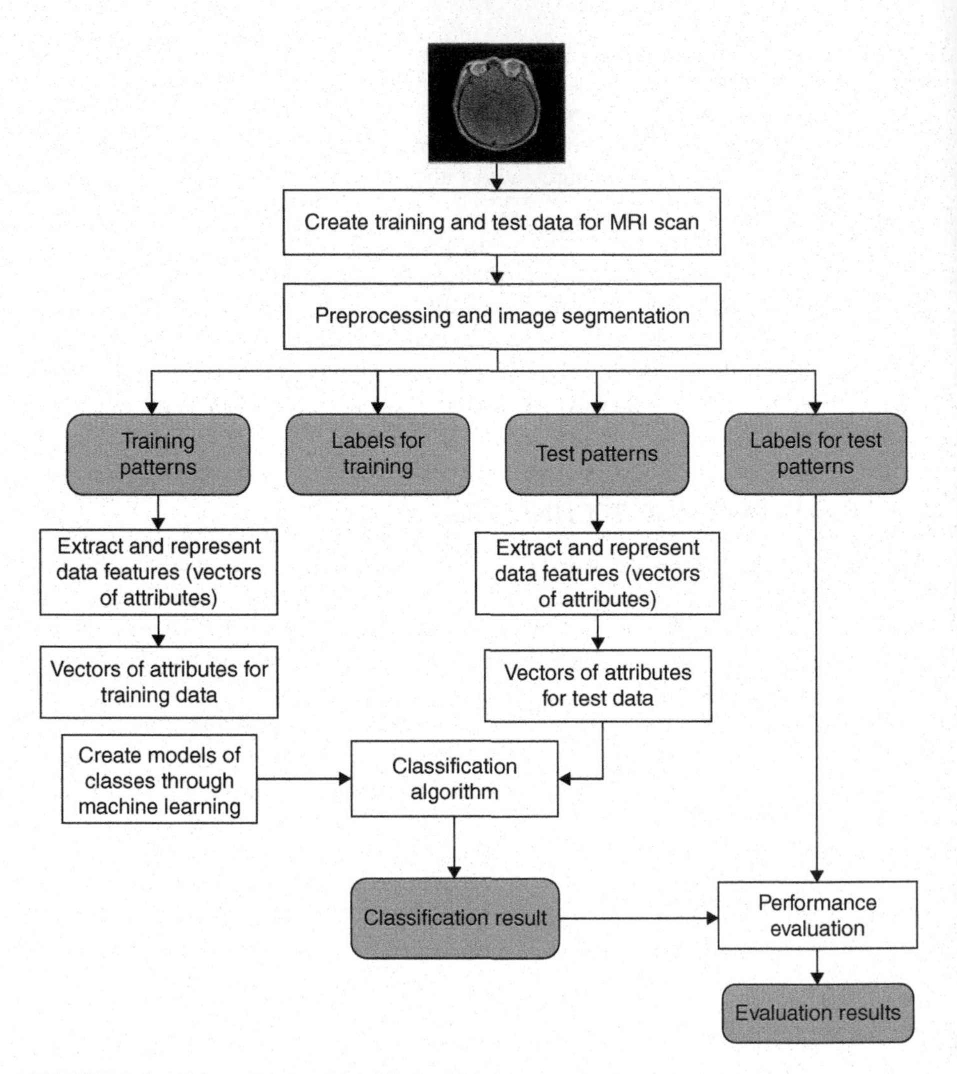

FIGURE 3.1 Pattern Recognition Methodology.

the data. Data collection is usually followed by a preprocessing step to clean and standardize the data [24]. Once the data are well defined, the next step is to extract and represent the data characteristics in the form of vectors, followed by the development of category models through machine learning. The expert must choose one of the pattern recognition techniques (algorithms), such as classification, clustering and regression, depending on the type of label output (categorical labels or real-valued labels), whether learning is supervised or unsupervised, and whether the pattern algorithm is statistical or nonstatistical. Finally, assessment criteria such as bootstrapping and cross-validation are used to progress the performance evaluation of pattern recognition algorithm tests.

3.3.1 Preprocessing Algorithms for MRI scans

Preprocessing images is the initial step of retrieving images to ensure the reliability of the subsequent steps [25]. The images obtained from different modalities cause many problems, such as low resolution and distortion, which reduces the precision of the results obtained. Preprocessing image techniques are important in order to remove noise and increase the image quality and make the segmentation results more accurate and use redundancy in images. The preprocessing stage is a shift in image data that smooth unnecessary twists, enhances any image or highlights essential facts for further processing. The basic reason for applying correction is to minimize or decrease the impact of errors or anomalies in object darkness values that may be a containment point in one's ability to translate or quantitatively plan and examine remotely observed computerized objects. Preprocessing [26] plays an important role because of noisy, inconsistent, and incomplete data. It is one of the necessary preliminary steps to acquire the high accuracy of the steps. MRI images consist of objects, patient-specific artifacts and artifacts dependent on equipment; others are artifacts of circle, staircase, and volume effect. Before analyzing all of these, preprocessing procedures will remove them. We have proposed various approaches to de-noise the image. The following algorithms are used to preprocess the image [27].

3.3.1.1 Noise Removal

Noise reduction algorithm is the mechanism by which noise from the object is eliminated or reduced. Noise reduction algorithms [28] minimize noise visibility by smoothing the entire image from areas close to contrast boundaries.

3.3.1.2 Gabor Filter

Gabor filter is an edge detection filter. Gabor filters' frequency and orientation representations are close to those of the human visual system and have been found to be particularly suitable for representing texture and discriminating against it [29]. A two-dimensional (2D) Gabor filter is a Gaussian kernel function that is modulated by a sinusoidal plane wave in the spatial domain. Gabor functions can model simple cells in the visual cortex of mammalian brains. In the human visual system, therefore, object processing with Gabor filters is considered to be close to perception.

3.3.1.3 Median Filter

A nonlinear filtering technique is the median filter, often used to remove noise [30]. Such noise reduction is a traditional preprocessing stage, such as edge detection on an image, to improve the results of later processing. Median filtering is commonly used in digital image processing as it preserves edges while eliminating noise under certain conditions. The median filter's main idea is to run through the input signal, replacing each input with the median of the neighboring entry. Neighbors' pattern is called the "window" that slides through the entire signal, entry by entry. The most visible window for one-dimensional (1D) signals is just the first ones that precede it.

3.3.1.4 Image Enhancement

Image enhancement is the preprocessing process for improving the quality and information content of original data [31]. Common practices include improvement of contrast, spatial filtering, and slicing of density. Contrast enhancement or stretching is done through linear transformation that expands the original gray level range. Spatial filtering strengthens spatial features such as fault, shear zones, and lineaments that occur naturally. Density slicing transforms the continuous gray tone range into a series of intervals of density marked by a separate color or symbol to represent different characteristics.

3.3.2 Segmentation Algorithms for MRI Scans

To determine objects and boundaries in images, the idea of image segmentation depends on dividing a digital image into multiple parts. Segmentation refers to converting an image's presentation to be simple, precise, and easier to analyze. For clinical diagnosis, segmentation of the visual picture plays a vital role. It can be considered a difficult issue because medical images often have poor contrasts, different types of noise, and missing or diffuse boundaries [32–34]. The brain anatomy can be detected and scanned by brain imaging techniques such as MRI or CT scan. Compared to CT scans, MRI scan is considered the best in the diagnosis and detection of AD.

The segmentation of the image can be divided into two basic types: local segmentation which is related to specific part or area of the image and global segmentation which is related to segmentation of the entire image and consists of a large number of pixels [35].

Image segmentation algorithms are constructed based on one of the two basic image intensity value properties: discontinuity and similarity [36]. The segmentation method in the formal classification decomposes the processed image based on the changes in frequency, such as edges and corners. The second one is based on splitting an image into related regions due to a set of predefined criteria. Therefore, as shown in Figure 3.2, there are many segmentation strategies that can be commonly used, such as threshold methods, edge-based methods, region-based methods (splitting, increasing, and merging), and clustering methods (Fuzzy C-means clustering and k-means clustering,). Image segmentation has many challenging issues, such as developing a unified approach that can be applied to all image and application types. Even selecting a suitable technique for a specific type of image is a difficult issue.

Therefore, there is no universally accepted procedure for segmentation of images. So, image processing and computer processing remain a challenging problem in image processing and computer vision fields [37].

3.3.2.1 Old-School Image Segmentation Methods

3.3.2.1.1 Threshold Methods

Thresholding methods are the simplest methods for image segmentation. These methods divide the pixels of the image by their level of intensity. For images of lighter artifacts than context, these approaches are used. Such methods can be chosen

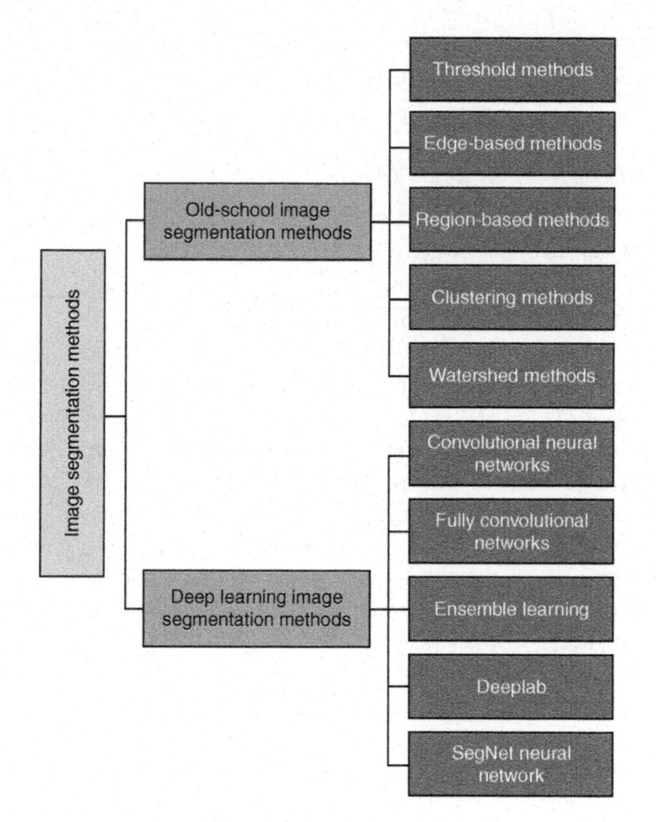

FIGURE 3.2 Image Segmentation Techniques.

manually or automatically, that is, they can be based on prior knowledge or image feature data. There are three forms of thresholding [38]:

1. *Global thresholding*: This is done by using an appropriate threshold value T. This value of T will be constant for the whole image. On the basis of T, the output image can be obtained from the original image $p(x, y)$ as follows:

$$q(x,y) = \{\{1, if\ p(x,y) > T\ 0,\ if\ p(x,y) \le T\} q(x,y) \tag{3.1}$$

   Global thresholding have two famous methods: Otsu and Kapur [39].
2. *Variable thresholding*: In this type of thresholding, the value of T can vary over the image. This can further be of two types:
   a. Local threshold: In this the value of T depends on the neighborhood of x and y.
   b. Adaptive threshold: the value of T is a function of x and y.
   Savala [40], Niblack [41], and Bernsen [42] are the methods included in local thresholding.

3. *Multiple thresholding:* In this type of thresholding, there are multiple threshold values like T0 and T1. By using these, the output image can be computed as follows:

$$q(x,y) = m,\ if\ p(x,y) > T1\ n, if\ p(x,y) \leq T10,\ if\ p(x,y) \leq T0 \tag{3.2}$$

3.3.2.1.2 Edge-Based Methods

Edge-based segmentation relies on image data discontinuities to locate segment boundaries before evaluating the enclosed region [43]. The problem $\{m,\ if\ p(x,y) > T1\ n,\ if\ p(x,y) \leq T10,\ if\ p(x,y) \leq T0$ with this approach is that edge profile is not usually known in practice. In addition, the profile also varies significantly along the edge induced by shading and texture. Normally symmetrical simple step edge is assumed due to these difficulties and the edge detection is done on the basis of a gradient of maximum intensity. The identified boundary is rarely complete. Therefore, edge linking is usually required to fill gaps. In order to achieve segmentation, boundary data are sometimes combined with region growing. Regional edges can be defined by the local limit of the gradient operator's magnitude, the second-order Laplacian operator's zero crossing, or the sue of morphological erosion and dilation operators.

3.3.2.1.2.1 GRADIENT OPERATOR-BASED EDGE DETECTION

By using the Prewitt or Sobel convolution masks [44], vertical and horizontal elements of gradient operator are often implemented as finite difference formulas. They reflect numerous compromises between noise robustness and response sharpness.

3.3.2.1.2.2 LAPLACIAN OF GAUSSIAN ZERO-CROSSING EDGE DETECTION

In 1980, Marr and Hildrethw invented Laplacian of Gaussian zero-crossing [45], who combined Gaussian filtering with the Laplacian. This algorithm is not often used in machine vision. The Laplacian is an isotropic 2D representation of a picture's second spatial derivative. An image's Laplacian highlights regions of rapid change in intensity and is therefore often used to detect edges. Usually the operator takes as input a single gray-level image and produces another gray-level image as output.

3.3.2.1.2.3 CANNY EDGE DETECTION

The Canny edge detection method [46] aims to locate the edges of objects where the frequency changes rapidly and is optimal in a precise mathematical sense but more difficult to implement than methods based on Prewitt or Sobel operators. The canny detector, combined with hysteresis monitoring, which involves two thresholds, aims to track borders between poorly defined objects as well as hard edges and avoids soft edges that are not related to stronger edges.

3.3.2.1.3 Region-Based Methods

The region-based segmentation [47] divides an image into similar/homogeneous areas of connected pixels by applying the criteria of homogeneity/similarity between candidate pixel sets. With respect to certain characteristics or calculated properties, such as color, brightness, and/or texture, each of the pixels in a region is identical. Failure to change the criterion for homogeneity/similarity would result in unexpected results. The following are some of them:

- The segmented region might be smaller or larger than the actual region.
- Over- or under-segmentation of the image.
- Fragmentation.

3.3.2.1.3.1 REGION GROWING

Region growing algorithms as discussed in Figure 3.3 start with one or more pixels, called seeds, and then grow regions around them based on specified criteria of homogeneity. If the adjacent pixels are identical to the seed, they are combined into the region; often the decision is based on a statistical test. The process continues until a predefined condition of termination has been reached. Region splitting and merging using quadtrees is an alternative approach to forming homogeneous regions.

3.3.2.1.4 Clustering Methods

Clustering complies with certain process classification requirements and laws [48]. The clustering method of the feature space is used to segment the pixels with the corresponding feature space points in the image space. The feature space is segmented according to their aggregation in the feature space and then mapped back to the original image space to get the effect of segmentation. In other words, it can be considered as the partition of data set into subsets so that some common properties should be displayed in the data in each subset. Proximity may be the properties according to some given measure of distance or other means of measurement. There are many clustering methods such as k-means clustering or fuzzy clustering, each of which has its own advantages.

3.3.2.1.4.1 K-MEANS ALGORITHM

One of the most commonly used clustering algorithms is the k-means clustering algorithm. Its basic idea is to collect the samples according to the distance in various clusters. The closer the two points are, the closer they get to the goal of clustering the

```
Region growing algorithm (reproduced from [47])
While all the pixels in image are not visited;
Choose an unlabeled pixel p_k;
Set the region's mean to intensity of pixel p_k;
Consider unlabeled neighboring pixel p_kj; If(pixel's intensity - region's mean) < threshold;
a. Affect the pixel p_kj; to the region labeled by k.
b. Update the region's mean and go back to 3;
 Else k = k + 1 and go back to 1.
End If
End While
```

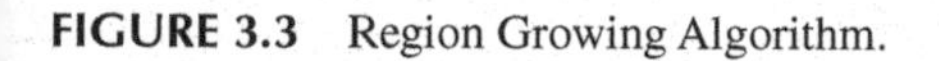

FIGURE 3.3 Region Growing Algorithm.

K-means segmentation algorithm (Reproduced from [49])
(1) Randomly select K initial clustering centers;
(2) Calculate the distance from each sample to each cluster center, and return each sample to the nearest clustering center;
(3) For each cluster, with the mean of all samples as the cluster of new clustering centers;
(4) Repeat steps (2) to (3) until the cluster center no longer changes or reaches the set number of iterations [21].

FIGURE 3.4 K-means Segmentation Algorithm.

compact and independent clusters. The k-means implementation method is shown in Figure 3.4.

The advantage of the k-means clustering algorithm is that it is fast and simple, and for large data sets it is highly efficient and scalable. And the complexity of its time is similar to linear and ideal for large-scale data sets mining. The disadvantage of k-means is that it has no explicit selection criteria for its clustering number k and is hard to estimate. Second, from the k-means algorithm context, it can be seen that each iteration of the algorithm goes through all the samples, so the algorithm's time is very costly.

3.3.2.1.4.2 FUZZY C-MEANS ALGORITHM

One of the methods used to classify a given set of data into a very similar group is the fuzzy c-means algorithm [50]. Therefore, an image's pixel value can belong to more than one cluster. There is a value called membership value for each cluster for each pixel of an image, which determines the degree of share in each cluster of that particular point. So for all clusters, the membership matrix is a matrix composed of each pixel's membership value. In other words, it performs segmentation by classifying fuzzy pixels in the sense that pixels can be in multiple classes with membership varying from 0 to 1. Let us consider a finite set of n number of data X={x1,x2,...xn}. Fuzzy c-means algorithm divides the data set X into a group of c fuzzy cluster based on some specified conditions. It is an iterative process that is based on minimization of the objective function. The algorithm for fuzzy c-means algorithm is given in Figure 3.5.

3.3.2.1.5 Watershed Segmentation

A watershed is the ridge dividing different river system drained areas. The watershed is a technique of segmentation based on morphological gradients. The image gradient map is known to be a relief map in which different gradient values suit different heights. The water level will rise above the basins if we punch a hole in each local minimum and immerse the entire map in water. A dam is built between them when two different bodies of water meet. The progress continues until all points are submerged in the map. Finally, the entire image is segmented by the reservoirs that are then called watersheds and are referred to as catchment basins for the segmented areas.

Fuzzy C means segmentation algorithm (Reproduced from [51])
Step 1: Initialize number of cluster and membership function matrix υ.
Step 2: Find value of center for each cluster using the formula given below

$$??_? = \frac{\bar{\upsilon}_?^{??} - ??^{??}_{??}{}^{??}{}_?}{\bar{\upsilon}_?^{??} - ??^{??}_{??}} \quad (3)$$

Step 3: Calculate the error or cost function, and check if it is lower than the given specific threshold value or improvement over previous iteration.
Step 4: If it is satisfy than it will cluster the data.
Step 5: If it is not satisfied, then update the membership matrix using the relation given below and continue the algorithm again

$$??_{???} = \frac{??}{\bar{\upsilon}_{??}^{??} -_{??}^{=} \frac{??_{???}}{??_{???}}^{\frac{??}{??-??}}_{=}} \quad (4)$$

FIGURE 3.5 Fuzzy C-means Algorithm.

Watershed segmentation algorithm (Reproduced from [53])
Step 1: Compute segmentation function
Step 2: Compute gradient magnitude using derivative operator
Step 3: Compute foreground markers
Step 4: Compute background markers
Step 5: Modify the segmentation function to have minimum values at the foreground and background marker locations.

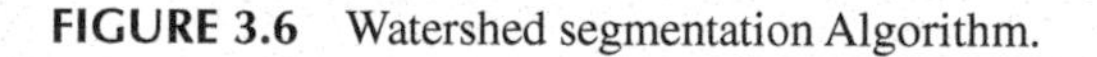

FIGURE 3.6 Watershed segmentation Algorithm.

A catchment basin is the geographical area draining into a river or reservoir. The watershed algorithm applies these ideas to the processing of grayscale images so that a variety of image segmentation problems can be solved [52]. The steps of the watershed segmentation algorithm are shown in Figure 3.6.

3.3.2.1.6 *Deep Learning Image Segmentation Methods*

Deep learning has become more essential in tackling more advanced challenges with image segmentation. There are several deep learning architectures used for segmentation.

3.3.2.1.6.1 CONVOLUTIONAL NEURAL NETWORKS (CNNS)

CNN [54] image segmentation involves feeding object segments as input into a CNN that tags the pixels. The CNN is unable to process the entire image at once. It scans the image, looking at a small multi-pixel "filter" every time until the entire image has been mapped.

3.3.2.1.6.2 Fully Convolutional Networks (FCNs)

Standard CNNs have layers that are completely connected and cannot manage various input sizes. FCNs [55] use convolutional layers to process different input sizes and can operate more quickly. The final output layer has a large receptive field and matches the image height and width, whereas the number of channels matches the number of classes. The convolution layers identify each pixel to determine the image background, including the image position.

3.3.2.1.6.3 DeepLab

One of DeepLab's key motivations [56] is to perform image segmentation while helping to monitor signal decimation, reducing the number of samples and the amount of data the network needs to process. Another motivation is to enable multi-scale learning of contextual features by aggregating image features at various scales. DeepLab uses a residual neural network (ResNet) [57] pre-trained by ImageNet to extract features. Instead of standard convolutions, DeepLab uses atrocious (dilated) convolutions. The varying dilation levels of each convolution allow multi-scale situational information to be captured by ResNet block.

3.3.2.1.6.4 SegNet Neural Network

An architecture based on deep encoders and decoders, also known as semantic pixel-wise segmentation. It involves encoding the input image in low dimensions and then recovering it in the decoder with the capabilities of orientation invariance. This creates a segmented image at the end of the decoder.

Table 3.1 shows the strengths and weaknesses of segmentation techniques

3.3.3 Feature Selection and Extraction Algorithms for MRI Scans

Feature extraction is an important step in computer-assisted brain abnormality diagnosis using MRI [58–60]. Feature extraction is the process of reducing image data size by obtaining the required information from the segmented image. One of the major problems when performing the analysis of complex data is the number of variables involved. Analysis with a large number of variables generally requires a large amount of memory and computation power or a classification algorithm that overfits the training sample and generalizes poorly to new samples.

Feature selection [61] is the technique used to select a subset of appropriate features to construct robust learning models by eliminating most obsolete and redundant functionality from the data.

Feature selection (FS) algorithms [61–62] take up another dimension reduction method by searching for the "best" least subset of the original features without transforming the data into a new set of dimensions. Feature selection is a fairly well-posed question in the sense of supervised learning. The aim may be to determine features that are correlated with class label [63] or predictive. The goal may be to select features that will build the most accurate classifier. The object is less well posed in unsupervised selection of features and is therefore a much less explored field. The following algorithms are used to select and extract the most important features from the image.

TABLE 3.1
Segmentation Techniques Strengths and Weaknesses

Segmentation Technique	Strengths	Weaknesses	After Segmented
Thresholding technique	• Simple calculation and faster running speed • In particular, the segmentation effect can be obtained when the target and the context are strongly contrasted [46].	• Precise results for object segmentation problems are difficult to obtain when there is no substantial gray scale difference or a large overlap of the gray scale values in the image.	
Region based	• The speed is very fast. • It performs well with noisy image.	• No appropriate thresholds or seeds were found, mainly due to unknown and erratic noise. Poor contrast • Weak boundaries that are inherent to medical images. • Time-consuming problem.	
Edge based	• Easy to implement • Easy to understand	• It is not suitable with very noise image. • It is not suitable for images whose boundaries are very small.	
Watershed technique	• Simplicity • Speed • Complete division of the image.	• Over segmentation • Sensitivity to noise • Poor detection of significant areas with low-contrast boundaries • Poor detection of thin structures.	
Clustering methods	• Fast • Suitable with medical image.	• Misclassification in noise-affected images and coincident clusters. • Using all pixels in the image and this increases the time of segmentation.	
Deep learning	• Solve the overfitting problem because the network architecture works on large data sets • Get high performance due to the deeper network.	• It spends long time to train the network.	

3.3.3.1 Discrete Wavelet Transform (DWT)

The wavelet is an effective computational tool for extracting information, and it has become the method of choice in many medical image analysis and classification problems[64]. The main advantage of wavelets is to extract image features in different directions and scales as they provide localized time frequency information of a specially beneficial signal for classification[65],[66]. The DWT is a linear transformation operating on a data vector whose length is an integer power of 2, converting it into a vector of the same size, which is numerically different. This divides information into different components of the frequency and then studies each component with the resolution corresponding to its size. The basic feature extraction procedure consists of:

- Decomposing the image using DWT into *N* levels using filtering and decimation to obtain the approximation and detailed coefficients
- Extracting the features from the DWT coefficients.

The features extracted from the DWT coefficients of ultrasonic test signals are considered useful features for input into classifiers due to their effective time and frequency representation of nonstationary signals.

3.3.3.2. Gray Level Co-Occurrence Matrix (GLCM)

The GLCM is a simple statistical tool used to derive textural features from the pixel relationships by examining the gray level's spatial dependency in an image [67]. It is a powerful high-performance technique that uses a smaller number of gray levels to shrink the size of GLCM, resulting in a reduction in the algorithm's computational cost [68].

A GLCM is a matrix where the number of rows and columns is equal to the number of gray levels, G, in the image [69]. The matrix element P $(i, j \mid \Delta x, \Delta y)$ is the relative frequency with which two pixels, separated by a pixel distance $(\Delta x, \Delta y)$, occur within a given neighborhood, one with intensity 'i' and the other with intensity 'j'. The matrix element P $(i, j \mid d, \theta)$ contains the second-order statistical probability values for changes between gray levels 'i' and 'j' at a particular displacement distance d and at a particular angle (θ). Using a large number of intensity levels G implies storing a lot of temporary data, that is, a $G \times G$ matrix for each combination of $(\Delta x, \Delta y)$ or (d, Θ). The GLCMs are very sensitive to the scale of the texture samples on which they are measured because of their large dimensionality. The number of gray levels is therefore also increasing. For four different gray grades, the GLCM matrix formulation can be clarified with the example shown in Figure 3.7. A pixel offset (a reference pixel and its immediate neighbor) is used here. If the window is wide enough, it is possible to use a smaller offset. The top left cell is filled with the number of times the combination 0, 0 occurs, that is, how much time a pixel with gray level 0 (neighbor pixel) falls to the right of another pixel with gray level 0 (reference pixel) within the image area. To extract the characteristics of texture statistics from remote sensing images, Haralick [70] defines some of the textural features measured from the probability matrix. These features are given in Table 3.2 with its calculations.

Neighbour pixel value ---> ref pixel value:	0	1	2	3
0	0,0	0,1	0,2	0,3
1	1,0	1,1	1,2	1,3
2	2,0	2,1	2,2	2,3
3	3,0	3,1	3,2	3,3

FIGURE 3.7 GLCM Matrix Formulation.

3.3.3.3 Nonnegative Matrix Factorization (NMF)

Patero and Tapper developed NMF in 1994[71]. It became popular after a 1999 publication by Lee and Seung, proposing a simple multiplicative update algorithm to find meaningful parts-based facial image representation [72]. Since then, in the field of pattern recognition, NMF has become a widely used tool for multivariate data analysis. One of the main challenges of NMF is developing fast and efficient algorithms which produce nonnegative (W, H) factors that minimize the objective function[73]. The Euclidean distance between X and WH and KL diverges. KL-based cost function is expressed as:

$$D_{NMF}(X \| WH) \triangleq \sum_{i,j}\left(x_{ij} \ln \frac{x_{ij}}{\sum_k w_{ik}h_{kj}} + \sum_k w_{ik}h_{kj} - x_{ij} \right) \tag{3.3}$$

This expression can be minimized by applying multiplicative update rules subject to $W, H \geq 0$.

NMF is a relatively recent approach in which nonnegative entries decompose data into two factors. There are at least two reasons as to why the entries are nonnegative. The first reason comes from neurophysiology, where the visual perception neuron firing rate is nonnegative. The second reason comes from the field of image processing, where the intensity of images has nonnegative values.

3.3.3.4 Principal Component Analysis (PCA)

PCA is considered one of the most powerful tools to extract effective features from a data set of high dimensions [74]. Its main objective is to minimize the dimensions of the d-dimensional data set to a k-dimensional subspace (where $k < d$) by preserving most of the relevant information to improve computational efficiency [75]. By calculating the correlation between variables in terms of main components, it reduces the dimensionality of data.

The central idea behind PCA is to find in the data [76] an orthonormal array of axes pointing to the direction of maximum covariance. It is often used in representing facial images. The idea is to find the orthonormal base vectors, or the individual vectors, of a series of images' covariance matrix, with each image being viewed in a high-dimensional space as a single point. The facial images are supposed to form a

TABLE 3.2
GLCM Features

No.	Feature	Formula	Description
1	Contrast	$\sum_{i,j=0}^{N-1} p_{i,j}(i-j)^2$	Contrast measures the intensity variation between the reference pixel and neighbor pixel.
2	Correlation	$\sum_{i,j=0}^{N-1} p_{i,j}\left[\frac{(i-\mu_i)(j-\mu_j)}{\sqrt{(\sigma_i^2)(\sigma_i^2)}}\right]$	Correlation measures how the reference pixel is related with its neighbor pixel.
3	Dissimilarity	$\sum_{i,j=0}^{N-1} p_{i,j}\lvert i-j\rvert$	
4	Energy	$\sum_{i,j=0}^{N-1} p_{i,j}^2$	Energy defines the measure of sum of squared elements. This measures the homogeneity. When pixels are very similar, the energy value will be large.
5	Entropy	$\sum_{i,j=0}^{N-1} p_{i,j}(-ln ln\ pi,j)$	Entropy is defined as a measure of uncertainty in a random variable. Its value will be maximum when all the elements of the co-occurrence matrix are the same.
6	Homogeneity	$\sum_{i,j=0}^{N-1} \frac{p_{i,j}}{1+(i-j)^2}$	
7	Mean	$\mu_i = \sum_{i,j=0}^{N-1} i.p(i,j)$, $\mu_j = \sum_{i,j=0}^{N-1} j.p(i,j)$	Mean defines the average level of intensity of the image or texture.
8	Variance	$\sigma_i^2 \sum_{i,j=0}^{N-1} p_{i,j}(i-\mu_i)^2$, $\sigma_j^2 \sum_{i,j=0}^{N-1} p_{i,j}(j-\mu_j)^2$	Variance defines the variation of intensity around the mean.

related subregion within the image space. The eigenvectors map the most important differences between faces and are compared to other techniques of comparison which presume that each pixel in an image is of equal importance. The steps of PCA algorithm are shown in Figure 3.8.

Principal Component Analysis (PCA) algorithm (Reproduced from [75])
Step 1: Get some data.
Step 2: Subtract the mean.
Step 3: Calculate the covariance matrix.
Step 4: Calculate the eigenvectors and eigenvalues of the covariance matrix.
Step 5: Choose components and form a feature vector.
Step 6: Derive the new data set.

FIGURE 3.8 PCA Algorithm.

Independent Component Analysis (ICA) algorithm (Reproduced from [78])
1. Center the data X to make its mean zero, and whiten it to give z.
2. Choose m, the number of independent components to estimate.
3. Choose initial values for the w_i, $i = 1,...,m$, each of unit norm. Orthogonalize the matrix **W** (=$\mathbf{A}^{-1}$) as in step 5.
4. For every $i = 1,...,m, w_i$? $E\{zg(wi^T z)\} - E\{g\_(wi^T z)\}w$, where $g(y) = \tanh(ay)$ $(1 = a = 2)$.
5. Do a symmetric orthogonalization of the matrix $\mathbf{W} = (w_1,...,w_n)^T$ by **W**? ($\mathbf{WW}^T$) **W**.
6. If not converged, go back to step 4.

FIGURE 3.9 ICA Algorithms.

3.3.3.5 Independent Component Analysis (ICA)

An effective blind signal separation technique, ICA has proven to be a powerful tool for analyzing neuro-image data[77]. It is one of the multivariate and data-driven techniques that allows MRI data sets to be explored to extract useful information about voxel relationships in local brain substructures. The algorithm illustrated in Figure 3.9.

3.3.3.6 Linear Discriminate Analysis (LDA)

LDA is used to extract the function and to distinguish samples of unknown classes from known classes based on training samples [79]. It results in a linear transformation of k-dimensional samples into an m-dimensional space ($m < k$) so that the samples are closely related to the same class; however, samples from different classes are far apart. This method maximizes the ratio of interclass variance to in-class variance in any set of data, thus ensuring the maximum theoretical separation in linear sense [80]. Because LDA requires effective directions for discrimination, it is the optimal classifier for specialized classes that are Gaussian distribution and have matrices of equal covariance. LDA requires a transformation matrix that maximizes the between-scatter matrix ratio to the within-scatter matrix in a certain sense.

The within-scatter matrix is defined as:

$$S_w = \sum_{i=1}^{k} \sum_{i=1}^{N_j} \left(y^i_{j-\mu_j} \right) \left(y^i_{j-\mu_j} \right)^T \tag{3.4}$$

where y_{ij} is the ith sample of class j, μ_j is the mean of class j, K is the number of classes, and N_j is the number of samples in class j. The between-scatter matrix is defined as:

$$S_b = \frac{1}{k}\sum_{i=1}^{k}(\mu_i - \mu)(\mu_i - \mu)^T \tag{3.5}$$

where μ is the mean of all classes. The goal is to maximize the between-class measure and minimize the within-class measure.

Table 3.3 shows the strengths and weaknesses of feature extraction techniques.

3.3.4 Feature Reduction of the AD Images Using Different Optimization Algorithms

Due to the difficulties of large-scale engineering issues, the optimization algorithms gained fame and attention. Therefore, optimization algorithms had been suggested to search for near-optimum problem solutions [81]. Optimization algorithms are stochastic methods of searching that simulate species' social behavior or natural biological evolution. There are various natural examples, such as how fish and birds make schooling and find their destination during migration, the cuckoo birds' aggressive breeding technique, how ants and bees find the shortest route to a food source, and how bats use echolocation to sense distance, and the difference between food/prey and background barriers. Various algorithms were developed to model these species' behavior. In this section, the five recent evolutionary optimization algorithms are studied and explained to extract the most significant features from three-dimensional (3D) MRI AD images.

These algorithms provide fast, robust, and almost optimal solutions to complex optimization problems [82, 83]. The genetic algorithm (GA) introduced in 1975 [84] is the first optimization algorithm. This model is based on Darwin's theory of natural crossover and recombination, mutation, and selection of 'the survival of the fittest.' There are numerous applications using GA techniques in science and engineering [85, 86]. GA has many advantages, such as its ability to handle complex issues and parallelism. Nonetheless, for a near-optimum solution to develop, GAs can require long processing time [86]. In 1960, the pattern search (PS) was developed as one of the direct search family. PS is an evolutionary technique that lies outside the scope of the standard optimization methods to solve a variety of optimization problems.

Generally PS has the advantage of being conceptually very simple, easy to implement, and computationally efficient [88]. The third algorithm is the simulated annealing (SA) that was presented in 1983[89].

The idea of SA came from the metal-processing annealing characteristics. The physical annealing process is enough slowly cooling a metal to adopt a low-energy, crystalline state. Various systems have used the SA optimizing technique [90]. The fourth algorithm is the particle swarm optimization (PSO), developed

TABLE 3.3
Feature Extraction Techniques' Strengths and Weaknesses

Feature Extraction Technique	Strengths	Weaknesses
DWT	• Finds discontinuities and irregularities of a signal and its derivatives • Finds break point location by wavelet ridge extrapolation • Denoise	• Computationally intensive • Its discretization, the discrete wavelet transform, is less efficient • It takes some energy to invest in wavelets to be able to choose the proper ones for a specific purpose, and to implement it correctly.
GLCM	• Easy to implement • Dives the exact feature of the medical image	• It can take large number of possible texture calculation because of image complexity and noise of an image. • Difficult to find the various parameters of GLCM matrixes.
NMF	• Reduces the large dimensionality of the input data	• Nonnegativity constraints can restrict correct clustering to only nonnegative data.
PCA	• Reduces the redundant features and large dimensionality of the image	
ICA	• No need a priori information • Useful tool for early diagnosis of SMRI data • Gives good performance when combined with SVM classifier	
LDA	• Searches for those vectors in the underlying space that are best discriminable among classes. • Attempts to express one dependent variable as a linear combination of other features or measurements	• When dealing with the image data, the image mertices must be first transformed into vectors that have high dimensionality. This leads to high computational cost.

in 1995 [91] and based on natural swarm behaviors such as fishing and bird schooling. Bat algorithm (BA) was developed in 2010 as a bio-inspired algorithms [92]. BA simulates bats' activity that has advanced echolocation capability. All optimization algorithms require a suitable form for each algorithm to represent the problem first. Then, to reach a near-optimum solution, the evolutionary search algorithm is applied iteratively. The following subsections provide a brief description of the above five algorithms.

Genetic algorithm (Reproduced from [86])
1. Encoding the objectives or cost functions.
2. Defining a fitness function.
3. Creating a population of individuals (solutions) is called a generation.
4. Evaluating the fitness function of all the individuals in the population.
5. Creating a new population by performing crossover and mutation, fitness-proportionate reproduction, etc., and replacing the old population and iterating again using the new population.
6. Decoding the results to obtain the solution to the problem.

FIGURE 3.10 Genetic Algorithm.

3.3.4.1 Genetic Algorithm

GA encodes the optimization function as bits arrays to represent chromosomes, genetic operators manipulating strings to find a near-optimal solution to the problem. This is done by the procedure shown in Figure 3.10 [85, 86].

GAs have three primary genetic operators: crossover, mutation, and selection [93]:

- **Crossover:** Exchanging parts of the solution in chromosomes or representations of solutions. The main role is to provide in a subspace a mix of solutions and convergence.
- **Mutation:** Changing of one solution randomly, which increases demographic diversity and offers a way to escape from the equilibrium of the local population.
- **Selection of the fittest, or elitism:** The use of high-fitness solutions to pass them on to the next generations, often performed in terms of selecting some form of the best solutions.

3.3.4.2 Simulated Annealing

SA is one of the most popular and earliest optimization algorithms that is a global optimization random search technique. It imitates the annealing process in the processing of materials when a metal cools and freezes in a crystalline state with minimal energy and larger crystal sizes to reduce the deficiencies in metallic structures. The method of annealing requires careful temperature control and its cooling rate, also referred to as the anneval plan. The SA algorithm's basic idea is to use random search as a Markov chain, which not only embraces changes that improve the objective function but also holds changes that are not ideal. For example, any improved movements or changes that decrease the value of the objective function (*f*) will be accepted in a minimization problem [90].

In the SA method, to simulate the heating process, a temperature variable is maintained and initialized to a high value. Then there are four basic phases: (1) generation of a new candidate point, (2) acceptance criterion, (3) reduction of the temperature, and (4) stopping criterion [94]:

1. The generation of a new candidate point is one of its key phases and should provide both a good search region exploration and a feasible point.
2. The acceptance criterion enables the SA algorithm not to be stuck in local solutions when searching for a global solution. For that matter, when an improvement in the objective function is checked, the system accepts points.
3. The temperature decreases slowly to zero during the iterative process. To determine a positive decreasing sequence, the control parameter, also known as the temperature or cooling schedule, must be modified. The control parameter is slowly reduced as the algorithm develops and the algorithm calculates better precision approximations to the optimum. The initial control parameter must be high enough (to search for promising regions) but not extremely high because the algorithm becomes too slow for a good performance of the algorithm.
4. The stopping criteria for the SA are based on the idea that if no further changes occur, the algorithm should be terminated. The usual stop criterion limits the number of function assessments or sets a lower limit for the control parameter value.

3.3.4.3 Pattern Search

The PS optimization technique is suitable for solving a variety of optimization problems, particularly those outside the scope of standard optimization methods. In concept, PS is flexible and very simple, easy to implement, and computationally efficient. PS algorithm depends on a sequence of points being calculated which may or may not be the optimal point. The algorithm starts with a mesh point being established around the given point. This point may be provided by the user or calculated from the algorithm's previous step. If the objective function is changed by a point in the mesh, this new point at the next iteration will be the current point. The algorithm is presented in Figure 3.11 [95].

3.3.4.4 Particle Swarm Optimization

A particle in GAs is similar to a chromosome. The PSO cycle does not create new parent birds. The population's birds only evolve their social behavior and their movement toward a destination accordingly. PSO imitates a flock of birds that chat while they migrate together. Each bird looks in a specific direction, and then they identify the bird in the best location when communicating together. Therefore, each bird speeds toward the best bird using a speed based on its current position. Then each bird explores the search space from its new local location and the process repeats until a desired destination is reached by the flock. It should be noted that the process involves both social interaction and intelligence so that birds can learn from their own experience (local search) and from the experience of others around them (global search) [82, 83, 91].

The process is initialized with a group of random particles (solutions), N. The ith particle is represented by its position as a point in an S-dimensional space, where S is the number of variables. Throughout the process, each particle i monitors three

Pattern Search Algorithm (Reproduced from [95])

PS starts at the initial point X_0 which is given by the user. At the first iteration, with a scalar of magnitude 1 called mesh size, the direction vectors are constructed as [0 1], [1 0], [–1 0], and [0 –1]. Then the PS adds the direction vectors to the initial point X0 to compute the mesh points: X_0 + [1 0], X_0 + [0 1], X_0 + [–1 0], and X_0 + [0 –1] as shown in Then, the PS calculates the objective function at each point in the mesh. Next, PS computes the objective function values until it finds one whose value is smaller than the objective function value of X_0. At this point, the poll is successful and the algorithm sets this point equal to X_1. Then, the PS goes to iteration 2 and multiplies the current mesh size by 2. The mesh at iteration 2 contains the following points: X_1 + 2*[1 0], X_1 + 2*[0 1], X_1 + 2*[–1 0] and X_1 + 2*[0 –1]. The algorithm polls the mesh points until it finds one whose value is smaller than the objective function value of X_1. This point is called X_2, and the poll is successful. Next, the algorithm multiplies the current mesh size by 2 to get a mesh size of 4 at the third iteration, and so on.

If in iteration 3 and none of the mesh points has a smaller objective function value than the value at X_2, the poll is called an unsuccessful poll. The algorithm does not change the current point at the next iteration, and X3 = X2. At the next iteration, the algorithm multiplies the current mesh size by 0.5, a contraction factor, so that the mesh size at the next iteration is smaller. The algorithm then polls with a smaller mesh size. The PS optimization algorithm will repeat the illustrated steps until it finds the optimal solution for the minimization of the objective function. The PS algorithm stops when any of the following conditions occurs:

1. The mesh size is less than the mesh tolerance.
2. The number of iterations performed by the algorithm reaches the value of maximum iteration number.
3. The total number of objective function evaluations performed by the algorithm reaches the value of maximum function evaluations.
4. The distance between the point found at one successful poll and the point found at the next successful poll is less than the specified tolerance.
5. The change in the objective function from one successful poll to the next successful poll is less than the objective function tolerance.

FIGURE 3.11 Pattern Search Algorithm.

values: its current position (X_i), the best position it reached in previous cycles (P_i), and its flying velocity (V_i). These three values are current position ($X_i =(x_{i1}; x_{i2};\ldots; x_{iS})$), best previous position ($P_i =(p_{i1}; p_{i2};\ldots; p_{iS})$), and flying velocity ($V_i =(v_{i1}; v_{i2};\ldots; v_{iS})$). The velocity update equation is shown in Andries [91]:

$$V_i = W \times V_i + C_1 \times R_{and} \times (P_{\text{best}} - X_i) + C_2 \times R_{and} \times (G_{\text{best}} - X_i) \tag{3.6}$$

where V_i is the velocity of each particle, i is the number of particles, W is the inertia weight, C_1, C_2 are learning constants, Rand is the random number between 0 and 1, P_{best} is the optimum position of each particle up to now, G_{best} is the optimum position of all particles up to now, and X_i is the present position of each particle. The position update equation of each particle point in particle swarm [96]:

$$\text{New position } X_i = \text{current position } X_i + V_i \tag{3.7}$$

3.3.4.5 Bat Algorithm

Some bats use echolocation to some extent; microbats are a famous example among all species as they make extensive use of echolocation, while megabats do not. Insectivores are the majority of microbats. Microbats use an echolocation type of sonar to track predators, avoid obstacles, and locate their roosting crevices in the night. These bats emit a very loud pulse of sound and listen to the echo that bounces back from the artifacts around. Their pulses vary in characteristics and depending on the species can be correlated with their hunting strategies. Most bats use short, frequency-modulated signals to sweep around an octave; others use echolocation signals with constant frequency more frequently. Their amplitude of the signal varies with species and often decreases with more harmonics. Studies have shown that microbats use the time delay from echo emission and detection, the time difference between their two ears, and the echoes' loudness differences to create a three-dimensional surrounding scenario. They can detect the distance and orientation of the target, the type of prey, and even the moving speed of the prey, such as small insects [97, 98].

3.4 PATTERN RECOGNITION ALGORITHMS

Starting from the acquisition of data and their preprocessing to the extraction and selection of an optimal vector of attributes, we need to perform the most important step of pattern recognition, which is the pattern recognition algorithm in the form of classifiers, clustering, regression, etc.

3.4.1 Classification Algorithms for MRI Scans

One of the main objectives of classification is to produce meaningful patterns from raw data, classify them according to their characteristics into different groups, and predict new patterns based on previous knowledge.

Classification of images is a major challenge for the tasks of image analysis. This challenge was related to using methods and techniques to exploit the results of image processing, the results of pattern recognition and methods of classification, and subsequently validating the image classification output into medical expert knowledge. The main objective of classifying medical images is not only to achieve high accuracy but also to distinguish the parts of the brain that are contaminated with the disease. For better clinical care, an automatic diagnostic technique with image data is needed in the future.

3.4.1.1 Support Vector Machine

An SVM classifier belongs to the group of supervised machine learning classifiers [99]. Supervised machine learning classifiers build a model based on historical data that can predict future instances. The available data set is usually divided into a train set and a test set for constructing these models. In a classification function, where each instance of a data set belongs to a certain class, a classifier uses the features of the train set instances to build a model based on those features that assign these instances to a certain class [100]. The result of the model will then be used to assign class labels to new instances where the feature values are known, but the class label is unknown. It is called supervised learning because the classes of instances in the train data are known and during training the model, it is continuously evaluated and adapted to make as few errors as possible. An SVM model's efficiency depends in part on its parameters. Based on their accuracy on the train data, the best parameters are selected. It is the most widely used machine learning classifier for the detection of AD [101] due to the strong generalization performance of SVMs for both linear and nonlinear data treatment.

Recent studies have frequently used the SVM algorithm to classify AD. Numerous studies have shown the importance of SVMs in discriminating between subjects with AD and CN subjects, many of which of used small data sets with MRI data [102].

3.4.1.2 Deep Learning

The area of artificial intelligence is important when machines are capable of performing tasks that typically require human intelligence. It includes machine learning, where machines can learn without human involvement through experience and acquire skills. Deep learning is a subset of machine learning where ANNs, human brain-inspired algorithms, learn from large quantities of data (see Figure 3.12).

Deep learning architectures, such as deep neural networks, Capsule Network (CapsNet), recurrent neural networks (RNNs) and CNNs, have been applied for the detection of AD.

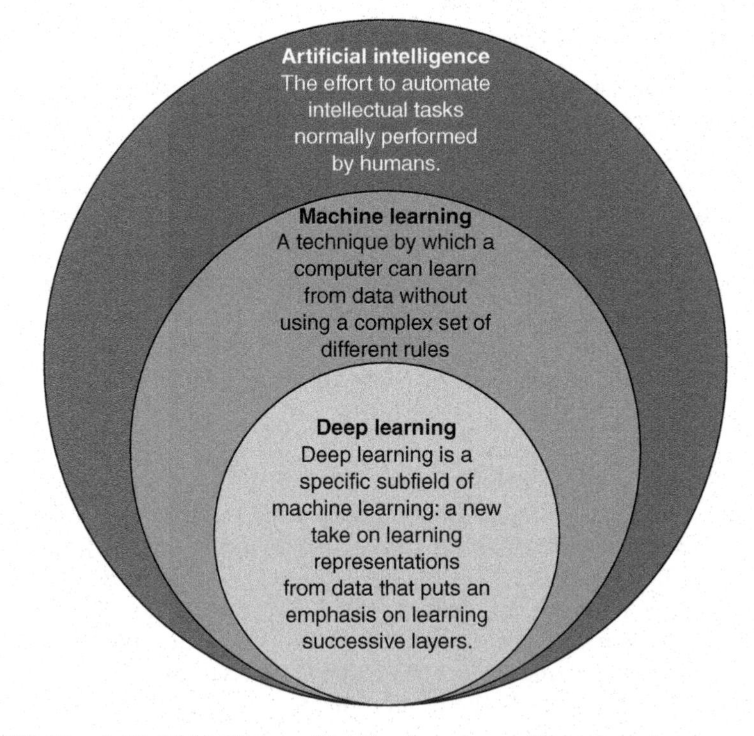

FIGURE 3.12 Artificial Intelligence, Machine Learning and Deep Learning.

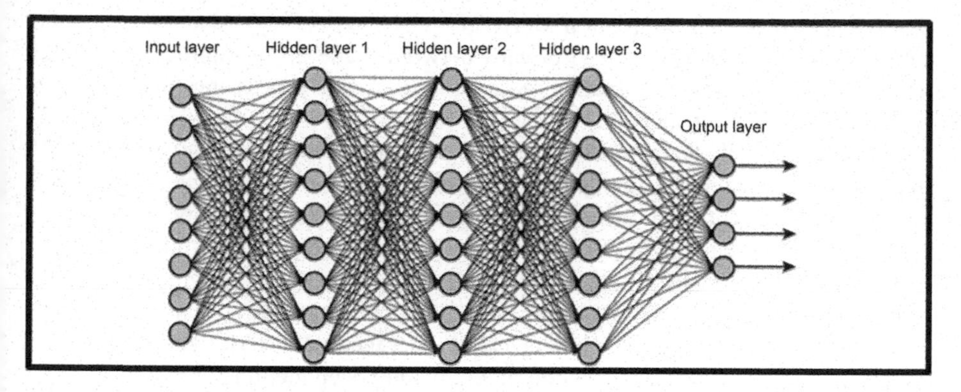

FIGURE 3.13 Deep Neural Network.

3.4.1.2.1 Deep Neural Networks (DNN)

An ANN with multiple layers between the input and output layers is a DNN [103–105]. The DNN finds the correct mathematical manipulation, whether it is a linear relationship or a nonlinear one, to turn the input into output. The network travels through the layers to measure each output's likelihood. Usually, DNNs are feed-forward networks where information flows from the input layer to the output layer without looping back as shown in Figure 3.13. First, the DNN creates a map of virtual neurons and assigns the connections between them to random numerical values, or "weights." The weights and inputs are multiplied and return an output between 0 and 1. If the network does not recognize a specific pattern correctly, then the weights would be changed by an algorithm. This allows the algorithm to make some parameters more influential until it determines the correct mathematical manipulation to process the data completely.

3.4.1.2.2 Recurrent Neural Network

An RNN [106] is a class of ANNs where connections between nodes form a directed graph along a temporal sequence. This allows it to exhibit temporal dynamic behavior. Unlike feedforward neural networks, RNNs can use their internal state (memory) to process sequences of inputs.

RNNs can take one or more input vectors and produce one or more output vectors and the output(s) is(are) influenced not only by weights applied on inputs like a regular NN, but also by a "hidden" state vector representing the context based on prior input(s)/output(s). So, the same input could produce a different output depending on previous inputs in the series. One of the main advantages of RNN is that it remembers each and every information through time. It is useful in time series prediction only because of the feature to remember previous inputs as well. This is called long short-term memory. Also, RNNs are used with convolutional layers to extend the effective pixel neighborhood. On the contrary, RNNs have many problems; for example, training an RNN is a very difficult task and it cannot process very long sequences if using Tanh or rectified linear unit (ReLu) as an activation function.

3.4.1.2.3 Convolutional Neural Network

CNN [107] is a deep neural feedforward network made up of multilayer artificial neurons with excellent performance in large-scale image processing. In contrast to traditional methods of manually extracting radiological image features, CNNs are used to automatically learn general features. CNN is a deep learning algorithm [108] that is capable of capturing an input image, assigning significance (learnable weights and biases) to different aspects/objects in the image, and separating them from each other. In a CNN, preprocessing is much smaller than in other classification algorithms.

CNNs are trained with a back propagation algorithm, consisting typically of multiple convolution layers, pooling layers, and fully connected layers, connecting to the output system through complete link layers or other methods [109]. CNNs have fewer connections and fewer parameters compared to other deep feedforward networks due to the weight of the sharing of the convolution kernel and are therefore easier to train and more common.

In Figure 3.14, CNN architecture involves a series of layers of convolution (CONV) and pooling (POOL) accompanied by a standard full neural network [110]. The input map converts with K filters (or kernels) to provide K function maps in the convolution layer. The pooling layer is performed after applying a nonlinear activation function (sigmoidal or linear rectified unit) to each feature graph. The learned features are the input of a fully connected neural network followed by a softmax layer performing the tasks of classification. Nevertheless, each component of the kernel matrix is more than once translated to the input image in a convolutional layer. The convolutional layers decompose stacks of predefined size filters that are converted with the layer's input. By setting the output of the pooling layer as the input of the next convolutional layer, the CNN depth can be increased.

3.4.1.2.4 Auto Encoder

An autoencoder is a three-layer ANN architecture that is used to learn unsupervised data and is capable of extracting data details from an input such as a data set or image, accessing input data in the form of "small parts" number, and extracting the hidden data structure [111]. As shown in Figure 3.15, in the middle there is an input (encoding) and an output (decoding) layer and a hidden layer, whereas the hidden layer contains more or less units for an incomplete and full representation, the input and output layers have equivalent units. They work by compressing the input into a latent space representation, and then reconstructing the output from this representation.

3.4.1.2.5 Capsule Network

The capsules in a CapsNet are generally groups of neurons [112]. These act in such a way that the activity vectors of these neurons represent different parametric poses, whereas the vector lengths represent the respective probability of a spatial feature being present.

CapsNet layers are substantially replaced by a more appropriate criterion known as "routing by agreement." Based on this criterion, the resulting outputs generated in the first layer are transmitted to the next layer parent capsules, even though the capsules' coupling coefficient is not identical. All the capsules here try to perceive the parent capsules' output. The coupling coefficient between these two capsules is

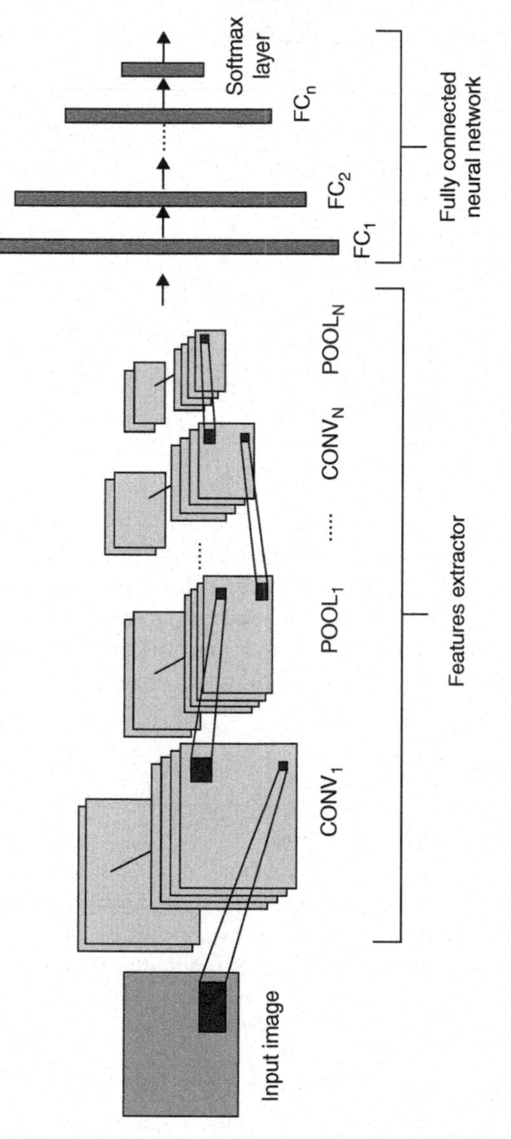

FIGURE 3.14 CNN Architecture.

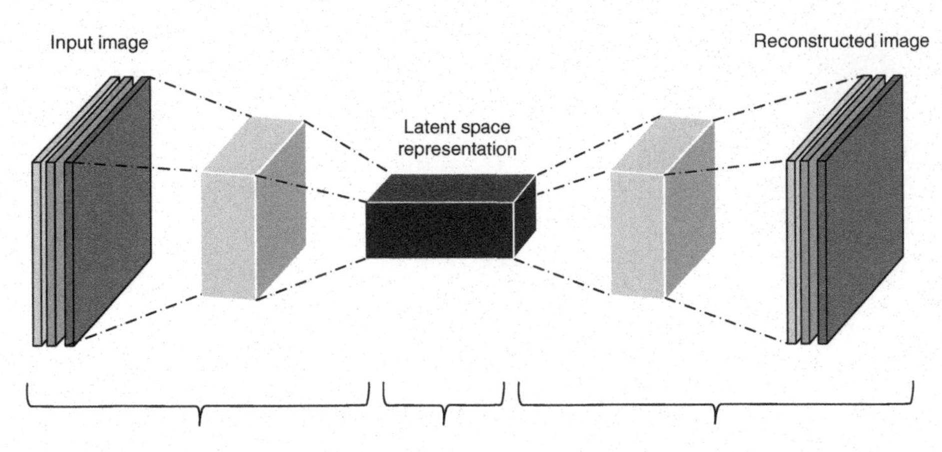

FIGURE 3.15 Autoencoder Representation.

increased based on predictive information to the parent capsules' actualized outputs. Thus, if we consider *ui* as the outputs of capsule *i*, its detection for parent capsule *j* is calculated by the following formula:

$$u_{j|i} = W_{ij} U_i$$

where $U_{j|i}$ represents the prediction vector of output of the *j*th capsule in a higher level, which is calculated by capsule *i* in the subsequent layer. W_{ij} is the weighted coefficient matrix that is learned in the backward process. Thus, on the basis of the degree of conformations among below layer and the parent capsules, the coupling coefficient C_{ij} can be computed from the following equation:

$$C_{ij} = \frac{exp\left(b_{ij}\right)}{\sum_{k}^{i} exp\left(b_{ik}\right)}$$

where b_{ij} is the probability of log for determining if capsule *i* should be linked to the capsule *j*; also, it is initialized to zero at the very start of the procedure. Hence, the input vector to the parent capsule S_j will be computed as follows:

$$S_j = \sum_{i}^{j} C_{ij} U_{j|i}$$

CapsNets can handle robust image transitions and rotations effectively and has the ability to learn quickly even for small data sets. It is also capable of handling large data sets with low training turns and small sample sizes, which is the reason why it has succeeded (Table 3.4).

TABLE 3.4
Classification Techniques' Strengths and Weaknesses

Classification Techniques	Strengths	Weaknesses
Deep learning	• Feature engineering can be automatically executed inside deep learning model • Can solve complex problems • Flexible to be adapted to new challenge in the future (or transfer learning can be easily applied) • High automation. Deep learning library (Tensorflow, Keras, or MATLAB, etc.) can help users build a deep learning model within seconds (without the need of deep understanding)	• Needs huge amount of data • Expensive and intensive training • Overfitting if applied into uncomplicated problems • No standard for training and tuning model • It's a blackbox, not straightforward to understand inside each layer
Convolutional neural network (CNN)	• CNNs have a fewer connections and small number of parameters due to the weight of the convolution kernel sharing.	• CNNs are mostly connected to the presence of pooling layer.
Support Vector Machine (SVM)	• SVM is a powerful classification algorithm.	• It gives poor performance and does not directly provide probability estimates.

3.5 CONCLUSIONS

An early detection of AD is important for those affected by the disease and their environment as well as for drug developers to test new treatments. With the advance of artificial intelligence and machine learning techniques, pattern recognition attracts more attention for the detection of AD. It has become one of the major research subjects in medical imaging and diagnostic radiology. This chapter shed the light on MRI because it plays an essential role in the analysis of medical brain images. Then it discussed the methodology of pattern recognition. The different preprocessing, segmentation, feature extraction, optimization, and classification algorithms used to diagnose AD are explained in detail.

The study presents a comparison protocol of different image segmentation, feature extraction, and classification techniques. This study shows that deep learning is one of the most powerful tools used in recent years for the detection of AD. Deep learning can solve complex problems to be adapted to new challenge in the future. Deep learning uses many libraries such as Tensorflow and Keras in Python to build a deep learning model within seconds without the need of deep understanding. Deep learning has many challenges to overcome in order to be successful, such as (1) overfitting if applied on a small amount of data – therefore, the bigger the data, the better the performance – and (2) time consuming.

REFERENCES

1. Iman Beheshtia, Hasan Demirelb, Hiroshi Matsudaa, "Classification of Alzheimer's disease and prediction of mild cognitive impairment-to-Alzheimer's conversion from structural magnetic resource imaging using feature ranking and a genetic algorithm", *Computers in Biology and Medicine* 83, 109–119, 2017.
2. Yubraj Gupta, Ramesh Kumar Lama, Goo-Rak Kwon, "Prediction and classification of Alzheimer's disease based on combined features from apolipoprotein-E genotype, cerebrospinal fluid, MR, and FDG-PET imaging biomarkers", *Frontiers in Computational Neuroscience*, 13, Article 72, 2019.
3. Andrew E. Budson, Paul R. Solomon, "Chapter 4 – Alzheimer's disease dementia and mild cognitive impairment due to Alzheimer's disease", *Memory Loss,* Alzheimer's Disease, and Dementia (2nd edn.), Copyright: © Elsevier, **eBook ISBN:** 9780323316118, pp. 47–69, 2016.
4. Keith A. Johnson, Nick C. Fox, Reisa A. Sperling, William E. Klunk, "Brain imaging in Alzheimer disease", Cold Spring Harbor Perspectives in Medicine 2(4): a006213, 2012.
5. Xiaojing Long, Lifang Chen, Chunxiang Jiang, Lijuan Zhang, "Prediction and classification of Alzheimer disease based on quantification of MRI deformation", *Plos One.* 2017. DOI: 10.1371/journal.pone.0173372
6. Helena Aidos, João Duarte, Ana Fred, "Identifying regions of interest for discriminating Alzheimer's disease from mild cognitive impairment", **Date of Conference** 27–30 Oct. 2014, *IEEE International Conference on Image Processing (ICIP)*, 2014. DOI: 10.1109/ICIP.2014.7025003
7. M. Latha, S. Arun, "Detection of ROI for classifying Alzheimer's disease using Mr. Image of Brain", *International Journal of Innovative Technology and Exploring Engineering (IJITEE)* 8(5), 2019. ISSN: 2278–3075
8. Luís Gustavo Ribeiro, Geraldo Busatto, Filho, "Voxel-based morphometry in Alzheimer's disease and mild cognitive impairment: Systematic review of studies addressing the frontal lobe", *Dement & Neuropsychol.* 10(2): 104–112, 2016. DOI: 10.1590/S1980-5764-2016DN1002006
9. Daniel Schmitter, Alexis Roche, "An evaluation of volume-based morphometry for prediction of mild cognitive impairment and Alzheimer's disease", *NeuroImage: Clinical,* 7: 7–17, 2015.
10. Hakim C. Achterberg, Lauge Sørensen, Frank J. Wolters, "The value of hippocampal volume, shape, and texture for 11-year prediction of dementia: A population-based study", *Neurobiology of Aging* 81: 58–66, September 2019.
11. Emilie Gerardin, Gaël Chételat, Marie Chupin, "Multidimensional classification of hippocampal shape features discriminates Alzheimer's disease and mild cognitive impairment from normal aging", *NeuroImage* 47(4): 1476–1486. 2009. DOI: 10.1016.
12. L Sørensen, M Nielsen, "Ensemble support vector machine classification of dementia using structural MRI and mini-mental state examination", *Journal of Neuroscience Methods* 302: 66–74, 2018.
13. Yubraj Gupta, Kun Ho Lee, "Early diagnosis of Alzheimer's disease using combined features from voxel-based morphometry and cortical, subcortical, and hippocampus regions of MRI T1 brain images", *Plos One* 2019. DOI: 10.1371/journal.pone.0222446
14. Xiangyu Ma, Zhaoxia Li, Bin Jing, "Identify the atrophy of Alzheimer's disease, mild cognitive impairment and normal aging using morphometric MRI analysis", *Frontiers in Aging Neuroscience*, volume 8, Article 243, 18 October 2016.

15. Stefan Klöppel, Cynthia Stonnington, Carlton Ch, "Automatic classification of MR scans in Alzheimer's disease", *Journal of Neurology* 2008. DOI:10.1093/brain/awm319.
16. Carlos Aguilar, Eric Westman, J-Sebastian Muehlboeck, "Different multivariate techniques for automated classification of MRI data in Alzheimer's disease and mild cognitive impairment", *Psychiatry Research: Neuroimaging*, 212(2): 89–98, 2013.
17. Iman Beheshti, Hasan Demirel, Hiroshi Matsuda, "Classification of Alzheimer's disease and prediction of mild cognitive impairment-to-Alzheimer's conversion from structural magnetic resource imaging using feature ranking and a genetic algorithm", *Computers in Biology and Medicine* 83: 109–119, 2017.
18. Mary Ellen Koran, 2019, "Neuroimaging and Alzheimer's disease", PhD thesis, Stanford University Medical Center, Stanford, CA.
19. Prashanthi Vemuri, Clifford R Jack Jr , "Role of structural MRI in Alzheimer's disease", *Alzheimer's Research and Therapy*, 2: 23, 2010. DOI: 10.1186/alzrt47
20. Mina Park, Won-Jin Moon, "Structural MR imaging in the diagnosis of Alzheimer's disease and other neurodegenerative dementia: Current imaging approach and future perspectives", *Korean Journal of Radiology* 2016. DOI: 10.3348/kjr.2016.17.6.827
21. Christian Salvatore, Antonio Cerasa, Isabella Castiglioni, "MRI characterizes the progressive course of AD and predicts conversion to Alzheimer's dementia 24 months before probable diagnosis", *Frontiers in Aging Neuroscience* 2018. DOI: 10.3389/fnagi.2018.00135
22. Cai Tang, DX Ding, LL Zhang, XY Cai, Q Fang, "Magnetic resonance imaging relaxation time in Alzheimer's disease", *Brain Research Bulletin* 140: 176–189, June 2018.
23. Srinivasan Nagaraj, G Narasinga Rao, K Koteswararao, "The role of pattern recognition in computer-aided diagnosis and computer-aided detection in medical imaging: A clinical validation", International Journal of Computer Applications 8(5): 41–60, October 2010.
24. SB Kotsiantis, D Kanellopoulos, PE Pintelas, "Data preprocessing for supervised leaning", *International Journal of Computer Science* 1(2), 2006.
25. P Chinmayi, L Agilandeeswari, M Prabukumar, "Survey of image processing techniques in medical image analysis: Challenges and methodologies", International Conference on Soft Computing and Pattern Recognition, pp. 460–471, 2017.
26. R Beaulah Jeyavathana, R Balasubramanian, A Anbarasa Pandian, "A survey: Analysis on pre-processing and segmentation techniques for medical images", *International Journal of Research and Scientific Innovation III(VI)*, 113–120, June 2016.
27. N Shameena, Rahna Jabbar, "A study of preprocessing and segmentation techniques on cardiac medical images", *International Journal of Engineering Research & Technology* 3(4), April 2014.
28. Sambit Satpathy, Mohan Chandra Pradhan, Subrat Sharma, "Comparative study of noise removal algorithms for denoising medical image using LabVIEW", *International Conference on Computational Intelligence and Communication Networks*, At: JABALPUR Volume: 978-1-5090-0076-0/15, 2015.
29. A Bosnjak,G Montilla, V Torrealba, "Medical images segmentation using Gabor filters applied to echocardiographic images", *Computers in Cardiology* 25: 457–460, 1998.
30. Youlian Zhu, Cheng Huang, "An improved median filtering algorithm for image noise reduction", *International Conference on Solid State Devices and Materials Science*, pp. 609–619, 2012.
31. Gabriel Babatunde Iwasokun, Oluwole Charles Akinyokun, "Image enhancement methods: A review", *British Journal of Mathematics & Computer Science* 4(16): 2251–2277, 2014.

32. Eman Abdel-Maksoud, Mohammed Elmogy, Rashid Al-Awadi, "Brain tumor segmentation based on a hybrid clustering technique", *Egyptian Informatics Journal*, 16(1): 71–81, 2015.
33. EA Zanaty, Said Ghoniemy, "Medical image segmentation techniques: An overview", *International Journal of Informatics and Medical Data Processing* 1(1): 16–37, 2016.
34. KJ Shanthi, DK Ravish, M Sasikumar, "Image segmentation an early detection to Alzheimer's disease", Annual IEEE India Conference (INDICON), 2013.
35. Dilpreet Kaur, Yadwinder Kaur, "Various image segmentation techniques: A review", *International Journal of Computer Science and Mobile Computing* 3(5): 809–814, May 2014.
36. Hiba Jabbar, Abdulwahid Aleqabi, "A hybrid approach for image segmentation", *Journal of Kerbala University*, 10(2), 2012.
37. R Dass, Devi S. Priyanka, "Image segmentation techniques", *Int J Electron Commun Technol* 3(1): 66–70, 2012.
38. Yu-Jin Zhang, "An overview of image and video segmentation in the last 40 years", Proceedings of the 6th International Symposium on Signal Processing and Its Applications 2006. DOI: 10.4018/978-1-59140-753-9.ch001
39. Pawan Patidar, Manoj Gupta, Sumit Srivastava, Ashok Kumar Nagawat, "Image denoising by various filters for different noise", *International Journal of Computer Applications* 9(4), November 2010.
40. Yi Yang, Sam Hallman, Deva Ramanan, Charless C. Fowlkes, "Layered object models for image segmentation", IEEE Transactions on Pattern Analysis and Machine Intelligence, DOI:10.1109/TPAMI.2011.208, 2010.
41. Rajesh C Patil, AS Bhalchandra, "Brain tumour extraction from MRI images using MATLAB", *International Journal of Electronics, Communication & Soft Computing Science and Engineering* 2(1), 2012.
42. KR Nicer Navid , KC James, "A Review of Different Segmentation Techniques Used in Brain Tumor Detection", *International Journal of Scientific & Engineering Research,* 7(2), February 2016.
43. Shubhashree Savant, "A review on edge detection techniques for image segmentation", *International Journal of Computer Science and Information Technologies*, 5(4): 5898–5900, 2014.
44. Mamta Joshi, Ashutosh Vyas, "Comparison of Canny edge detector with Sobel and Prewitt edge detector using different image formats", *International Journal of Engineering Research & Technology*, ISSN: 2278-0181, ETRASCT' 14 Conference Proceedings, 133–137, 2014.
45. Dharampal, Vikram Mutneja, "Methods of image edge detection: A review", *Journal of Electrical & Electronic Systems* 2015. DOI: 10.4172/2332-0796.1000150
46. NP Revathy, S Janarthanam, T Karthikeyan, "Optimal edge perservation in volume rendering using canny edge detector", *International Journal of Scientific & Engineering Research,* 4(6), 2013.
47. Shilpa Kamdi, RK Krishna, "Image segmentation and region growing algorithm", *International Journal of Computer Technology and Electronics Engineering* 2(1), 2019.
48. Nameirakpam Dhanachandra, Khumanthem Manglem, Yambem Jina Chanu, "Image segmentation using K-means clustering algorithm and subtractive clustering algorithm", Procedia Computer Science 54 (2015) 764–771, Eleventh International Multi-Conference on Information Processing, 2015.
49. Xin Zheng, Qinyi Lei, Run Yao, Yifei Gong, Qian Yin, "Image segmentation based on adaptive K-means algorithm", *EURASIP Journal on Image and Video Processing* 2018.

50. Nameirakpam Dhanachandra, Yambem Jina Chanu, "A survey on image segmentation methods using clustering techniques", European Journal of Engineering Research and Science 2(1), 2017.
51. Xin-Bo Zhang, Li Jiang, "An image segmentation algorithm based on fuzzy C-means clustering", *International Conference on Digital Image Processing,* 2009. DOI: 10.1109/ICDIP.2009.15
52. Tara Saikumar, P Yugander, PS Murthy, B Smitha, "Image segmentation algorithm using watershed transform and fuzzy C-means clustering on level set method", *International Journal of Computer Theory and Engineering*, 5(2), 2013.
53. D Selvaraj, "A review on tissue segmentation and feature extraction of MRI brain images", *International Journal of Computer Science & Engineering Technology* 4, 2013.
54. G Urban, M Bendszus, F Hamprecht, J Kleesiek, "Multi-modal brain tumor segmentation using deep convolutional neural networks", *Proceedings of MICCAI BRATS (Brain Tumor Segmentation) Challenge*, Boston, 2014.
55. G Zeng, G Zheng, "Multi-stream 3D FCN with multi-scale deep supervision for multi-modality isointense infant brain MR image segmentation", *IEEE 15th International Symposium on Biomedical Imaging*, pp. 136–140, 2018.
56. Liang-Chieh Chen, George Papandreou, Iasonas Kokkinos, Kevin Murphy, Alan L Yuille, "DeepLab: Semantic image segmentation with deep convolutional nets", *Atrous Convolution, and Fully Connected CRFs*, 2017.
57. Aly ValliamiAmeet Soni, "Deep Residual Nets for Improved Alzheimer's Diagnosis", the 8th ACM International Conference, DOI: 10.1145/3107411.3108224, 2017.
58. Fermin Segovia, JM Go´ rriz, J Ramı´rez, D Salas-Gonzalez, Ignacio A´lvarez, Diego Salas-Gonzalez, R Chaves, "A comparative study of feature extraction methods for the diagnosis of Alzheimer's disease using the ADNI database", *Neurocomputing* 75(2012): 64–71.
59. Seyyid Ahmed Medjahed, "A comparative study of feature extraction methods in images classification", *International Journal of Image, Graphics and Signal Processing*, 3: 16–23, 2015. DOI: 10.5815/ijigsp.2015.03.03
60. P Soumya Balan, Leya Elizabeth Sunny, "Survey on feature extraction techniques in image processing", *International Journal for Research in Applied Science & Engineering Technology*, 6(III), 2018.
61. K Baskar, D Seshathiri, "A survey on feature selection techniques in medical image processing", *International Journal of Engineering Research & Technology*, ISSN: 2278-0181, 174-177, 2018.
62. Girish Chandrashekar, Ferat Sahin, "A survey on feature selection methods", *Computers and Electrical Engineering,* 40(2014): 16–28.
63. Mohamed M Dessouky, Mohamed A Elrashidy, Taha E Taha, Hatem M Abdelkader, "Effective features extracting approach using MFCC for automated diagnosis of Alzheimer's disease", *International Journal of Data Mining and Knowledge Engineering*, 6(2), 2014.
64. Heba Mohsen, El-Sayed A El-Dahshan, El-Sayed M El-Horbaty, Abdel-Badeeh M Salem, "Intelligent methodology for brain tumors classification in magnetic resonance images", *International Journal of Computers* 11, 2017.
65. DR Nayak, R Dash, B Majhi, "Brain MR image classification using two-dimensional discrete wavelet transform and AdaBoost with random forests", *Neurocomputing* 177: 188–197, 2016.
66. AB Al-Khafaji, "Classification of MRI brain images using discrete wavelet transform and K-NN", *International Journal of Engineering Sciences & Research Technology* 4(11), November 2015.

67. B Thamaraichelvi, G Yamuna, "Gray level co-occurrence matrix features based classification of tumor in medical images", *ARPN Journal of Engineering and Applied Sciences* 11(19), 2016.
68. P Mohanaiah, P Sathyanarayana, L GuruKumar, "Image texture feature extraction using GLCM approach", *International Journal of Scientific and Research Publications*, 3(5), May 2013.
69. Jayashri Joshi, AC Phadke, "Feature extraction and texture classification in MRI", *Special Issue of IJCCT* 2 (2–4), 2010.
70. Robert M Haralick, K Shanmugam, Its'hak Dinstein, "Textural features for image classification", *IEEE Transactions on Systems, Man, and Cybernetics,* 1973.
71. P Paatero, U Tapper, "Positive matrix factorization: A nonnegative factor model with optimal utilization of error estimates of data values", *Environmetrics* 5(2): 111–126, 1994.
72. Ioan Buciu, "Non-negative matrix factorization, a new tool for feature extraction: Theory and applications", *International Journal of Computers, Communications & Control* III(Suppl Issue): pp. 67–74, 2018.
73. Nicolas Sauwen, "Unsupervised and semi-supervised non-negative matrix factorization methods for brain tumor segmentation using multi-parametric MRI data", *Kasteelpark Arenberg* 10 box 2446, B-3001, 2016.
74. RM Vidhyavathi, "Principal component analysis (PCA) in medical image processing using digital imaging and communications in medicine (DICOM) medical images", *International Journal of Pharma and Bio Sciences*, 8(2): 598–606, 2017. DOI:10.22376/ijpbs.2017.8.2.b.598–606
75. Archana H Telgaonkar, Sachin Deshmukh, "Dimensionality reduction and classification through PCA and LDA", *International Journal of Computer Applications* 122(17): 4–8, 2015.
76. Dibyadeep Nandi, Amira S Ashour, Sourav Samanta, Sayan Chakraborty, Mohammed AM Salem, Nilanjan Dey, "Principal component analysis in medical image processing: A study", *International Journal of Image Mining* 1(1): 65–86, 2015. DOI: 10.1504/IJIM.2015.070024
77. Martin J McKeown, Terrence J Sejnowski, "Independent component analysis of fMRI data: Examining the assumptions", *Human Brain Mapping* 6: 368–372, 1998.
78. Wenlu Yanga, Ronald LM Luib, Jia-Hong Gaoc, Tony F Chand, Shing-Tung Yaub, "Independent component analysis-based classification of Alzheimer's disease MRI data", *Journal of Alzheimer's Disease* 24(4): 775–783, 2011. DOI: 10.3233/JAD-2011–101371
79. Heba Mohsen, El-Sayed A El-Dahshan, El-Sayed M El-Horbaty, Abdel-Badeeh M Salem, "Classification of brain MRI for Alzheimer's disease based on linear discriminate analysis", *Egyptian Computer Science Journal* 41(3), 2017.
80. S Balakrishnama, A Ganapathiraju, "Linear discriminant analysis – A brief tutorial", *Institute for Signal and Information Processing*, 18, 1998.
81. Mohan Allam, M Nandhini, "A study on optimization techniques in feature selection for medical image analysis", *International Journal on Computer Science and Engineering* 9(3), 2017.
82. Ashraf Darwish, Gehad Ismail Sayed, Aboul Ella Hassanien, "Meta-heuristic optimization algorithms based feature selection for clinical breast cancer diagnosis", *Journal of the Egyptian Mathematical Society* 26(3), 2018.
83. E Elbeltagi, T Hegazy, D Grierson, "Comparison among five evolutionary-based optimization algorithms", *Advanced Engineering Informatics* 19: 43–53, 2005.
84. Melanie Mitchell, "Genetic algorithms: An overview", *Computer Science, Mathematics Published in Complexity*, 1(1): 31–39, 1995. DOI: 10.1002/cplx.6130010108

85. L Haldurai, T Madhubala, R Rajalakshmi, "A study on genetic algorithm and its applications", *International Journal of Computer Sciences and Engineering* 4(10), 2016.
86. Harsh Bhasin, Surbhi Bhatia, "Application of genetic algorithms in machine learning", *International Journal of Computer Science and Information Technologies*, 2(5): 2412–2415, 2011.
87. R Hooke, TA Jeeves, "Direct search solution of numerical and statistical problems", *Journal of the Association of Computing Machinery* 8: 212–229, 1961.
88. Michael Wetter, Jonathan Wright, "Comparison of a generalized pattern search and a genetic algorithm optimization method", Eighth International IBPSA Conference, 2003.
89. L Ingber, "Simulated annealing: Practice versus theory", *Mathematical and Computer Modelling* 18(11): 29–57, 1993.
90. LM RasdiRere, Mohamad Ivan Fanany, Aniati Murni Arymurthy, "Simulated annealing algorithm for deep learning", *Procedia Computer Science* 72: 137–144, 2015.
91. Andries Engelbrecht, "Particle swarm optimization: Velocity initialization", 2012 IEEE Congress on Evolutionary Computation, 2012. DOI: 10.1109/CEC.2012.6256112
92. Pei-Wei Tsai, Jeng-Shyang Pan, Bin-Yih Liao, Ming-Jer Tsai, Vaci Istanda, "Bat algorithm inspired algorithm for solving numerical optimization problems", *Applied Mechanics and Materials* 148–149: 134–137, 2012.
93. M Tabassum, K Mathew, "A genetic algorithm analysis towards optimization solutions", *International Journal of Digital Information and Wireless Communications* 4: 124–142, 2014.
94. Tobias Uhlig, Oliver Rose, "Simulation-based optimization for groups of cluster tools in semiconductor manufacturing using simulated annealing", Proceedings of the 2011 Winter Simulation Conference (WSC), Phoenix, AZ IEE, 2011.
95. JS Al-Sumait, AK AL-Othman, JK Sykulski, "Application of pattern search method to power system valve-point economic load dispatch", *Electrical Power and Energy Systems* 29: 720–730, 2007.
96. Peter Wilson, H Alan Mantooth, "Model-based optimization techniques", *Model-Based Engineering for Complex Electronic Systems*, 2013.
97. SX Yang, A Gandomi, "Bat algorithm: A novel approach for global engineering optimization", *International Journal for Computer-Aided Engineering and Software* 29: 464–483, 2012.
98. Mohamed M Dessouky, Mohamed A Elrashidy, "Feature extraction of the Alzheimer's disease images using different optimization algorithms", *Journal of Alzheimer's disease & Parkinsonism* 2016. DOI: 10.4172/2161-0460.1000230
99. Gidudu Anthony, Hulley Greg, Marwala Tshilidzi, "Classification of images using support vector machines", 2007.
100. Le Hoang Thai, Son Hai Tran, Thanh Thuy Nguyen, "Image classification using support vector machine and artificial neural network", *International Journal of Information Technology and Computer Science* 5: 32–38, 2012.
101. Luiz K Ferreira, Jane M Rondina, Rodrigo Kubo, Carla R Ono, Claudia C Leite, "Support vector machine-based classification of neuroimages in Alzheimer's disease: Direct comparison of FDG-PET, rCBF-SPECT and MRI data acquired from the same individuals", *Revista Brasileira de Psiquiatria 2017*. DOI: 10.1590/1516-4446-2016-2083
102. Jesse Verheijen, "Classification and conversion prediction of Alzheimer's disease based on brain glucose metabolism using support vector machines", Master Thesis Data Science, Tilburg, the Netherlands, 2017.

103. Taeho Jo, Kwangsik Nho, Andrew J Saykin, "Deep learning in Alzheimer's disease: Diagnostic classification and prognostic prediction using neuroimaging data", *Frontiers in Aging Neuroscience*, 2019.
104. Garam Leel, Kwangsik Nho, Byungkon Kang, Kyung-Ah Sohn, Dokyoon Kim, "Predicting Alzheimer's disease progression using multi-modal deep learning approach", PMCID: PMC6374429, DOI: 10.1038/s41598-018-37769-z, *Scientific Reports* 9, Article number: 1952, 2019.
105. Hongming Lia, Mohamad Habesab, David AWolkb, Yong Fan, "A deep learning model for early prediction of Alzheimer's disease dementia based on hippocampal magnetic resonance imaging data", *Alzheimer's & Dementia*, 15(8): 1059–1070, August 2019.
106. Hojjat Salehinejad, Sharan Sankar, Joseph Barfett, Errol Colak, Shahrokh Valaee, "Recent advances in recurrent neural networks", *Computer Science, Neural and Evolutionary Computing*, 2018.
107. Yechong Huang, Jiahang Xu, Yuncheng Zhou, Tong Tong, Xiahai Zhuang, "Diagnosis of Alzheimer's disease via multi-modality 3D convolutional neural network", *Frontiers in Neuroscience*, 31 May 2019. | DOI: 10.3389/fnins.2019.00509
108. Tianyi Liu, Shuangsang Fang, Yuehui Zhao, Peng Wang, Jun Zhang, "*Implementation of training convolutional neural networks*", 2015.
109. Alexander SelvikvågLundervold, Arvid Lundervold, "An overview of deep learning in medical imaging focusing on MRI", *Med Phys* 29: 102–127, 2019.
110. GB Vindhya, Mahera Alam, Medha Mansi, Muskan Kedia, D Anjal, "Prediction of Alzheimer's Disease using Machine Learning Technique", *International Research Journal of Engineering and Technology (IRJET)*, 7(5), 2020
111. Debesh Jha, Goo-Rak Kwon, "Alzheimer's disease detection using sparse autoencoder, scale conjugate gradient and softmax output layer with fine tuning", *International Journal of Machine Learning and Computing* 7(1), 2017.
112. KR Kruthikaa, Rajeswari, HD Maheshappa, "CBIR system using capsule networks and 3D CNN for Alzheimer's disease diagnosis", *Informatics in Medicine Unlocked*, 14: 59–68, 2019.

4 An Efficient Protein Structure Prediction Using Genetic Algorithm

Mohamad Yousef, Tamer Abdelkader, and Khaled El-Bahnasy

CONTENTS

4.1 THEORIES AND METHODS

Protein structure determination lab procedures carried out to define and determine the exact native structure of a given protein such as X-ray diffraction and NMR spectroscopy are time-consuming and expensive, and could be redone for multiple times due to their complex nature. Those disadvantages forced the development of computationally driven prediction techniques.
After the formation of a polypeptide, hydrogen bonds, salt bridges, or Vander Waals interactions between its atoms will cause the entire protein to have unique local structures.

These local structures are classified into two major classes: alpha helix and beta sheet. Alpha helix structures are the most occurring local structures. It has 3.6 amino acids per turn. In beta sheets, the polypeptide does not form a spiral coil. Instead, it zig-zags in an extended shape (see Figure 4.1).

4.1.1 THEORIES

Levinthal's paradox [1] states that there is no way for a protein structure to try and fold into all of its possible conformations to form its native structure because it will take a massively long time, but in fact proteins take only a few seconds or less to reach their native fold. This implies that every protein follows a folding pathway. In addition, Anfinsen's thermodynamic hypothesis [2] states that, for small globular proteins, the native structure is determined by the protein's amino acid sequence. This also infers that, at normal conditions (temperature and medium concentration, etc.), when folding process ends, the native structure is stable and has the lowest free energy. Levinthal's paradox and Anfinsen's hypothesis are the foundations of ab initio PSP.

Ab initio prediction, also known as free modeling, is preferred to be used if the target protein does not have a homologue (a homologue is a protein that is similar to the target protein by sequence) already existed in the biological databases. The task

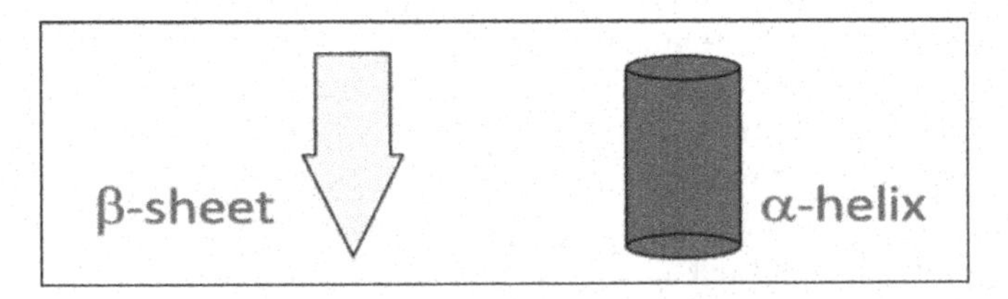

FIGURE 4.1 In any given ribbon diagram, the "spirals" or "cylinders" are alpha-helices and the "ribbons" or "arrows" are beta sheets.

of predicting a target protein's structure would be relatively easy if a homologue was found and high-quality structure can be assembled by copying the framework of the homologue(s) "solved" structure(s).

However, this procedure does not reveal any information about how and why a protein assumes its specific native structure. If no homologues are found, structures must be built from the scratch, and this defines the ab initio PSP concept.

Ab initio protein folding is considered a global optimization problem where the goal is to find the values of the dihedral angles for a given protein structure which contribute into that structure's stability and balance, i.e., having the global or near-global minimum potential energy, expressed in Kcal/mol.

4.1.2 Protein Structure Prediction (PSP) Methods

4.1.2.1 MODELLER

Formerly written in FORTRAN 90 and then re-implemented using Python, MODELLER runs on UNIX, windows, and MAC computers via scripts written in the Python. It does not provide any graphical user interface. MODELLER is a software used for creating homologous protein structure models for proteins that does not have experimentally determined three-dimensional (3D) structures yet. It utilizes the satisfaction of spatial restraints method assisted by nuclear magnetic resonance (NMR) spectroscopy data. Using the NMR data, a set of geometrical measures are used to produce probability density functions for each atom's location in the protein [3, 4].

4.1.2.2 SWISS-MODEL

Developed by the Swiss Institute of Bioinformatics (SIB) [5], it is a web server to build protein structure models using comparative approach. It is accessible via the ExPASy web server and program Deep View [6].

Its comparative approach uses options like BLAST (Basic Local Alignment Search Tool) and PSI-BLAST (Position-Specific Iterative Basic Local Alignment Search Tool) for template identification.

4.1.2.3 3D-JIGSAW

A web server that produces 3D models for proteins using comparative approach. In version 3.0, templates are identified using HMM and the returned alignments are used to generate the final models [7, 8].

4.1.2.4 ESyPred3D

A modeling web server that uses a homology/comparative method to predict the protein structures. It implements four steps:

1. Identify structure homologs done by searching multiple databases.
2. Target template alignment.
3. Model building and optimization using Modeller.
4. Model evaluation.

In CASP4 contest, it was found that alignment strategy of EsyPred3D is better than PSI-BLAST alignment.

In CASP3, models generated by EsyPred3D were among the best of experiments[9].

4.1.2.5 RaptorX

Rapid protein threading by operation research predicts 3D structures by an innovative linear programming method. RaptorX employs a statistical knowledge-based technique to design a new threading scoring function [10].

4.1.2.6 HHpred

It is a web-based server for protein homology detection and structure prediction. Input to HHpred can be amino acid sequence or a multiple sequence alignment. It uses a novel approach that conducts a pair-wise alignments of profile hidden Markov models (HMMs). It also uses a variety of databases like SCOP (Structural Classification of Proteins), Pfam, and PDB (Protein Data Bank). HHpred performs fast and well for single domain and for multi-domain query sequences and can be used to predict functional information of a protein from homolog proteins using various sequence-based search tools like BLAST, FASTA, or PSI-BLAST [11, 12, 13].

4.1.2.7 BHAGEERATH-H

It was a hybrid between homology and ab initio methods. The web server produces five structures for the input target sequence. The web server takes longer time to complete for sequences of length greater than 100 residues [14].

Structure evaluation is performed using energy-based empirical scoring function [15] and it selects 100 lowest energy structures. At the end, only five structures are selected from the 100 models by using solvent accessible surface areas (SASA). The web server is no longer available.

4.1.2.8 I-TASSER

I-TASSER is a web-based protein structure prediction tool that employs profile–profile threading alignment (PPA) [16] and Threading ASSEmbly Refinement (TASSER) program [17]. The query sequence is aligned to a selected library of PDB structures to search for the potential structures by four methods: PPA, HMM [18], PSI-BLAST profiles, and the Needleman–Wunsch and Smith–Waterman alignment algorithms. The unaligned regions (e.g., loops) are built by ab initio modeling, while the aligned regions after threading are used to build the main structure [19, 20].

4.1.2.9 Genetic Algorithm in the Two-Dimensional (2D) Hydrophobic-Polar Model

Genetic algorithm (GA) is introduced to find the lowest energy conformation for some standard HP (Hydrophobic-Polar) protein sequences [21].

The 2D HP model [22] implements the important components of protein folding. Every protein is represented by a sequence of amino acids. Each amino acid is represented in the sequence by one of the two types: either H (hydrophobic or non-polar) or P (hydrophilic or polar). This sequence is plotted on a 2D square lattice [23]. This method is not reliable because it does not generate real protein structures – like the ones found in PDB – which makes its evaluation process impossible.

4.1.2.10 QUARK

QUARK is a web server for ab initio PSP and protein peptide folding; it builds the correct protein structure using its amino acid sequence as an input. QUARK was the number one server in free modeling (FM) category in CASP9 (Critical Assessment of Structure Prediction 9) and CASP10 contests [24, 25]. QUARK is not a 100% ab initio method because it uses a fragment assembly approach, in which tiny fragments (1–20 residues long taken from known PDB structures) are joined to build the final structure by replica-exchange Monte Carlo search with assistance of an atomic-level knowledge-based force field [26, 27]. It accepts peptide sequences less than 200 amino acids long. In addition, QUARK users cannot submit multiple jobs at once.

4.1.2.11 PEP-FOLD2

Also known as PEP-FOLD 2.0, it is an ab initio PSP web server aimed at carrying out the process of PSP using amino acid sequences as an input. It is based on structural alphabet (SA) letters to construct the conformations of four consecutive residues and combines the predicted series of SA letters to a greedy algorithm and a coarse-grained force field. It may result in unconnected disulfide bonds in the all-atom representation even if the cysteines are near each other. It accepts sequences ranged from 9 to 36 residues [28, 29]. For an unknown reason, this method is prone to failure. It may require resubmitting the job multiple times.

4.1.2.12 PEP-FOLD3

Also known as PEP-FOLD 3.5, it is a faster and more stable version of PEP-FOLD2. Although it can deal with disulfide bonds, it cannot achieve results better than PEP-FOLD2. PEP-FOLD2 should be used for such peptides [30, 31, 32].

4.2 THE PROPOSED METHOD: 3DPROFOLD

It is a desktop application that integrates GA search algorithm with ECEPPAK energy calculation program to find the best conformation of a protein using its amino acids sequence only, which makes it a pure ab initio method. It does not use neither PDB templates nor fragment assembly [33].

The proposed solution employs GA [34]. GA is an adaptive heuristic search algorithm based on the evolutionary ideas of natural selection and genetics. It was introduced by John Holland in the mid-1970s but became popular in the late 1980s [35] due to its ability to solve different hard computational problems. This method was reintroduced into biology, and to structural biology problems particularly, because of its resemblance with the laws of biological environments in the 1990s.

The basic idea behind the GA search method is to generate a population of chromosomes (solutions). Then, this population will be used to produce a set of successive generations by manipulating those chromosomes using genetic operations. The population size is kept unchanged through the whole process by eliminating in a way that gives bigger chance of survival to more fit solutions, while preserving diversity within the population. This indicates that the algorithm must utilize a fitness function that is used to evaluate the fitness of each solution as a numerical value. Possible solutions are represented as chromosomes "set of successive values" and will be manipulated by three genetic operators: selection, crossover, and mutation.

We implemented two models: the first one is a basic GA-driven model that utilizes Ramachandran plot dihedral angles and three different crossover operators. The other is an integration between the basic model and the ECEPPAK software which utilizes – in addition to the aforementioned features – a checkup feature that ensures the integrity and stability of the produced chromosomes.

4.2.1 Basic Model

See Figure 4.2

4.2.1.1 Encoding

- Input: a given protein's amino acid sequence.
- Description: each chromosome will be represented by a set of values that are the dihedral angles (also called internal coordinates) – ranging from −180° to 180° – that describe the degrees of freedom for each amino acid in the 3D space. Each amino acid shares three dihedral angles –phi (Φ), psi (Ψ), and omega (ω) – which are the main chain angles and each amino acid differs in the number of side chain angles chi (χ): $\chi 1, \chi 2 \ldots \chi 5$.

To minimize the search space, the initial population generation is not totally random. It follows the Ramachandran plot which was constructed after a huge set of experiments. It illustrates the preferred confirmations (Φ, Ψ) for each of the 20 amino acids found in a number of various experimentally determined protein structures [36, 37, 38, 39, 40, 41, 42, 43].

- Output: encoded chromosome.

4.2.1.2 Selection

- Input: a set of encoded chromosomes
- Description: in each generation, a portion from the current population is chosen to produce a new generation of population. Parent solutions are chosen based on their quality, where the most qualified solutions, measured by a fitness function "energy function," have a higher likelihood to be selected. Most selection methods are based on random selection (stochastic methods). They are designed to allow for a few numbers of lower quality solutions to be selected. This aids in maintaining the diversity of solutions, avoiding early convergence on unreliable solutions. One of the well-investigated selection methods is the tournament selection.

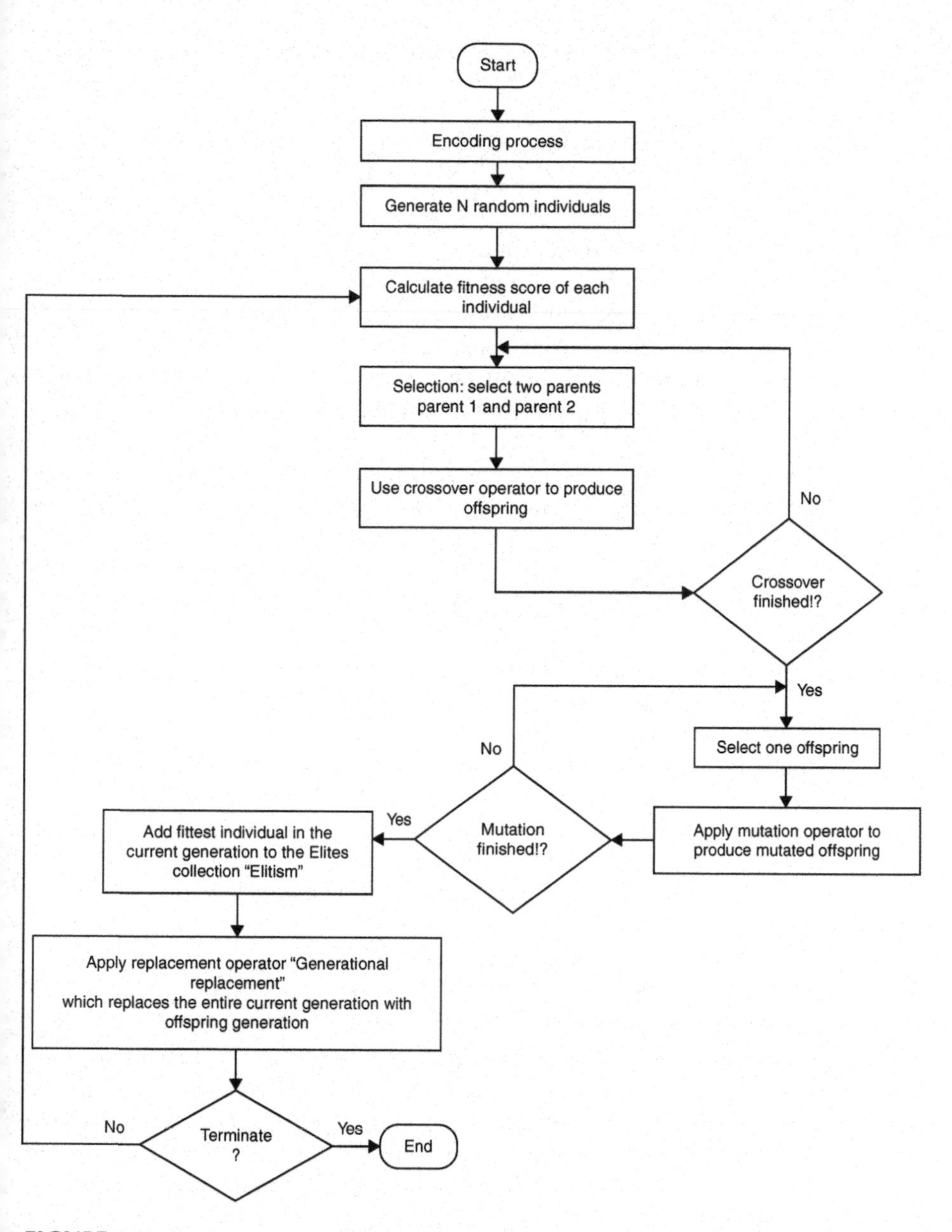

FIGURE 4.2 Implemented PSP – Basic approach [33].

Tournament selection involves running several tournaments (or rounds) among the population of chromosomes. The winner of each tournament (the one with the best fitness "lowest free energy") is selected to be a part of the crossover operation. Selection pressure is easily adjusted by changing the tournament factor "k." The larger the tournament factor is, the lesser the chance that weak individuals will be selected [44], which ultimately leads to loss of diversity [45]. It has been shown by our experiments through different runs that $k = 2$ is the best choice [45].

- Output: two parent chromosomes ready for crossover operation.

4.2.1.3 Crossover

- Input: a pair of parent chromosomes.
- Description: the next phase is to produce a new generation of chromosomes. A pair of parents is selected to perform crossover. A pair of children chromosomes will be produced by exchanging the genes of the parents' chromosomes. By producing a pair of solutions using crossover, the newly created chromosomes share the traits of their parents. Parents are selected in pairs without repetitions and the process repeats until the size of the new generation of population reaches the size of the previous generation which will form the next generation of chromosomes. In most cases, the average fitness of the population will be enhanced by this operation, since only the best chromosomes from the first generation are selected for breeding along with a small portion of less fit solutions for reasons mentioned earlier.

Three different versions of the crossover operators are implemented to prevent the early convergence on weak solutions:

- One-point crossover: select one gene randomly called the cutting point "Cp" and exchange all the genes afterward.
- Two-point crossover: randomly select two cutting points and exchange all genes in between.
- Uniform crossover: exchange every gene with probability 0.5.

4.2.1.4 Mutation

- Input: an encoded chromosome.
- Description: to guarantee that the chromosomes are not all identical to each other, we permitted for a slight chance of mutation. Looping through all the genes, the single units that build up a chromosome, of all chromosomes, and if a certain gene is chosen for mutation, you can either alter it by a small magnitude or change it entirely. The probability of mutation "mutation rate" lies usually between 0.001 and 0.1.
- Output: a mutated chromosome.

4.2.1.5 Structure Refinement

This step is used in the integrated approach and not in the basic one.

- Input: an encoded chromosome.

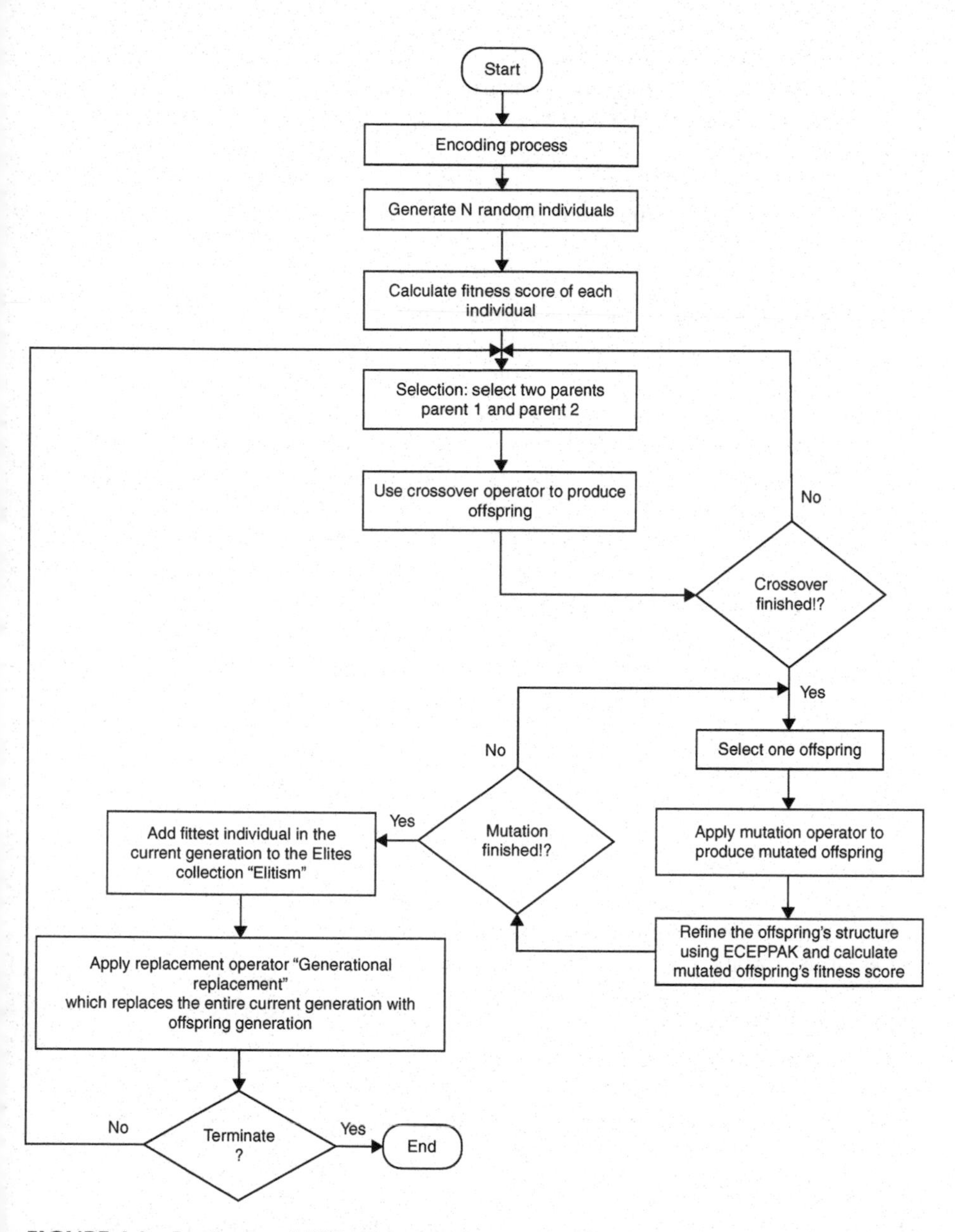

FIGURE 4.3 Implemented PSP – Integrated approach [33].

- Description: the structures predicted by the basic approach, GA alone, are not reliable "as will be shown later." The randomness of the algorithm might be one of the reasons; also the crossover operator is blindly shuffling the angle values without considering the structure's state of stability. One measure of protein stability is its free potential energy. High free energies could be an indication of a very unstable structure.

As a result, the basic approach skeleton is modified where a refinement step is added to the prediction process to help in ensuring the stability of a given protein structure by incorporating the free energy minimization feature provided by ECEPPAK package [46].

- Output: a refined chromosome.

4.2.1.6 Elitism

- Input: the best chromosome in each generation.
  Description: the best individual – i.e. having the smallest potential free energy – in each generation will be added into a final list of candidate solutions. Those will be compared to the native structure found in the PDB repository and the candidate with the highest similarity score should be selected as the best structure, and thus the solution structure for the given protein sequence input.
- Output: the elites list which contains the best chromosome in every generation.

4.2.1.7 Chromosome Evaluation

- Input: an encoded chromosome.
- Description: each chromosome will be assigned a fitness score which is the free potential energy calculated by the following force field function provided by ECEPPAK package:

$$\boldsymbol{Etot = Ees + Enb + Etor + Eloop} \tag{4.1}$$

where:

Etot = Total conformational energy (fitness score).
Ees = Electrostatic energy.
Enb = Nonbonded energy.
Etor = Torsional energy.
Eloop = Loop-distortion energy.

- Output: fitness score of the given chromosome.

4.2.1.8 Termination

This prediction process is repeated until a fixed number of generations have been reached.

4.2.2 Integrated Model

Figure 4.3 illustrates the integration between Genetic algorithm and ECEPPAK

4.3 EXPERIMENTAL RESULTS

In this section, we will compare the quality of the basic approach against the hybrid/integrated one. We will also compare the integrated model with a group of well-known ab initio prediction methods.

4.3.1 Results of PSP Basic Model versus Integrated Model

Using the peptide sequence of the PDB entry 1Q2K Figure 4.4:

> "AACYSSDCRVKCVAMGFSSGKCINSKCKCYK" as a test case, different runs have been performed with different population sizes (50,60,100) and number of generations (50,60,100) using both approaches with a crossover rate = 0.7 "ideal" and a mutation rate = 0.001. Then, the candidate structures were superimposed against the native structure found in PDB using TM-Align software to measure their structural similarity.

4.3.1.1 Results of Basic Model

Next are the results obtained from using basic model which uses genetic algorithm only – see Figure 4.5 which shows the alignment between the native structure and predicted structure.

4.3.1.2 Results of Integrated Model

Next are the results obtained from using genetic algorithm combined with ECEPPAK – see Figure 4.6 which shows the alignment between the native structure and predicted structure.

From Table 4.1, Figures 4.7 and 4.8, the TM-scores indicate that GA alone produced a solution with a maximum score of 0.239. Tables 4.2, 4.4 and 4.6 show that root-mean-square deviation (RMSD) values are less than 4 Angstroms which is a good indicator. Table 4.3 shows the success of the integrated approach in predicting the structure of 1Q2K with a score equal to 0.46.

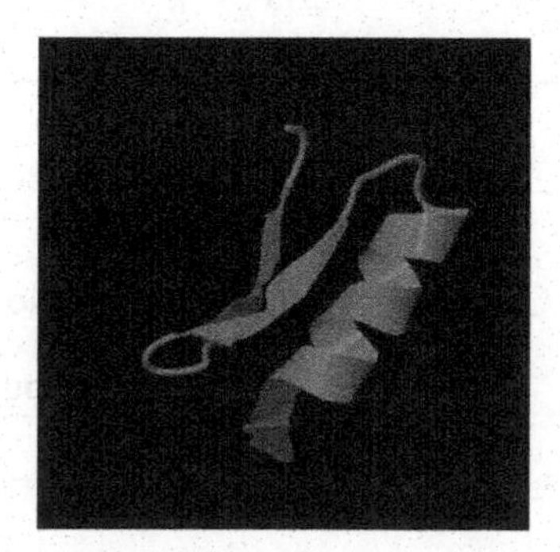

FIGURE 4.4 1Q2K native three-dimensional view.

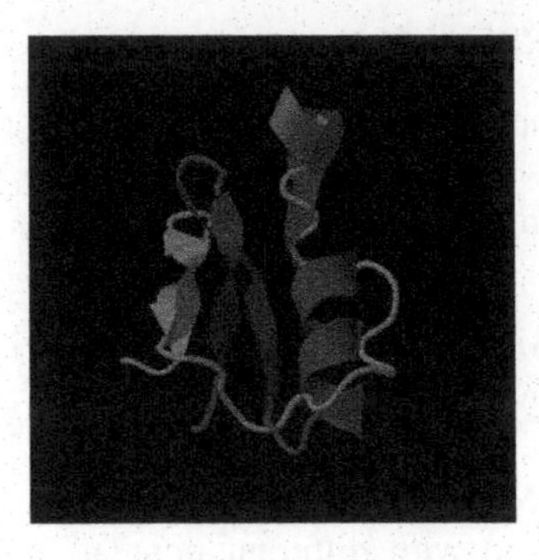

FIGURE 4.5 The predicted structure superimposed against the native one.

TABLE 4.1
TM-Scores of Structures Obtained from Basic Model "GA Only" Runs [33]

	Population Size		
Number of Generations	**50**	**60**	**100**
50	0.239	0.229	0.226
60	0.21	0.229	0.226
100	0.21	0.229	0.22

TABLE 4.2
RMSDs of Structures Obtained from Basic Model "GA Only" Runs [33]

	Population Size		
Number of Generations	**50**	**60**	**100**
50	3.81	1.91	1.56
60	2.58	1.91	1.56
100	2.58	1.91	1.56

TABLE 4.3
TM-Scores of Structures Obtained from Integrated Model Runs [33]

	Population Size		
Number of Generations	**50**	**60**	**100**
50	0.4	0.34	0.31
60	0.39	0.35	0.425
100	0.42	0.44	0.46

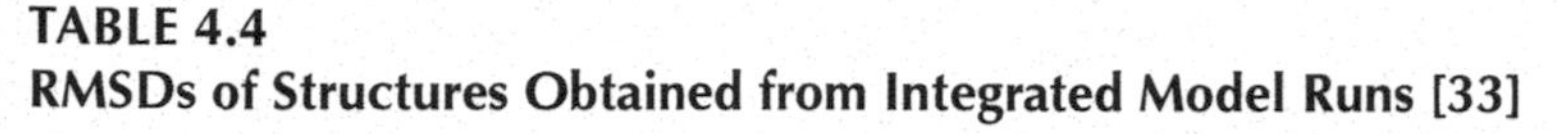

TABLE 4.4
RMSDs of Structures Obtained from Integrated Model Runs [33]

	Population Size		
Number of Generations	**50**	**60**	**100**
50	1.88	2.99	2.26
60	2.4	2.01	2.3
100	2.2	1.75	2.25

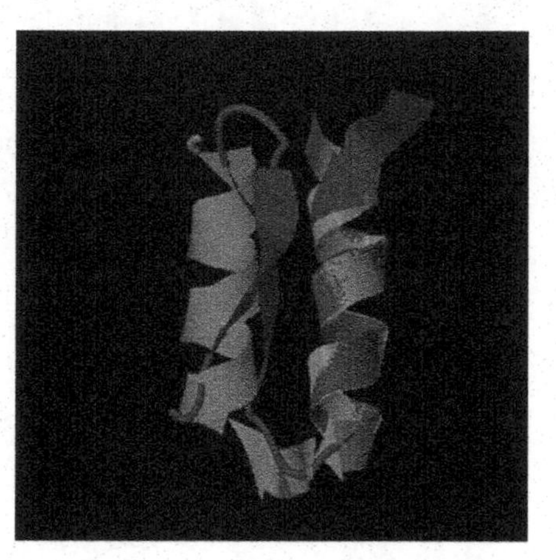

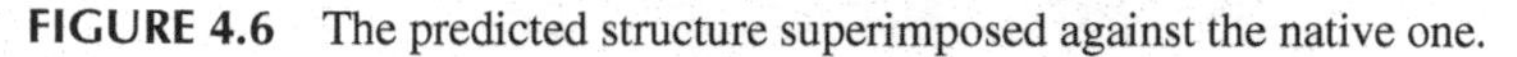

FIGURE 4.6 The predicted structure superimposed against the native one.

Table 4.3 also shows that the increase in population and generation numbers is proportionate to the improvement of the predicted structure, and if the population size is kept unchanged while the number of generations is increasing, the results tend to be significantly improved while this is not the case in the basic approach.

4.3.2 3dProFold Compared to Other Prediction Methods

The results were obtained from a set of 48 experiments conducted as running three prediction trials using the same method for one structure each time and then choosing the best TM-score see Figure 4.9 [47] out of the three trials as the result and its respective RMSD value see Figure 4.10. [48]

Note: The predicted structure is considered to be the same as the native one if 0.5 <= TM-Score <= 1 (the closer to 1 the better) and its RMSD should be nearly equal to 3Å.

From the previous chart, 3dProFold never came last compared to the other methods in predicting proteins structures.

From Tables 4.5 & 4.7 and Figure 4.11, the TM-scores show that the 3dProFold method surpassed the other methods in predicting the structures of 1BH0 and 1Q2K

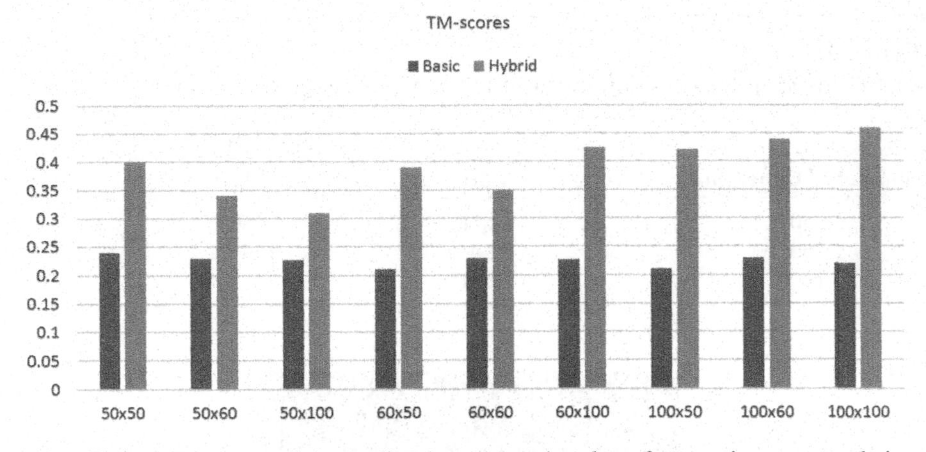

FIGURE 4.7 TM-scores of the predicted structures (number of generations vs. population size) [33].

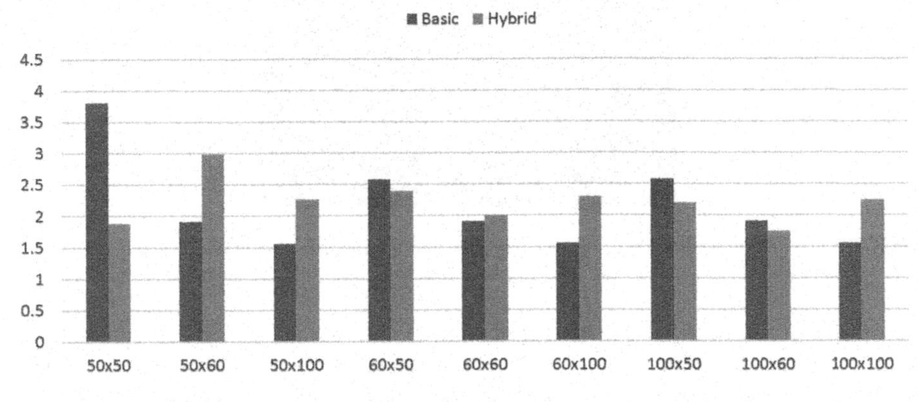

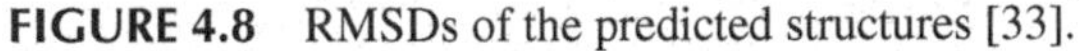
FIGURE 4.8 RMSDs of the predicted structures [33].

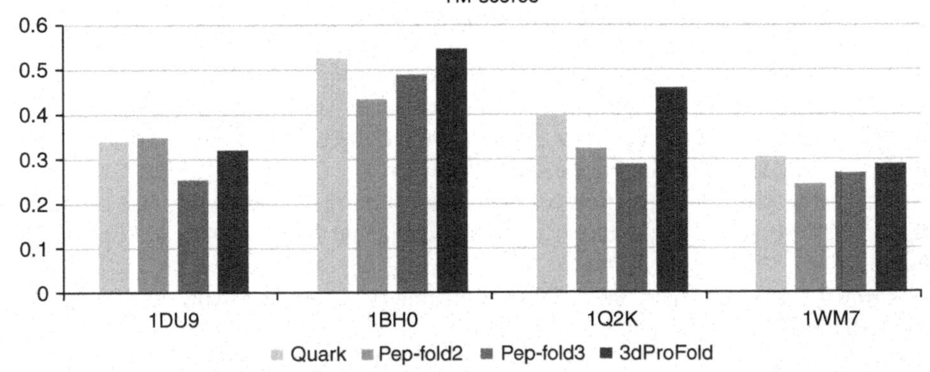

FIGURE 4.9 TM-scores of the predicted structures.

TABLE 4.5
TM-Scores: Each Cell Represents the Best TM-Score of Three Prediction Trials

PDB_ID	QUARK	Pep-Fold2	Pep-Fold3	3dProFold
1DU9	0.34	0.35	0.256	0.32
1BH0	0.527	0.435	0.49	0.545
1Q2K	0.4	0.326	0.29	0.46
1WM7	0.306	0.245	0.27	0.289

TABLE 4.6
RMSD Values

PDB_ID	QUARK	Pep-Fold2	Pep-Fold3	3dProFold
1DU9	2.22	2.67	2.04	3.17
1BH0	1.17	1.21	1.86	1.07
1Q2K	2.1	1.98	2.67	2.25
1WM7	2.57	2.23	2.89	2.04

TABLE 4.7
Time Consumption in Terms of Hours

PDB_ID	QUARK	Pep-Fold2	Pep-Fold3	3dProFold
1DU9	14	0.5	0.2	5
1BH0	4	0.5	0.25	6
1Q2K	3	0.53	0.2	9
1WM7	13	0.36	0.1	4

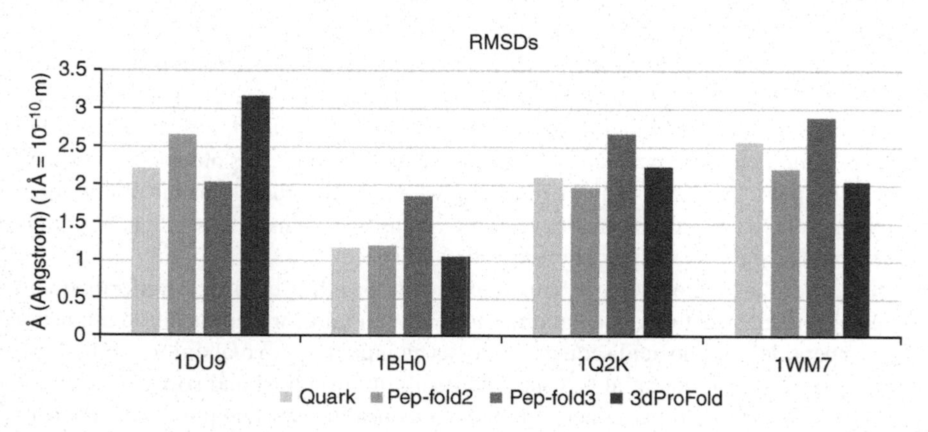

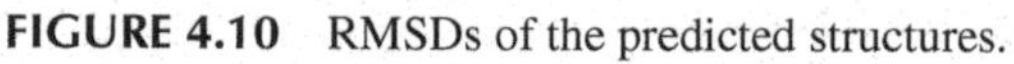
FIGURE 4.10 RMSDs of the predicted structures.

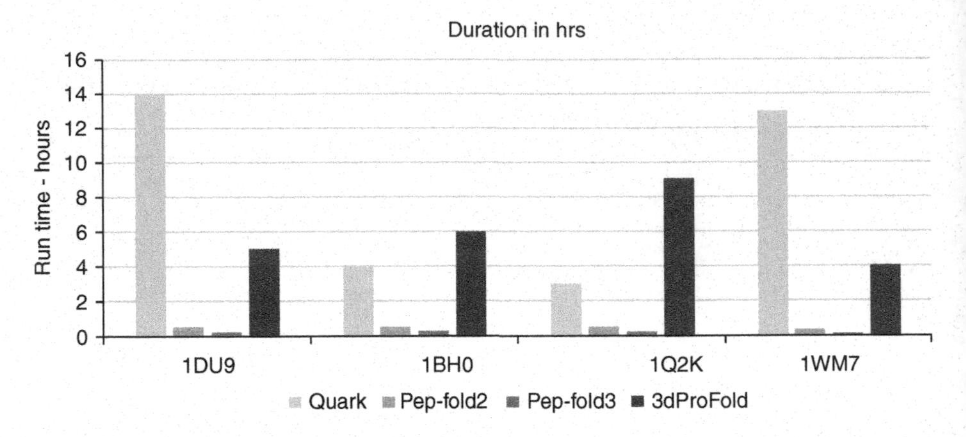

FIGURE 4.11 Time consumed in hours.

but took a longer time in relation to them. In structure 1DU9, PEP-FOLD2 has predicted its structure in 0.5 hr with a slight difference in TM-score ahead of 3dProFold and QUARK which took very long to predict its structure (14 hr). 1WM7 structure prediction results show that 3dProFold is as near as QUARK in terms of structural similarity and it took 3dProFold shorter time compared to QUARK.

In Table 4.6, all the predicted structures have RMSDs values equal to 3Å, which is an additional indicator of good accuracy shared among the methods.

The time consumption of PEP-FOLD2 and PEP-FOLD3 is much smaller than the other methods, but their accuracies are not guaranteed to be high. Both QUARK and 3dProFold may forsake time in favor of accuracy. The long time consumed by 3dProFold method is attributed to the overhead of Ramachandran plot feature implemented.

4.4 CONCLUSION

The objective of this work was to fold a given protein primary structure "sequence" into its near-optimal 3D structure without the use of any helping templates.

GA is powerful in solving many scientific problems and has a promising potential in solving PSP problem. However, because of crossover operator the generated structures may be noisy compared to the native structure in terms of similarity. To solve this problem a checkup was required to ensure that the protein's atoms are balanced in the 3D space. This was done by checking whether the structure needs to minimize its energy due to the collisions between the atoms and their false arrangement, thus leading to the stability of the structure in the 3D space.

In 3dProfold method, GA is implemented to search a compact conformational space of refined structures in an attempt to find optimal/near-optimal structure using a given peptide's amino acid sequence only as an input (de novo/ab initio prediction), because of the great potential GA has and its ability to model and solve a variety of problems. However, the generated structures may be distorted and noisy. An enhancement step was added to confirm that the protein structures are at rest in the 3D space.

We implemented two de novo approaches of PSP: basic PSP and integrated PSP. First, the basic approach was implemented to test the feasibility of GA as a protein structure predictor. The results of this approach were promising but not reliable. This led us to enhance the basic approach by integrating it with the ECEPP package, which resulted in the development of 3dProFold method. Both approaches were compared with each other by using the PDB sequence 1Q2K by running 18 experiments. The results showed that the integrated approach's "3dProFold" output is better than the basic one by a big margin.

To validate our method, we tested it against a collection of de novo-based PSP methods by conducting 48 experiments. The results showed that 3dProFold made a great attempt to predict the structures of 1DU9, 1BH0, 1Q2K, and 1WM7.

In the integrated approach, when making the number of generations constant and increasing the population size, we are searching for an optimal solution without proper balance between exploration "searching pressure" and exploitation "chromosomes generation", thus leading the algorithm to lower its searching pressure.

To asses our results, we used the TM-align tool. The software compares the generated 3D structures against the native structures found in the PDB repository using TM-score and RMSD.

Even conducting a run with large numbers of generations and population size, respectively, "1000x1000" using the basic approach, GA was only good in predicting 1Q2K's backbone torsional angles with a TM-Score of 0.32 and an RMSD score of 2.63 Å but failed to predict the sidechain torsional angles which are very important in determining the different types of secondary structures that define the local parts "domains" of a given protein.

Both Ramachandran plot and the three crossover versions were implemented to cover the absence of:

1. Surface hydration model – with solvent and atomic hydration parameters that are optimized using nonpeptide data (the ECEPPAK uses solvation parameters file "srfopt.set" for this feature).
2. Volume hydration model (the ECEPPAK uses solvation parameters file "volume.set" for this feature).
3. Electrostatically driven Monte Carlo (EDMC) calculations which have shown its consumption for a lot of time, nearly 1–2 weeks to predict a small peptide chain of 31 residues "1Q2K", and its low-quality produced conformations. Also, the work of Barreraet al. [49] has shown that EDMC calculations option in ECEPPAK produced low-quality structures compared to native structure.

Our future work will be focused on enhancing performance and reducing time consumption of 3dProFold by applying CUDA Graphical processing unit (GPU) technology.

With all the things proteins do to keep our body functioning and healthy, they can be harmful, damaging, and involved in many diseases in many ways. The better we understand protein folding mechanisms and pathways, the more novel proteins can be designed to combat the disease-related proteins and fix or even destroy them.

REFERENCES

1. Levinthal C. "Are there pathways for protein folding?" *Journal of Medical Physics*, 65(1): 44–45, 1968.
2. Anfinsen CB. "The principles that govern the folding of protein chains," *Science*, 181(4096): 223–230, 1973.
3. Gibrat JF, Madej T, Bryant SH. "Surprising similarities in structure comparison," *Current Opinion in Structural Biology*, 6: 377–385, 1996.
4. Yan R, Wang X, Huang L, Yan F, Xue X, Cai W. "Prediction of structural features and application to outer membrane protein identification," *Scientific Reports*, 5: 11586, 2015.
5. Tramontano A, Leplae R, Morea V. "Analysis and assessment of comparative modeling predictions in CASP4," *Proteins*, 5: 22–38, 2001.
6. Martí-Renom MA, Stuart AC, Fiser A, Sánchez R, Melo F, et al. "Comparative protein structure modeling of genes and genomes," *Annu Rev Biophys Biomol* Struct 29: 291–325, 2000.
7. Laskowski RA, MacArthur MW, Moss DS, Thornton JM. "PROCHECK – A program to check the stereochemical quality of protein structures," *J. Appl. Cryst*, 26: 283–291, 1993.
8. Sim EU-H, Er C-M, "Structure-to-function computational prediction of a subset of ribosomal proteins for the small ribosome subunit," *International Journal of Bioscience, Biochemistry and Bioinformatics*, 10.17706, 2015.
9. Lambert C, Léonard N, De Bolle X, Depiereux E. "ESyPred3D: Prediction of proteins 3D structures," *Bioinformatics*, 18: 1250–1256, 2002.
10. Källberg M, Wang H, Wang S, Peng J, Wang Z, et al. "Template-based protein structure modeling using the RaptorX web server," *Nat Protoc*, 7: 1511–1522, 2012.
11. Meiler J, Baker D. "Rapid protein fold determination using unassigned NMR data," *Proc Natl Acad Sci* USA, 100: 15404–15409, 2003.
12. Wright B, et al. "GRID and docking analyses reveal a molecular basis for flavonoid inhibition of Src family kinase activity," *Journal of Nutritional Biochemistry*, 26(11): 1156–1165 2015.
13. Smith TF, Waterman MS. "Identification of common molecular subsequences," *Journal of Molecular Biology*, 147: 195–197, 1981.
14. Zhou H, Zhou Y. "Single-body residue-level knowledge-based energy score combined with sequence-profile and secondary structure information for fold recognition," *Proteins*, 55: 1005–1013, 2004.
15. Zhou H, Zhou Y. "SPARKS 2 and SP3 servers in CASP6," *Proteins*, 61(Suppl 7): 152–156, 2005.
16. Skolnick J, Kolinski A. "A unified approach to the prediction of protein structure and function," In: Richard A Friesner (Ed.), *Advances in Chemical Physics, Computational Methods for Protein Folding* (vol. 120). New York, NY: John Wiley & Sons. Inc., 2002.
17. Floudas CA, Fung HK, McAllister SR, Monnigmann M, Rajgaria R. "Advances in protein structure prediction and de novo protein design: A review," *Chemical Engineering Science*, 61: 966–988, 2006.
18. Zhang Y, Skolnick J. "Tertiary structure predictions on a comprehensive benchmark of medium to large size proteins," *Biophys J*, 87: 2647–2655, 2004.
19. Wu S, Zhang Y. "LOMETS: A local meta-threading-server for protein structure prediction," *Nucleic Acids Res*, 35: 3375–3382, 2007.
20. Yang J, Zhang Y. "I-TASSER server: New development for protein structure and function predictions," *Nucleic Acids Research*, 43(W1): W174–W181, 2015.

21. Unger R, Moult J. “Genetic algorithms for protein folding simulations,” *J. Mol. Biol.*, 231: 75–81, 1993.
22. Lau KF, Dill KA. “Theory of protein mutability and biogenesis,” *Proc. Nat. Acad. Scie.*, 87: 638–642, 1990.
23. Halm E. “Genetic algorithm for predicting protein folding in the 2D HP model,” 2007. http://www.liacs.nl/assets/Bachelorscripties/09-EyalHalm.pdf.
24. http://predictioncenter.org/casp9/CD/data/html/groups.server.fm.html.
25. http://predictioncenter.org/casp10/groups_analysis.cgi?type=server&tbm=on&tbm_hard=on&tbmfm=on&fm=on&submit=Filter.
26. Xu D, Zhang Y. “Ab initio protein structure assembly using continuous structure fragments and optimized knowledge-based force field,” *Proteins*, 80: 1715–1735, 2012.
27. Xu D, Zhang Y. “Toward optimal fragment generations for ab initio protein structure assembly,” *Proteins*, 81: 229–239, 2013.
28. Maupetit J, Derreumaux P, Tufféry P. “PEP-FOLD: An online resource for de novo peptide structure prediction,” *Nucleic Acids Res.*, 37(Web Server issue): W498–W503, 2009. doi:10.1093/nar/gkp32.
29. Maupetit J, Derreumaux P, Tuffery P. “A fast and accurate method for large-scale de novo peptide structure prediction,” *J Comput Chem.*, 31(4):726–738, 2010. doi:10.1002/jcc.21365
30. Lamiable A, Thévenet P, Rey J, Vavrusa M, Derreumaux P, Tufféry P. “PEP-FOLD3: Faster de novo structure prediction for linear peptides in solution and in complex,” *Nucleic Acids Res.*, 44(W1): W449–W454, 2016.
31. Shen Y, Maupetit J, Derreumaux P, Tufféry P. “Improved PEP-FOLD approach for peptide and miniprotein structure prediction,” *J. Chem. Theor. Comput.*, 10: 4745–4758, 2014.
32. Thévenet P, Shen Y, Maupetit J, Guyon F, Derreumaux P, Tufféry P. “PEP-FOLD: An updated de novo structure prediction server for both linear and disulfide bonded cyclic peptides,” *Nucleic Acids Res.*, 40: W288–W293, 2012.
33. Yousef M, Abdelkader T, ElBahnasy K. “A hybrid model to predict proteins tertiary structure,” *12th International Conference on Computer Engineering and Systems (ICCES)*, Cairo, 2017, pp. 85–91. doi:10.1109/ICCES.2017.8275282
34. Holland JH. *Adaptation in Natural and Artificial Systems*. Ann Harbor, MI: The University of Michigan Press , 1975.
35. Goldberg DH. *Genetic Algorithms in Search, Optimization and Machine Learning*. Reading, MA: Addison-Wesley, 1985.
36. Ramachandran, GN, Ramakrishnan C, Sasisekharan V. “Stereochemistry of polypeptide chain configurations,” *Journal of Molecular Biology*, 7: 95–99, 1963. doi:10.1016/S0022-2836(63)80023–6
37. Morris AL, MacArthur MW, Hutchinson EG, Thornton JM. “Stereochemical quality of protein structure coordinates,” *Proteins: Structure, Function, and Genetics*, 12(4): 345–364, 1992. doi:10.1002/prot.340120407
38. Kleywegt GJ, Jones TA. “Phi/psi-chology: Ramachandran revisited,” *Structure*, 4(12): 1395–1400, 1996. doi:10.1016/S0969-2126(96)00147-5
39. Hooft RWW, Sander C, Vriend G. “Objectively judging the quality of a protein structure from a Ramachandran plot,” *Comput Appl Biosci.*, 13(4): 425–430, 1997. doi:10.1093/bioinformatics/13.4.425
40. Hovmöller S, Zhou T, Ohlson T. “Conformations of amino acids in proteins,” *Acta Crystallographica D.*, 58(Pt 5): 768–776, 2002. doi:10.1107/S0907444902003359
41. Lovell SC, Davis IW, Arendall WB, De Bakker PIW, Word JM, Prisant MG, Richardson JS, Richardson DC. “Structure validation by Ca geometry: ϕ,ψ and Cß deviation,”

Proteins: Structure, Function, and Genetics, 50(3): 437–450, 2003. doi:10.1002/prot.10286
42. Anderson RJ, Weng Z, Campbell RK, Jiang X. "Main-chain conformational tendencies of amino acids," *Proteins*, 60(4): 679–689, 2005. doi:10.1002/prot.20530
43. Mannige R. "An exhaustive survey of regular peptide conformations using a new metric for backbone handedness (h)," *Peer J.*, 5: e3327, May 2017. doi:10.7717/peerj.3327
44. Miller B, Goldberg D. "Genetic algorithms, tournament selection, and the effects of noise," *Complex Systems*, 9: 193–212, 1995.
45. Blickle T, Thiele L. "A comparison of selection schemes used in evolutionary algorithms," *Evolutionary Computation*, 4(4): 361–394, December 1996. doi:10.1162/evco.1996.4.4.36
46. Scheraga HA, Ripoll DR, Liwo A, Czaplewski C. *User Guide ECEPPAK and ANALYZE Programs,* Cornell University, 1983.
47. Zhang Y, Skolnick J. "TM-align: A protein structure alignment algorithm based on TM-score," *Nucleic Acids Research*, 33: 2302–2309, 2005.
48. Yousef M, Abdelkader T, El-Bahnasy K. "Performance comparison of ab initio protein structure prediction methods," *Ain Shams Engineering Journal*, 2019.
49. Barrera Guisasola EE, Masman MF, Enriz RD, et al. *Cent. Eur. J. Chem.*, 8: 566, 2010. https://doi.org/10.2478/s11532-010-0015-

5 Evaluating the Effectiveness of Healthcare Services by Using the Method of Data Envelopment Analysis

Vitalina Babenko

CONTENTS

5.1 INTRODUCTION

5.1.1 Healthcare System Efficiency

One of the main issues of the economic analysis in the field of medicine is to increase the efficiency of the healthcare system. The economic analysis is considered as a method of assessment of the costs and benefits, determination of the potential of the healthcare system and its implementation, etc.

The problem of the effectiveness of the healthcare system is common for the development of any country: the health of the nation, saving and prolongation of human lives, and influences from various fields of activity and social institutions Solving the problem of the health care system to improve efficiency is defined as a complex task. It covers many aspects such as the availability of medicines for the population, the level of service, industrial equipment, the qualifications and wages of health workers, and health financing.

To increase the efficiency of public administration in healthcare, adequate methods were used to assess the effectiveness of the implemented guidelines, taking into account regional specifics and international experience in this field. Many forms of systems of public health protection organization from all over the world were investigated. Their formation and development were examined by taking into account the influence of economic, political, cultural, historical, moral, and ethical factors. Examples of various models of health systems from every corner of the world are given. Moreover, the fact that a similar level of socioeconomic development does not always mean a similarity of health systems was established. For example, developed countries use various models of medical systems: liberal (the United States of America), corporate (Japan), social democratic (Scandinavian countries), etc.

The fact that not only socioeconomic conditions affect the health of the population, but also the health of society, in a large measure, affects the main factors of its development (economic, social, psychological, etc.) is considered. The deterioration of public health indicators leads to the so-called economic losses of society (economic damage), which can be direct and indirect.

When studying this material, participants will become familiar with the types of healthcare costs – direct and indirect. The direct costs include the costs of providing medical care: outpatient, inpatient, spa treatment, research work, training, along with social insurance benefits for temporary disabled, disability pension, etc. Indirect economic losses include losses due to a decrease in labor productivity, morbidity, or underproduced products and a decrease in national income at the national level, as a result of temporary or permanent disability or death of a person of working age. Moreover, indirect economic losses are many times higher than direct economic damage due to morbidity. According to researchers, direct economic losses account for about 10% of the total economic damage due to illnesses, and around 90% are indirect losses.

When studying healthcare management, attention must be given to the issue of the impact of health on the development of society. For this, various criteria (coefficients) of effectiveness are considered. From a general point of view, efficiency is considered as achieving the greatest (at a given level of development) result from the amount of all possible costs. It should be noted that efficiency in healthcare does not mean the necessity to reduce costs; on the contrary, it involves an achievement of the maximal result by using those resources that are within the system.

1. One of the main issues of the economic analysis in the field of medicine is to increase the efficiency of the healthcare system.
2. The main social indicators of the level of development of a country are fertility, mortality, natural growth rates, time for doubling the population, growth and population growth rates, etc.

The results of a healthcare system, unlike investing in it, are difficult to measure in money. When solving economic problems in healthcare, specialists will be able to analyze the received or possible effects from the social, medical, and economic points of view. We will familiarize them with the concept of the effectiveness of healthcare systems, performance indicators and criteria, study methods for assessment of the medical, social, and economic effectiveness of the healthcare system, economic effect and efficiency, and direct and indirect costs.

5.2 LITERATE REVIEW

In order to form foreign economic activity (FEA) of the country in the sphere of healthcare, it is necessary to study the effectiveness of healthcare functioning, as the timely detection of problem factors allows to adapt to difficult conditions of changing of foreign economic environment of the country. Flexibility and timely forming of FEA directions are integral factors of preserving the existing and identifying new competitive advantages and, consequently, maintaining or increasing competitiveness.

A significant number of works are dedicated to the study of the effectiveness of integrated healthcare (IHC). IHC focuses on coordinated and integrated health service delivery. The World Health Organization (WHO) defines it as "the management and delivery of health services so that clients receive a continuum of preventive and curative services, according to their needs over time and across different levels of the health system." IHC is also known as coordinated care, comprehensive care, transmural care, and seamless care and has been considered as a solution to fragmented and silo forms of healthcare delivery, which do not take into account patient needs and which lack communication, connectivity, and continuity of care between sectors (Nikpay et al. 2017).

The study of the effectiveness of health systems was carried out by a group of scientists (Suter et al. (2017)). These scientists have discovered many tools for measuring the quality of care for the patients, interaction of the patient, and efficiency of the "team." The researchers identified the existing gap between the tools for measuring the main components, supporting integrated treatment. The authors suggest that the continuation of progress toward integrated care depends on our ability to assess the success of strategies at different levels of management.

The level of effectiveness of health services, particularly mental health services, depends to a large extent on the level of development of the country. This issue has been studied by Semrau et al. (2015). Their research was focused on 'Emerging mental health systems in LMICs' (Emerald) program. The program focused on creating the potential of researchers, policymakers, and planners, as well as increasing the level of service for users and carers supporting mental health promotion. Emerald also regards stigma and discrimination as one of the main barriers to access and successful delivery of health services.

But the issue of quantifying efficiency remains open. Multidimensional methods, such as regression analysis, method of comparative analysis, and expert estimation method, are used for efficiency analysis. However, despite their significant number and certain advantages, most of these methods are based on the calculation of parameters that do not take into account long-term prospects, but only provide an opportunity to summarize the available information. That is why there is a necessity to use a new method giving an opportunity to deliver a complex assessment of activity in the sphere of medical services.

5.3 RESEARCH METHODS

As an example of research method, it was suggested to use the method of comparative analysis, that is, data envelopment analysis (DEA). The methodology of DEA is based on the linear programming for determining the relative efficiency of an economic entity (enterprise) through the implementation of the manufactured products.

According to this interpretation, each set of resources (market inputs) is characterized by a maximum production, and the actual values of market outputs represent the degree of achievement of this maximum. Economic entities that provide maximum market outputs per unit of market inputs acquire the status of the "standard" and form a "threshold of productivity." The task of the analysis is to compare these objects by the efficiency of using their resource base and determining the distance between them and the "threshold of productivity." DEA method is used for this – a relatively new method for measuring performance. An important stage in the evolution of approaches to the measurement of the effectiveness was the research of Farrell (1957). Concerning the concept of economic efficiency, the researcher suggested that its essence should be regarded as the ratio of actual efficiency and the maximum possible one (Du 2016). In his study, Farrell (1957) estimated the efficiency of a unit of final product with one input and one output parameter. This idea was further developed by Charnes et al. (1978), which reformulated it as a task of mathematical programming.

DEA method is based on the use of linear programming machine. It eliminates the influence of the executor on determining the weight of each market input and output, eliminating the risk of subjectivity in the assessment. The efficiency criterion in the DEA method is achievement of Pareto's optimum, which is determined by the maximum possible production volume for the existing technological level and supply of resources. DEA method allows to define an aggregate indicator for each object under study using market inputs to market outputs, to take into account the environmental factors not limited to a functional form of the relationship between inputs and outputs, to identify the priority directions of productivity growth, and to evaluate the necessary changes in market inputs/outputs that would allow the object to be brought to the limit of efficiency.

The first DEA model was developed by Charnes et al. (1978). The further development of DEA models is characterized by a two-vector approach according to the magnitude of production. If the productivity of enterprises increases in proportion to the volumes of expended resources, the line on which the research enterprises must be located sets the constant return scale (CRS) for them. However, if with an increase in the amount of the resource its return is reduced, the margin of production capacity will look like a curve. In this case, the question is about variable return to scale (VRS). The first vector represents CPR models, according to which the measure of performance is based on an optimally balanced relationship between market inputs and market outputs. The evaluation is carried out in coordinates from 0 (minimum efficiency) to 1 (maximum efficiency). The diagnosis of productivity growth involves a search for alternative options for maximizing the efficiency indicator to 1.

A significant progress in the use of DEA has been achieved over the past 15 years. The use of DEA is appropriate when testing hypotheses. DEA model can be used to assess a plurality of countries, for example, in the process of analyzing the country's health effectiveness. The main features of the economy of service delivery, economies of scale, the logic of the service structure serve to test the model, as well as statistical tests to check the statistical model developed to replicate some basic data generation process.

The analysis of various types of efficiency, taking into account the constant and variable magnitude of the scale, makes it possible to analyze the medical services of countries, the level of efficiency, to find a rational ratio of resources and their minimum volumes that are necessary for the production of a unit of production.

5.4 CALCULATION OF THE COST-EFFECTIVENESS OF THE HEALTHCARE SYSTEM ON THE EXAMPLE OF LIFE EXPECTANCY

Let us discuss modern techniques for calculating the effectiveness of healthcare systems. It is essential to get familiar with the DEA technique and the features of the choice of factor indicators for calculating the effectiveness of the healthcare system. We will analyze the effectiveness using the DEA method and evaluate the results.

Assessing the effectiveness of the health system is a complex task, which involves the ability to measure the costs and results of the healthcare system. Economic efficiency is considered as a direct or indirect effect of population health indicators on macroeconomic indicators, for example, GDP, national income, and indicators of social and economic growth.

To calculate the economic efficiency of the functioning of the healthcare system, the average life expectancy is taken as the main result indicator. The average life expectancy is considered as the resulting factor and an integral indicator of the successful development of society, as well as a necessary component of well-being and the global public good. It has been proved that national healthcare system plays the main functional role in maintaining health, the state of human labor resources. The economic and intellectual potential of a nation depends on it. Life expectancy at birth is an important indicator of the health status of the population, the effectiveness of the healthcare system, and the availability of medical services in the country.

Various types of effectiveness, in particular, medical, social, and economic ones, are considered. Medical efficiency should be manifested in the achievement of a certain result in the field of public health, in preventive measures, in the diagnosis and treatment of various pathologies, along with some social aspects – the level of satisfaction of the population with the quality and availability of medical care. Economic efficiency has a direct or indirect impact on indicators that reflect the health of a country's population, as well as on macroeconomic indicators such as GDP, national income and indicators of social and economic growth.

The focus group of the study included European countries: Austria, Spain, Italy, France, Netherlands, and countries of Northern and Eastern Europe. The tendency of increasing life expectancy at birth in these countries for the period 2008–2018 was studied. A quantitative assessment of the difference of the average life expectancy of the population in these countries was given. For the basis we have taken the highest and lowest values for the countries under consideration in the period 2008–2018.

The following factors were used as indicators to assess the economic efficiency of the healthcare system: total expenditures on the healthcare branch (percentage of GDP), total expenditures on healthcare per capita, private expenditures on healthcare as a percentage of total expenditure on healthcare, and the number of hospital beds per 100.000 people. The utilization of these factor indicators for the resulting (average life expectancy) made us able to analyze the effectiveness of the functioning of healthcare systems.

The DEA method was used to measure the effectiveness of the health care system. This made it possible to analyze the efficiency of medical services in the studied countries, find a measure of efficiency, a rational ratio of financial, human and other types of resources and their minimum volumes required to improve efficiency.

The calculations are based on the DEA method, which was selected as a tool for evaluating the efficiency of healthcare funding. DEA is a computing method for the quantitative analysis of the functioning environment, based on the use of linear programming. Most often, this method is used to measure the efficiency of healthcare, but initially it was used for the assessment of production efficiency and its productivity. As DEA modeling has become a new tool for assessing the "technical" efficiency of public sector decision-making, these models have been actively used to assess efficiency and quality in the private sector. Later, DEA models were used for performance and quality assessments also in many sectors, in particular in the health care system.

The DEA method under consideration includes a principle of extracting information from observations that differs from regression analysis. So, in comparison to the parametric approach, the purpose of which is to average the data within one regression model, the DEA method allows students to construct the Pareto optimal boundary of all decisions, taking into account each individual observation. In parametric analysis, the researcher tries to find a relatively universal "recipe" that describes the phenomena under study and their interrelationships. In nonparametric analysis (mathematical programming), any averaging is abandoned. That is, the DEA proposes variables that are individual for each, rather than constants, weights the sample units, and compares each observation for effective and ineffective solutions.

Studies of the effectiveness of health systems around the world using the DEA method have shown that achieving the greatest efficiency does not necessarily occur due to an increase in the total cost of the healthcare system (in% of GDP). Some developed countries often take advantage of the minor advantages that modern technologies offer for the development of medicine, health insurance, and other factors.

5.5 DEA METHOD

We have chosen the DEA method as a tool to evaluate the effectiveness of the healthcare financing. DEA is an analysis of the operating environment. It is based on the use of the linear programming. Most often this method is used for measurement of the healthcare effectiveness, but initially its development involved the assessment of production efficiency and its productiveness.

The method is based on the construction of the efficiency of frontier. It measures the performance of other investigated objects. This is shown in Figure 5.1.

As shown in the graph, there are only points that lie under the efficiency curve. If there was such an efficiency value, the coordinate of which was located above the curve, it would be more efficient. In this case, the efficiency curve itself would shift, taking a new position.

It is worth noting that the benefits of DEA method in analyzing the effectiveness of healthcare system are varied:

- No need to define the production function explicitly.
- The possibility to disclose the ratios of the indicators under the study in more detail in comparison to applying alternative methods.

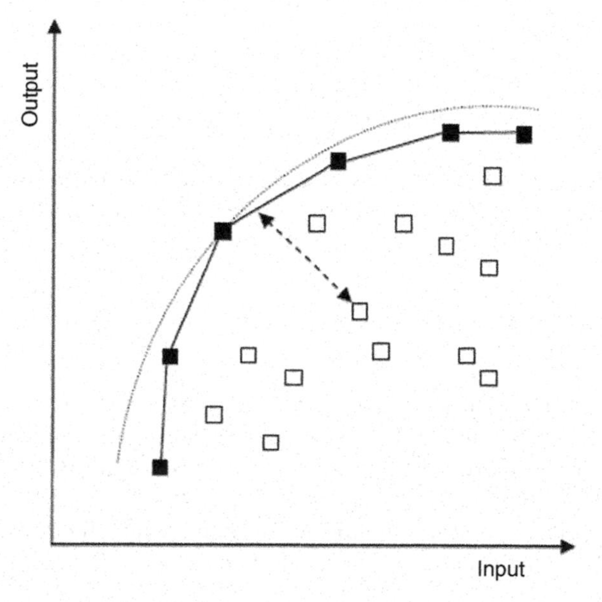

FIGURE 5.1 Graphic illustration of the construction of an effective cordon using the DEA method.

- Use of several input and output.
- The input and output measurement may belong to any quantifying figures.
- The researcher does not put weight limits on the indicators.
- The number of DNC (determines the number of calculations).
- Possible evaluation of the sources of inefficiency for the enterprises/systems.

5.5.1 Using DEA Method in the Research

For comparative analysis of the causes influencing the efficiency of the healthcare system functioning worldwide, we applied DEA method.

The average expectancy of life in countries worldwide is taken as the resulting indicator. Data processing was performed in the RStudio medium, using the dplyr and benchmarking libraries, which allows to solve the problem. To compare the countries, we have used the benchmarking technique that is a widespread method for interorganization and intercountry comparison.

To evaluate the efficiency of the medical enterprises applying DEA method, the following conditional indicators were defined:

- X: Inputs (indicators of medical services) of the object;
- Y: Outputs of the object (life expectancy);
- EFF: Farrell efficiency; (X,Y) of the object under the study;
- SLACK: A logical vector in which a certain component (e.g., costs) is true for an object when the scale effect is changeable and equal to 1; then for a particular object it is positive, but under the constant effect of the scale, the effectiveness is close to 0. These factors are the so-called object weaknesses that must be taken into account;
- Variable returns scale (VRS): Changeable effect of the scale;
- Constant returns scale (CRS): Constant effect of the scale;
- LAMBDA: The set of analogues for each object.

The evaluation according to the DEA method allowed us to use the statistical methods of scaling the data from countries where the extreme coefficients of substitution demonstrate observations as well as to obtain the evaluation of the errors.

5.5.2 Assessment of the Effectiveness of Healthcare Expenditures (% Out of GDP)

Grounding on the empirical data on the share of the total healthcare expenditures (total healthcare expenditures out of GDP) and life expectancy, there was the boundary of the healthcare efficiency (technological curve), which is used to evaluate the results of each country (see Figure 5.2).

The calculations point at the significant diversity of the efficiency assessment in 53 countries under the study either for continuous (CRS) or variable (VRS) effects (Table 5.1).

As can be seen, there are only four countries with efficiency 1, which are located in Figure 5.2 on the curve of the efficiency (Andorra, San-Marino, Monako, and Turmenistan), three countries with efficiency from 0.7 to 0.8, and seven countries

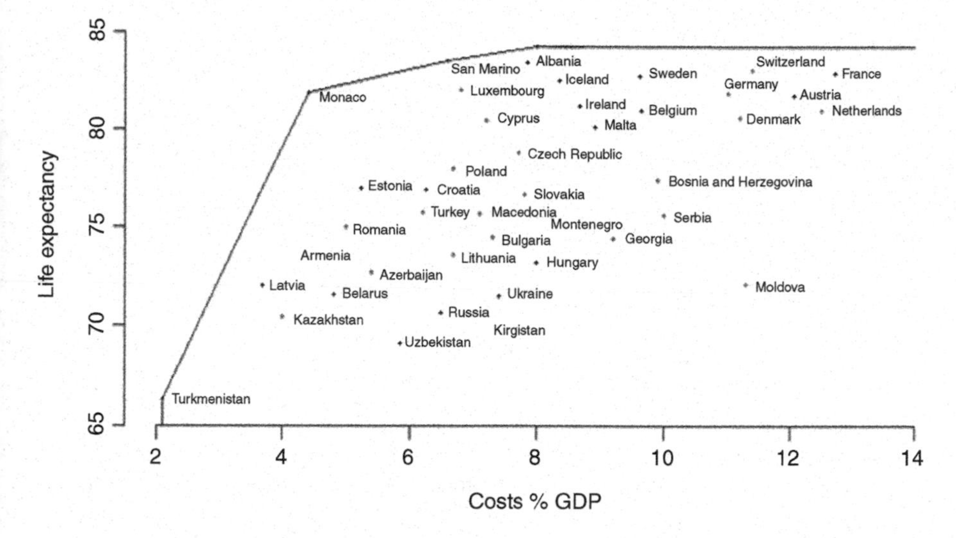

FIGURE 5.2 The curve of the healthcare efficiency according to the indicators of the share of healthcare expenditures out of GDP for countries worldwide. (Figure created by the author).

TABLE 5.1
The Value of the Healthcare Efficiency According to the Indicator of the Share of the Total Healthcare Expenditures Out of GDP for the Countries Worldwide

Efficiency Values, Interval	Number of Countries	Relative Number of Countries (%)
[0,2; 0,3)	1	1.9
[0,3; 0,4)	8	15.1
[0,4; 0,5)	19	35.8
[0,5; 0,6)	11	20.8
[0,6; 0,7)	7	13.2
[0,7; 0,8)	3	5.7
[0,8; 0,9)	0	0
[0,9; 1)	0	0
1	4	7.5

Source: Calculated by the author.

with efficiency from 0.6 to 0.7. We must note that the effectiveness of the healthcare measures in Ukraine on the basis of the total healthcare expenditures share out of GDP is 0.42. Thus, there exists an enormous potential to improve the efficiency of this category of healthcare measures for a number of countries.

5.5.3 Evaluation of the Healthcare Expenditures Efficiency (Per Capita)

We analyzed the efficiency of the share of the healthcare out of GDP per capita over the world (Figure 5.3).

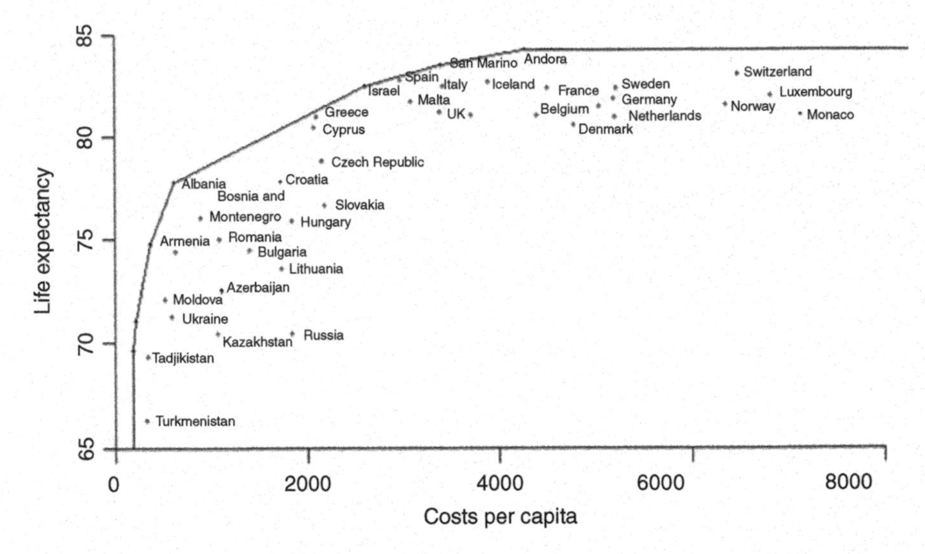

FIGURE 5.3 Healthcare efficiency curve according to the indicator of the share of total healthcare expenditures out of GDP per capita for countries worldwide. (Figure created by the author.)

TABLE 5.2
The Values of the Healthcare Efficiency According to the Indicator of the Share from the Total Healthcare Expenditures out of GDP Per Capita for Countries Worldwide and Ukraine

Efficiency Values, Interval	Number of Countries	Relative Number of Countries (%)
[0,1; 0,2)	3	5.7
[0,2; 0,3)	5	9.4
[0,3; 0,4)	11	20.8
[0,4; 0,5)	9	17.0
[0,5; 0,6)	8	15.1
[0,6; 0,7)	3	5.7
[0,7; 0,8)	3	5.7
[0,8; 0,9)	2	3.8
[0,9; 1)	2	3.8
1	7	13.2

Source: Calculated by the author.

Among the 53 countries under study, there is a significant diversity of assessment of the efficiency either for constant (CRS) or for variable (VRS) effect. According to calculations, the minimal efficiency is 0.11, the maximum efficiency is 1, and the average efficiency is 0.546. Below are the results of calculating DEA (Table 5.2).

According to the indicator of the share for the total healthcare expenditures out of GDP per capita, there are seven countries with efficiency 1 (Andorra, San- Marino,

Israel, Albania, Armenia, Kyrgyzstan, and Turkmenistan), which are shown in Figure 5.3 on the curve of the efficiency, four countries with efficiency from 0.8 to 1, and six countries with efficiency from 0.6 to 0.8. We must note that the efficiency of the healthcare measures according to the total expenditures on the healthcare out of GDP per capita for Ukraine is 0.38, which indicates to the extremely low efficiency of these healthcare measures according to this indicator.

5.5.4 Evaluation of the Effectiveness of Healthcare Expenditures (Share of Private Expenditures out of Total Healthcare Expenditures)

We analyzed the efficiency of the private share out of total healthcare expenditures (Figure 5.4).

The minimal efficiency of healthcare services according to the private share is 0.07, the maximum efficiency is 1, and the average efficiency is 0.297. The results of the calculations are presented in Table 5.3.

5.5.4.1 Conclusion

According to the indicator of the private share out of total healthcare expenditures, there are three countries with efficiency 1 (Andorra, San-Marino, and Netherlands), which are shown in Figure 5.4 on the curve of the efficiency, two countries with efficiency from 0.7 to 0.9, and two countries with efficiency from 0.5 to 0.6. We must note that the effectiveness of the chosen measures on the healthcare for the post-Soviet countries according to the indicator of the personal share out of total healthcare expenditures is 0.11, which points out to the extremely low effectiveness of these measures.

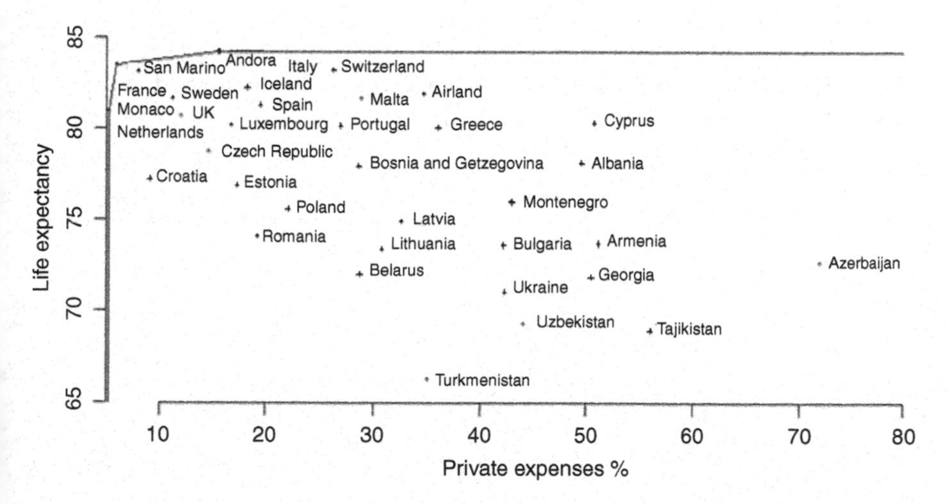

FIGURE 5.4 Health service efficiency curve in terms of private health spending (% of total health spending). (Figure created by the author.)

5.5.5 Evaluation of the Efficiency of the Healthcare Branch Functioning (Number of Hospital Beds per 100.000 Inhabitants)

We analyzed the efficiency of the healthcare measures grounding on the provision of hospital beds (its number per 100.000 inhabitants) (Figure 5.5).

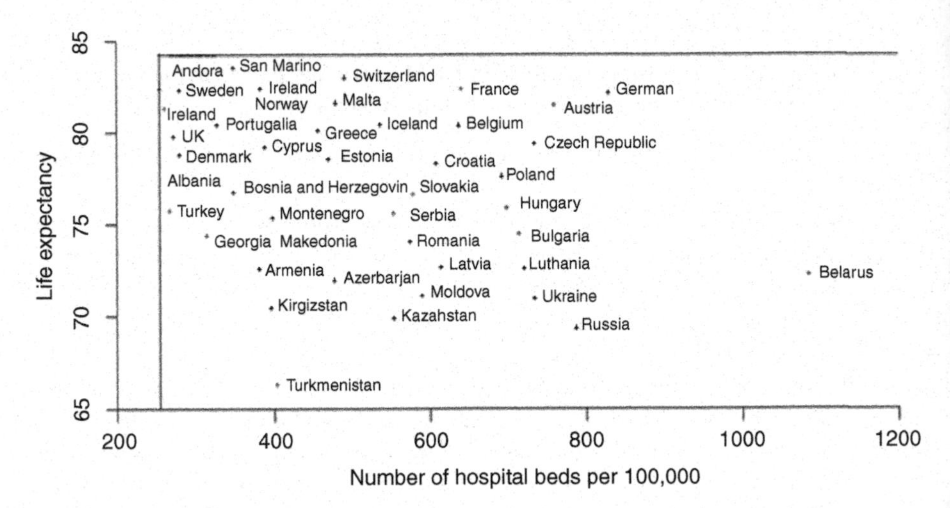

FIGURE 5.5 The curve of the efficiency of medical services in terms of the number of hospital beds per 100.000 inhabitants. (Figure created by the author.)

TABLE 5.3
Values of the Healthcare Efficiency According to the Indicator of the Private Share Out of Total Healthcare Expenditures Worldwide and in Ukraine (%)

Efficiency Values, Interval	Number of Countries	Relative Number of Countries (%)
[0; 0,1)	4	7.5
[0,1; 0,2)	20	37.7
[0,2; 0,3)	11	20.8
[0,3; 0,4)	8	15.1
[0,4; 0,5)	3	5.7
[0,5; 0,6)	2	3.8
[0,6; 0,7)	0	0
[0,7; 0,8)	1	1.9
[0,8; 0,9)	1	1.9
[0,9; 1)	0	0
1	3	5.7

Source: Calculated by the author.

TABLE 5.4
The Values of Efficiency of Healthcare Services According to the Indicator of the Number of Hospital Beds per 100.000 Inhabitants Worldwide and in Ukraine

Efficiency Values, Interval	Number of Countries	Relative Number of Countries (%)
[0,1; 0,2)	1	1.9
[0,2; 0,3)	4	7.5
[0,3; 0,4)	14	26.4
[0,4; 0,5)	6	11.3
[0,5; 0,6)	11	20.8
[0,6; 0,7)	2	3.8
[0,7; 0,8)	6	11.3
[0,8; 0,9)	5	9.4
[0,9; 1)	3	5.7
1	1	1.9

Source: Calculated by the author.

The average effectiveness of the healthcare services level according to the indicator of the number of hospital beds per 100.000 inhabitants is equal to 0.541, the maximum efficiency is 1, and the average efficiency is 0.116. The results of the calculations are presented in Table 5.4.

An analysis of the efficiency curve in terms of the number of hospital beds per 100.000 inhabitants (Figure 5.5) showed that there is one country with an efficiency of 1, three countries with an efficiency of 0.9 to 1, five countries with an efficiency of 0.8. to 0.9 and six countries with an efficiency of 0.7 to 0.8. The efficiency of healthcare in Ukraine in terms of the number of hospital beds is 0.27, which indicates the lowest efficiency.

Thus, according to the results of the calculations, we are able to make a list of countries with maximum efficiency of the healthcare system functioning according to diverse indicators (Table 5.5).

The results of the conducted analysis bring us to the conclusion that according to each indicator (the share of total healthcare expenditures out of GDP, the share of total healthcare expenditures out of GDP per capita, the private share out of total healthcare expenditures, and the number of hospital beds per 100.000 population), the most efficient is the healthcare system in Andorra, Monaco, and San-Marino. The healthcare systems in Switzerland, Israel, Spain, France, Iceland, and Luxemburg are also among the leaders.

TABLE 5.5
The Countries around the World with Maximum Efficiency of the Healthcare System Functioning According to the Diverse Indicators

Indicator	Countries
The share of the total healthcare expenditures out of GDP	Andorra
	San-Marino
	Monaco
	Turkmenistan
	Switzerland
	Israel
	Spain
	France
	Iceland
	Luxemburg
The share of the total healthcare expenditures out of GDP per capita	Andorra
	San-Marino
	Monaco
	Turkmenistan
	Switzerland
	Israel
	Spain
	France
	Iceland
The private share out of total healthcare expenditures	Andorra
	San-Marino
	Netherlands
	Switzerland
	Israel
	Luxemburg
The number of hospital beds per 100.000 inhabitants	Andorra
	San-Marino
	Switzerland
	Israel
	Iceland

Source: Calculated by the author

5.6 CONCLUSION

The study findings make the following conclusions:

1. The method of complex data analysis (DEA) is most often used in international comparisons of the effectiveness of government spending in various areas. DEA algorithm involves identifying the best combinations of values "costs – the result," which are accepted as reference for analyzed set of observations. The degree of proximity of actual values during all other observations

to the standard may be expressed in shares by taking values from 0 to 1 inclusive, where 1 corresponds to the value of the standard. Thus, the farther the value is from reference, the less effective position it characterizes. Therefore, the DEA method sets the scale for measuring effectiveness by demonstrating analysis optimization potential process.

2. The following indicators of health services will be considered as factor indicators: the share of total healthcare expenditures out of GDP, the share of total healthcare expenditures out of GDP per capita, the share of private expenditures out of total healthcare expenditures, and the number of hospital beds per 100,000 inhabitants.
3. It is worthy of note that the benefits of DEA method in analyzing the effectiveness of healthcare system are varied: no need to define the production function explicitly, the possibility to disclose the ratios of the indicators under study in more detail in comparison to applying alternative methods, the use of several inputs and outputs; the input and output measurement may belong to any quantifying figures, the researcher does not put weight limits on the indicators, the number of calculations, possible evaluation of the sources of inefficiency for the enterprises/systems.
4. The research has shown that the highest level of efficiency is not necessarily due to the large share of healthcare in the world GDP or other absolute indicators that characterize the development of the medical services industry. Certain countries use national peculiarities, in particular, minor advantages of the relatively small and highly specialized volume of the domestic healthcare market, the active use of modern medical technologies, including through the investment in healthcare infrastructure, widening of the forms of medical insurance, and other factors.

REFERENCES

Advance Data From Vital and Health Statistics No. 388. *Cdc.gov*. June 28, 2007. Retrieved from October 3, 2019.

Asgari, S. D., Haeri, A., & Jafari, M. (2017). Integration of Balanced Scorecard and Threestage Data Envelopment Analysis Approaches. Iranian Journal of Management Studies, 10(2), 527–550.

Babenko V., Boichenko O., Koniaieva, Y., 2019. Efficiency of human resource management in industrial automation enterprises with prospects of innovative susceptibility. *Advances in Economics, Business and Management Research. 6th International Conference on Strategies, Models and Technologies of Economic Systems Management (SMTESM 2019)*. Atlantis Press, Amsterdam, vol. 95, pp. 119–124. https://doi.org/10.2991/smtesm-19.2019.24

Babenko, V., Gaponova, E., Nehrey, M., Ryzhikova, N., Zaporozhets, E., 2019. Life expectancy of population of the country: the role of health services effectiveness. *Research in World Economy*, Vol. 10, No. 4 (Special Issue):86–91. https://doi.org/10.5430/rwe.v10n4p86

Babenko V., Mandych O., Nakisko O. 2018. Increasing the efficiency of enterprises through the implementation of IT-projects. *Transformational Processes the Development of*

Economic Systems in Conditions: Scientific Bases, Mechanisms, Prospects: Monograph. ISMA University, vol. 2:54–65.

Bautista, M., Nurjono, M., Wei Lim, Y., Dessers, E., Vrijhoef, H., 2016. Instruments measuring integrated care: A systematic review of measurement properties. *Milbank Quarterly*, 94:862–917. https://doi.org/10.1111/1468-0009.12233

Bem, A., Ucieklak-Jeż, P., Prędkiewic, P., 2014. Measurement of health care system efficiency. *Management Theory and Studies for Rural Business and Infrastructure Development*, 36(1):25–33. 10.15544/mts.2014.003

Busse, R., Stahl, J., 2014. Integrated care experiences and outcomes in Germany, the Netherlands, and England. *Health Affairs* (Milwood), 33(9):1549–1558. https://doi.org/10.1377/hlthaff.2014.0419

Care coordination. *Agency for Healthcare Research & Quality*, 2015-05-01. Retrieved from October 15, 2019.

Charnes, A., Cooper, W.W., Rhodes, E., 1978. Measuring the efficiency of decision making units. *European Journal of Operational Research*, 2:429–444. Available online at: https://personal.utdallas.edu/~ryoung/phdseminar/CCR1978.pdf

Cooper, W., Seiford, L., Tone, K., 2007. Data Envelopment Analysis, 2nd edn. Springer.

Drummond, M., Sculpher, M., Claxton, K., Stoddart, G., Torrance, G., 2015. *Methods for the Economic Evaluation of Health Care Programs*. Oxford University Press.

Farrell, M., 1957. The measurement of productive efficiency. *Journal of the Royal Statistical Society. Series A*, 120(3):253–290.

Frandsen, B.R., Joynt, K.E., Rebitzer, J.B., Jha, A.K., 2015. Care fragmentation, quality, and costs among chronically ill patients. *The American Journal of Managed Care*, 21(5):355–362.

Ghiselline, P., Cialani, C., Ulgiati, S., 2016. A review on circular economy: The expected transition to a balanced interplay of environmental and economic systems. *Journal of Cleaner Production*, 114:11–32.

Gontareva, I., Maryna, B., Babenko, V., Perevozova, I., Mokhnenko, A., 2019. Identification of efficiency factors for control over information and communication provision of sustainable development in higher education institutions. *WSEAS Transactions on Environment and Development*, 15:593–604.

Hastings, S., Armitage, G., Mallinson, S., Jackson, K., Suter, E., 2014. Exploring the relationship between governance mechanisms in healthcare and health workforce outcomes: A systematic review. *BMC Health Services Research*, 14(1), 1. https://doi.org/10.1186/1472-6963-14-479

Liu, J., Mooney, H., Hull, V., Davis, S., Gaskell, J., Hertel, T., Li, S., 2015. Systems integration for global sustainability. *Science*, 347(6225), 1258832.

Lyngso, A., Godtfredsen, N., Host, D., Frolich, A., 2014. Instruments to assess integrated care: A systematic review. *International Journal of Integrated Care*, 14: 1–15. https://doi.org/10.5334/ ijic.1184

Medicare Reimbursements. *Dartmouth Atlas of Health Care*. Retrieved from October 19, 2019.

Nikpay, S., Freedman, S., Levy, H., Buchmueller, T., 2017. Effect of the Affordable Care Act Medicaid expansion on emergency department visits: Evidence from state-level emergency department databases. *Annals of Emergency Medicine*, 70(2):215–225. https://doi.org/10.1016/j.annemergmed.2017.03.023

Semrau, M., Evans-Lacko, S., Alem, A., Ayuso-Mateos, J., Chisholm, D., Gureje, O., Lund, C., 2015. Strengthening mental health systems in low-and middle-income countries: The Emerald program. *BMC Medicine*, 13(1), 79.

Soni, S.M., Giboney, P., Yee, H.F., 2016. Development and implementation of expected practices to reduce inappropriate variations in clinical practice. *Journal of American Medical Association*, 315(20):2163. https://doi.org/10.1001/jama.2016.4255. ISSN 0098-7484

Suter E., Oelke N.D., Dias da Silva Lima M.A., Stiphout M., Janke R., Witt R.R. et al., 2017. Indicators and measurement tools for health systems integration: A knowledge synthesis. *International Journal of Integrated Care*, 17(6):4. http://doi.org/10.5334/ijic.3931

UK's healthcare plummets on global efficiency tables. *The Daily Telegraph*, 9 October 2018. Retrieved from October 14, 2019.

UK's healthcare plummets on global efficiency tables. *The Daily Telegraph*, 9 October 2018. Retrieved from October 14, 2019.

Medicare Reimbursements. *Dartmouth Atlas of Health Care*. Retrieved from October 19, 2019.

6 Computer Simulation Study of Oscillation Mechanisms and Physical Properties of Nanosized Biostructures

P.J. Kervalishvili and T.N. Bzhalava

CONTENTS

> And Wuhan-400 has other, equally important advantages over most biological agents. For one thing, you can become an infectious carrier only four hours after coming into contact with the virus.
>
> *The Eyes of Darkness* by Dean Koontz, Berkley edition/July 1996

6.1 INTRODUCTION

Periodic change in various characteristics is common in biological systems. These are the so-called biological clocks: oscillations of biomacromolecules' concentrations, biochemical oscillations, rhythms of breathing, heart contractions, and periodic changes in body temperature, all the way up to population waves [1, 2].

Generally, all molecular systems show oscillatory behavior above the absolute zero, that is, normal molecular vibration, whose intensity depends on temperature. The energy for the vibration is provided by the metabolic processes as reaction enthalpy. The frequencies of the individual oscillating molecular groups in a given biomolecule depend on the type of atoms bound – primarily on the nature and polarity of the bonds, and secondarily on the adjacent molecules and the phase structure. The frequency pattern is typical of the substance under the prevailing condition [3, 4].

The excitation of vibrational states in monodispersive biological systems consisting of nanosized particles – for example, viruses – can have a significant impact on these systems up to their mechanical destruction [5]. The most efficient excitation of oscillations in such systems can be implemented with the resonant impact on the system, namely, the coincidence of the system eigenfrequency with a frequency of external influence. The use of electromagnetic (EM) radiation in the visible or near-infrared range for the efficient excitation of the vibrational modes of biological objects allows an increase in the radiation penetration into the sample. The biharmonic radiation of nanosecond duration as well as impulsive stimulated Raman scattering under femtosecond excitation [6, 7] can realize the coherent excitation of low-frequency Raman-active modes of different nanoparticles. The basic condition for the effective usage of biharmonic pumping for the efficient excitation of nanoparticle vibrations is the equality of the difference frequency and the eigenfrequency. For an exact eigenfrequency value calculation, a liquid drop model or an elastic sphere model [8, 9] can be used. Both approaches require some knowledge of the elastic characteristics of the nanoparticles and the environment. For the experimental eigenfrequency measurements, low-frequency Raman scattering can be used [10, 11]. Today there are a relatively small number of works in which the low-frequency Raman scattering by viruses in the liquid environment has been obtained experimentally.

Viruses are susceptible to the same kind of mechanical excitation. An experimental group from Arizona State University has recently shown that pulses of laser light can induce destructive vibrations in virus shells [12, 13].

The ability to detect rapidly, directly, and selectively individual virus particles has the potential to significantly impact healthcare, since it could enable diagnosis at the earliest stages of replication within a host's system. Simultaneous acquisition of the vibrational and electronic fingerprints of molecular systems of biological interest, at the interface between liquid media, or at the air/solid and air/liquid interfaces, is difficult to achieve with conventional linear optical spectroscopies due to their poor sensitivity to the low number of molecules or their maladjustment to water environment (infrared absorption), with the exception of polarization modulation infrared absorption spectroscopy. The shift in energy gives information about the vibrational modes in the system. Infrared spectroscopy yields similar but complementary information. Spontaneous scattering is typically very weak and as a result the main difficulty of this kind of spectroscopy lies in separating the weak inelastically scattered light from the intense Rayleigh scattered laser light. Viruses are assembled in the infected host cells of human, animals, or plants.

Because of viral breeding, the host cell dies. There are especially viruses that are breeding in the cell of the bacteria. Viruses spread in many different ways. Just as many viruses are very specific, as to which host species or tissue they attack, each species of virus relies on a particular propagation way. The microorganisms in the air may exist in three phases of bacterium aerosol-drop- shaped, drop nuclear, and dusty. We call bacterial aerosol a physical system that consists of tiny solid or liquid particles in the gaseous environment. Sum frequency generation spectroscopy and ultra-short pulsed lasers-based optical measurement methods are unique for the investigation of vibrational modes of different viruses and other pathogenic microorganisms, as well as for the study of the nature of their oscillation processes and parameters of oscillation. Nonlinear optics and its resonance technologies are a possible direction of organization for pathogenic microorganisms' treatment in their different living media [14, 15].

It is difficult to calculate what sort of push will kill a virus, since there can be millions of atoms in its shell structure. A direct computation of each atom's movements would take several hundred thousand gigabytes of computer memory. At the same time, the study of biostructure's physical characteristics, scattering and absorption properties, estimation of EM spectrum and resonance wave length ranges is important for the characterization of nano-micro-scaled particles and determination of the biostructure's unique spectral signatures, which is essential for bioagent detection and identification systems, and is a great challenge for real systems investigations.

Behavior of nano-micro-sized pathogenic microorganisms is selectively sensitive toward the EM field excitation. Estimation of vibration frequencies of microorganisms is the scope of investigations revealing the Raman-active low-frequency vibrational modes of viral capsids [16] and inactivation mechanisms for excitation of vibrational motions of virions resulted in mechanical resonances or breaking hydrogen bonds, respectively [17]. Also it is the objective of spectroscopy methods or atomistic molecular dynamics (MD) simulation studies giving opportunity to appreciate the wavenumbers corresponding to specific vibration bonds of functional groups and structures. Limited spectral ranges or operation parameters of experimental, spectroscopic, fluorescent, biochemical, and immunological techniques; long-term processes of sample preparation and measurements; and chemical or biological description of certain bonds and molecular structural fragments provoke the attempts for seeking new approaches and methods for the creation and analysis of complete spectral pictures of whole macromolecules, bio-cells, or bioparticles.

Elaboration of physical models of bioparticles as well as computer simulation study of (EM) near- and far-field distribution in the areas of particles and surrounded medium (air, aqua, and other liquids) should be a possible way for the investigation of physical properties of bioparticles of different morphology and origin.

6.2 METHOD AND APPROACH

The method of estimation of spectral response on EM field and particle interaction is based on solutions of electrodynamics two-dimensional (2D) or three-dimensional (3D) boundary tasks [18, 19]. Analytical expressions of EM fields are derived from rigorous solutions of Maxwell's and Helmholtz's equations and defined through the dimensionless parameters, diameters (d) over an excitation wavelength (λ). It makes possible to apply the classical well-known approach to sub-micro-particles characterization.

The proposed method is used for the investigation of viral particle's physical properties. EM spectrum and EM near- and far-field distribution are studied for viruses, having rod-like, prolate un-enveloped virions (e.g., Tobacco mosaic virus [TMV], bacteriophage M13). Electrodynamics (2D) solutions are applicable for TMV particle, the length of which is approximately 16 times greater than diameter. Helmholtz's equation in cylindrical coordinates is converted into three differential equations by using the variables separation method [20]. The equation with respect to radial $R(\xi)$ function has the following form:

$$\xi^2 R^{//}(\xi)+\xi R^{/}(\xi)+\left(\xi^2-m^2\right)R(\xi)=\frac{k^2}{k_q^2}\mu_q\xi^2 f\left(\xi/k_q\right)R(\xi) \tag{6.1}$$

where $\xi = k_q r$, $m = \pm 1, 2, \ldots$, "/" denotes the derivative with respect to an argument and $f(\xi/k_q)$ is the function of inhomogeneity, if dielectric permittivity is the function of radial direction (r) and written as $\varepsilon_q^{(r)} = \varepsilon_q - f(r)$. Wave vectors are defined by the formulas $k_q = k\sqrt{\varepsilon_q \mu_q}$ in (q) medium and in vacuum, $\varepsilon_o = 8{,}85.10^{-12}$ F/m, and $\mu_o = 1{,}26.10^{-6}$ H/m, where ω is an angular frequency of excitation plane wave, with electrical vector **E** parallel to the axis (z) of cylinder. Generally, dielectric permittivity $\varepsilon_q(\omega)$ and magnetic permeability $\mu_q(\omega)$ are complex values. Subscript (q) indicates the parameters and functions corresponding the core (q = 1), shell (q = 2), and surrounded medium (q = 3). Equation (6.1) could be solved by applying analytical or numerical methods relevant to $f(r)$. The fields in different areas are written as the sums of multipole waves [21] using the solutions of equation (6.1). According to the methodology of solving electrodynamics boundary problems, on the boundary surfaces of two mediums the components of electric (**E**) and magnetic (**H**) fields satisfy the necessary conditions on continuity of tangent components (E_z and H_φ). Also, radiation condition outside the area of particle ($kr \gg 1$), finiteness of the field inside the particle, as well as the condition for E_z component $(E_z \cdot grad\{\varepsilon_q - f(r)\}) = 0$ are taken into account while determining the EM field's expressions [22]. In a case when a medium is homogeneous, the function $f(r) = 0$ and equation (6.1) gets the form of Bessel's well-known equation [23]. Characteristics describing the ability of scattering of EM waves by the particles are known as the scattering cross-sections [20], and are used for studying the distribution of EM fields in the far (wave) zone and scattering properties of particles.

The characterization of bioparticles is based on the concept of considering the bio-object in physical point of view [24]. Virions, the extracellular infective forms of viruses, are modeled by the particles of different structures. We consider cylindrically shaped three structures: homogeneous, inhomogeneous through the radius of cylinder, and core-shell structure reflecting the properties of ribonucleic acids (DNA or RNA) of viruses and capsid's proteins. Shape, structure, and the set of geometrical, magnetic, and electrical characteristics are proposed as the main parameters for defining the particles' EM spectral properties. The advantage of simulation study of complex molecular systems such as virions, in contrast to measuring experiments associated with weak signals detection, is noteworthy.

6.3 RESULTS AND DISCUSSION

Computer simulation (based on MatLabR2013b software) was carried out for TMV particles characterization. Parameters of TMV particle were obtained from scientific publications based on different measuring techniques [25, 26]. The length of TMV

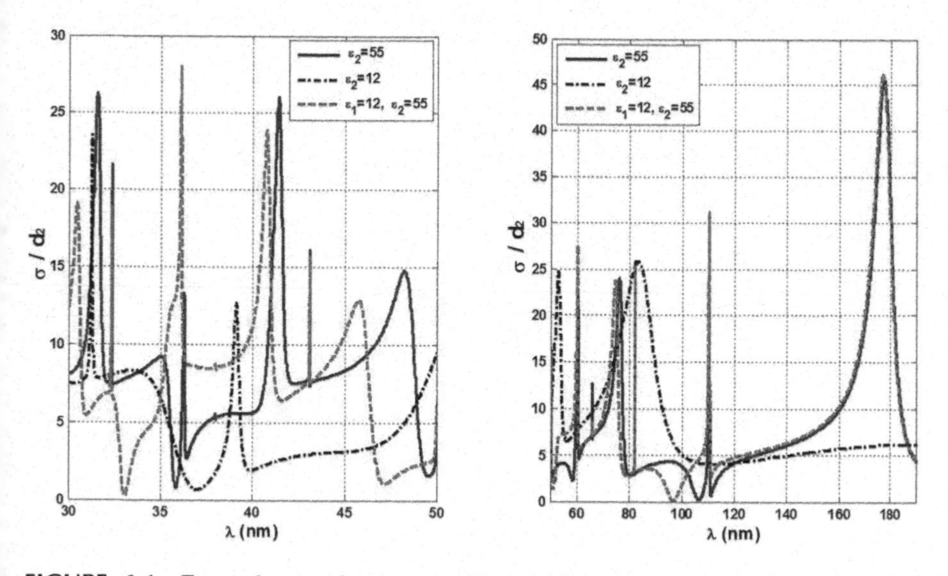

FIGURE 6.1 Forward scattering cross-section (σ/d_2) versus excitation wavelength (λ). Cylindrical model: diameter d_2 = 18 nm, dielectric permittivities ε_2 = 55 (solid), 12 (dash-dot); Core-shell model (dash): diameters d_2 = 18 nm (outer) and d_1 = 4 nm (inner), dielectric permittivities: ε_1 = 12 (core), ε_2 = 55 (shell); ε_3 = 1 (surrounding medium).

virion was 280–300 nm, and outer (d_2) and inner (d_1) diameters of capsid were 18 nm and 4 nm, respectively.

In this work, two models – homogeneous cylindrical (of diameter d_2) and homogeneous of core-shell structure (of diameters: outer d_2 and inner d_1) – were used for the simulation study of TMV virion. Computer simulation shows that expected resonant spectral response is observable on far-field ($r \gg 2d_2^2 / \lambda$) characteristics (Figures 6.1 and 6.2), and resonant vibrational frequencies of whole TMV particle may be associated with scattering cross-section maximums. Values and locations of maximums strongly depend on dielectric (Figure 6.1) and magnetic (Figure 6.2) parameters, and the greater the distance between the neighbor maximums the longer the wavelength's range is. The protein shell's portion of TMV particle is 19 times more than the portion of core containing the dsRNA; therefore, the shell's EM properties have significant effect on the formation of spectra, resonant values, and the upper limit of resonant wavelength ranges (Figure 6.1).

Near-field distribution presented in the form of isolines of EM field amplitudes (Figure 6.3) indicates the locations of energy maximums inside and outside of particle. Investigation of EM field distribution makes it possible to have insights into the vision of nano-bioparticles.

6.4 CONCLUSIONS

The method of estimation of EM field characteristics and resonant wavelength ranges based on computer simulation is developed and applied to nano-bioparticles

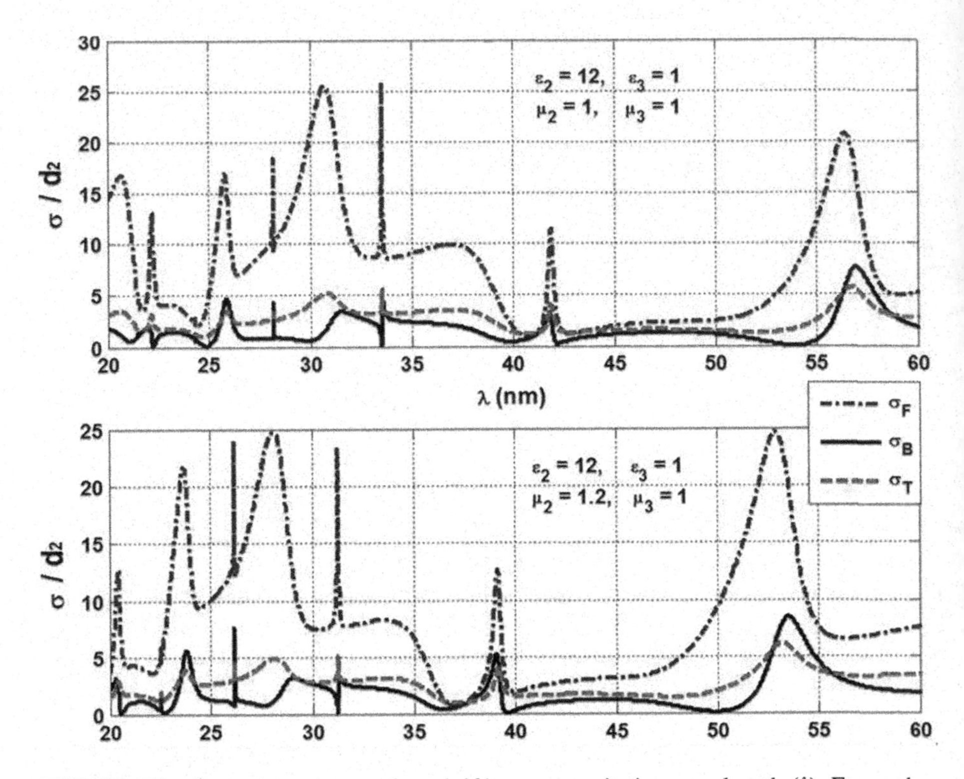

FIGURE 6.2 Scattering cross-sections (σ/d_2) versus excitation wavelength (λ). Forward σ_F (dash-dot); backward σ_B (solid); total σ_T (dash). Cylindrical model of TMV virion: diameter $d_2 = 18$ nm, dielectric permittivities of particle $\varepsilon_2 = 12$ and surrounding medium $\varepsilon_2 = 1$, magnetic permeabilities of particle $\mu_2 = 1.2$ (a), 1 (b) and surrounding medium $\mu_3 = 1$.

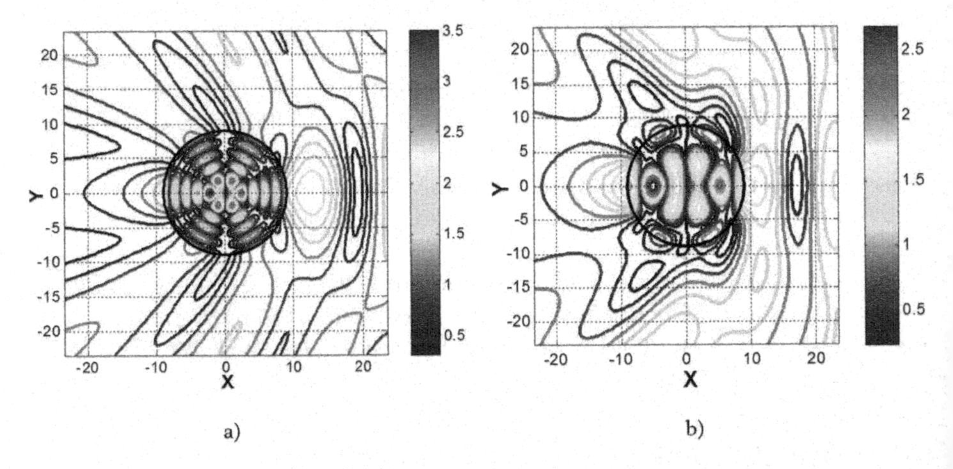

FIGURE 6.3 Isolines of EM field amplitudes for cylindrical model of TMV virion, in the range of ($-\lambda,+\lambda$). Diameter of cylinder: d_2 = 18 nm; dielectric permittivities: of cylindrical particle – $\varepsilon_2 = 55$(a), 12 (b), surrounding medium – $\varepsilon_3 = 1$, excitation wave length $\lambda = 23.5$ nm, (X,Y) plane is perpendicular to the axis of cylinder.

characterization. EM spectrum and near-field distribution based on structural and EM properties of un-enveloped virion of TMV are also presented. Data analysis revealed the strong dependence of field characteristics on EM plus geometrical parameters and wavelength in resonant wave range. The possibility of determination of resonant (own) frequencies of the entire system of molecules, like virion, is developed. A set of resonance wavelength is observed in ultraviolet (NUV-EUV) range of TMV particle's spectrum. Simulated EM spectra, measured or estimated in two (forward and backward) directions of wave scattering, introduce the specific signature of bioparticles of a given parameter. The given method, which relates to the field of computing and measuring of spectroscopic properties of bioparticles, includes determination of vibrational frequency of viruses [27] and is the basis of the new concept: estimation of unique vibration/oscillation properties of bio-objects and their original and specific "fingerprints" (characteristic vibrational frequency – CVF) of pathogenic microorganisms.

REFERENCES

1. Rubin A., Riznichenko G., Oscillations, Rhythms, and Chaos in Biological Systems. In: *Mathematical Biophysics*. Biological and Medical Physics, Biomedical Engineering. Springer, Boston, MA, 2014, pp. 25–33.
2. Frohlich H., Coherent Electric Vibrations in Biological Systems and the Cancer Problem. *Open Biochem J.*, 10, 2016, pp. 12–16.
3. Yang L., Hubbard T.A., Cockroft S.L., Can Non-Polar Hydrogen Atoms Accept Hydrogen Bonds? *Chem. Commun.*, 50, 2014, pp. 5212–5214.
4. Jaross W., Are Molecular Vibration Patterns of Cell Structural Elements Used for Intracellular Signaling? *The Open Biochemistry Journal*, 10(1), March 2016, pp. 12–16.
5. Yang S.-C., Lin H.-C., Liu T.-M., Efficient Structure Resonance Energy Transfer from Microwaves to Confined Acoustic Vibrations in Viruses. *Scientific Reports*, 5:18030, December 2015. DOI: 10.1038/srep18030
6. Zemskov K., Karpova O., Kudryavtseva A. et al., Stimulated Low-Frequency Raman Scattering in Tobacco Mosaic Virus Suspension. *Laser Physics Letters*, 13(8), May 2016. DOI: 10.1088/1612–2011/13/8/085701
7. Tcherniega N.V., Pershin S.M., Bunkin A.F. et al., Laser Excitation of Gigahertz Vibrations in Cauliflower Mosaic Viruses' Suspension. *Laser Physics Letters*, 15(9):095603, September 2018. DOI: 10.1088/1612-202X/aad28d
8. Ford L.H., Estimate of the Vibrational Frequencies of Spherical Virus Particles. *Phys. Rev. E*, 67, 2003, p. 051924.
9. Saviot L., Murray D.B., Mermet A., Duval E., Comment on Estimate of the Vibrational Frequencies of Spherical Virus Particles. *Phys. Rev. E.*, 69, 2004, pp. 023901–02391.
10. Painter P.C., Mosher L.E., Rhoads C., Low-Frequency Modes in the Raman Spectra of Proteins. *Biopolymers*, 21, 1982, pp. 1469–1472.
11. Fonoberov V.A., Balandin A.A., Low-Frequency Vibrational Modes of Viruses Used for Nanoelectronic Self-Assemblies. *Phys. Status Sol.* B, 241, 2004, pp. R67–R69.
12. Tsen S.W.D., Kingsley D.H., Poweleit C., Achilefu S., Soroka D.S., Wu T.C., Tsen K.T., Studies of Inactivation Mechanism of Non-Enveloped Icosahedral Virus by a Visible Ultrashort Pulsed Laser. *Virology Journal*, 11(20), 2014, pp. 1–9.
13. Dykeman, E.C., Atomistic Normal Mode Analysis of Large Biomolecular Systems: Theory and Applications. PhD Dissertation, Arizona State University, 2008, pp. 1–232. www users.york.ac.uk/~ecd502/files/eric_dykeman_thesis.pdf.

14. Kervalishvili P., Gotsiridze I., Oscillation and Optical Properties of Viruses and Other Pathogenic Microorganisms. NATO Science and Security Series – Physics and Biophysics. Springer, UK, 2016, pp. 169–186.
15. Kervalishvili P.J., Study of Vibrational Properties of Nanobioobjects by Optical Spectroscopy (Keynote). *The 5th Global Conference on Materials Science and Engineering*, November 8–11, 2016, Taipei, Taiwan.
16. Tama F., Brooks C.L. III., Diversity and Identity of Mechanical Properties of Icosahedral Viral Capsids Studied with Elastic Network Normal Mode Analysis. *J. Mol. Biol.*, 345, 2005, pp. 299–314.
17. Witz J., Brown F., Structural Dynamics, an Intrinsic Property of Viral Capsids. *Arch. Virol.*, 146, 2001, pp. 2263–2274.
18. Bohren C.F., Huffman D.R., *Absorption and Scattering of Light by Small Particles*. John Wiley & Sons Inc., New York, 1983, pp. 1–530.
19. Bzhalava T.N., Kervalishvili P.J., Study of Spectroscopic Properties of Nanosized Particles of Core-Shell Morphology. *J. Phys., Conf. Ser.*, 987, 2018, pp. 1–6.
20. Kervalishvili P.J., Bzhalava T.N., Computer Simulation Study of Physical Properties of Nanosized Biostructures. *11th Japanese-Mediterranean Workshop on Applied Electromagnetic Engineering for Magnetic, Superconducting Multifunctional and Nanomaterials*, Batumi Shota Rustaveli State University, July 16–19, 2019, Batumi, Georgia.
21. Ufimtsev P.Y., *Fundamentals of the Physical Theory of Diffraction*, 2nd edn. John Wiley & Sons, New York, May 2014. DOI:10.1002/9781118753767
22. Becherrawy T., *Electromagnetism: Maxwell Equations, Wave Propagation and Emission*. Wiley-ISTE, New York, July 2012, pp. 560.
23. Bowman F., *Introduction to Bessel Functions*, Dover Books on Mathematics. Dover Publications, October 2010, pp. 160.
24. Kervalishvili P.J., Bzhalava T.N., Investigations of Spectroscopic Characteristics of Virus-Like Nano-Bioparticles. *Amer. Jour. Cond. Matt. Phys.*, 6(1), 2016, pp. 7–16. DOI: 10.5923/j.ajcmp.20160601.02
25. Ermolina I., Morgan H., Green N., Milner J., Feldman Y., Dielectric Spectroscopy of Tobacco Mosaic Virus. *Biochimica et Biophysica Acta*, 1622, 2003, pp. 57–63.
26. Fumagalli L., Esteban-Ferrer D., Cuervo A., Carrascosa J.L., Gomila G., Label-Free Identification of Single Dielectric Nanoparticles and Viruses with Ultraweak Polarization Forces. *Nature Materials*, 11, 2012, pp. 808–816. DOI: 10.1038/nmat3369
27. Kervalishvili P., Computer Simulation Study of Bionanoparticles. *3rd International Computational Science and Engineering Conference*, October 21–22, 2019, Doha, Qatar.

7 Adapting Smartphone-Based Applications for Performance Improvement Metrics' Tracking in Healthcare Facilities as a Managerial Tool

Adriana Burlea-Schiopoiu and Koudoua Ferhati

CONTENT

7.1 INTRODUCTION

Healthcare is a fundamental need of every human being. In developing countries, the health care systems are mainly provided by the government with little or no charge besides the coverage of insurance programs provided by employers in both public and private sectors. However, this comes with many worries. The huge number of patients makes it difficult for the government hospitals to provide them with quality health care and to ensure that their management for the facilities is achieving the desired quality goals of performance, sustainability, and patient satisfaction [1].

Currently, progress in information technology (IT) field has certainly enhanced people's life style and standards. "Having the right technology can make life easier and healthier" [2]. Smart phones are utilized in healthcare sector in a very wide way, almost in all the specialties; as a result, people are making use of the beneficial mobile applications. A large number of health applications are used by patients in a personal way for following certain health situations and diseases, to localize hospitals and clinics, or to book an appointment. On the other hand, from doctors and practitioners to make diagnostics or to discuss with other professionals, smartphone compatibility has put even more powerful medical devices, which were previously found only in doctor's clinics and hospitals, directly into patients' hands. Visual acuity assessment, optic disc visualization (ophthalmoscope), inner ear visualization (otoscope), lung function (spirometer), heart function (electrocardiogram [ECG]), body sound analysis (stethoscope), and even sonography (ultrasound) can all now be conducted using an app or peripheral hardware [3]. However, from the managerial side, there is not much interest about creating such platforms or applications that could serve and support managers in making a clear vision of the facility's current situation; therefore, our aim in this chapter is to provide such a tool with all the information needed by managers to help them making decisions based on reliable data, setting strategic goals, and solving problems that cannot be found in an early phase unless we measure its causes in a frequent way. In addition, we desire to assess the effect of such a tool in the improvement of the quality and performance in the facility.

7.2 USING M-HEALTH IN HEALTHCARE SYSTEMS

Literature has shown that there is a great interest in integrating IT into healthcare systems, going from complex electronic health systems to mobile health applications, which presents a solution for many logistic and economic difficulties in quality insurance process. The majority of researchers have agreed that the development and implementation of a quality management system in healthcare organizations represents a revolutionary change for the organizations. Quality management affects the structure, core (internal and external), ownership and customer (patient–client) relationships, the quality system, and almost all other systems and segments of the organization. With that in mind, it is quite reasonable to speak that, in the last couple of decades, great progress has been made in organizing businesses, which has led to the situation where organizations are increasingly oriented to processes, rather than to the organizational structure [4].

The use of conventional mobile and wireless technologies to support health objectives is known as mobile health or m-Health [5]. The budding integration of m-Health in existing healthcare systems has been discussed and widely accredited in the literature of the last decade. Technological innovation and adoption have proved especially challenging for the healthcare industry, which increased pressure to lower the rising cost of healthcare while improving quality. Herzlinger [6] explained how entrepreneurs and technology companies are focusing on providing tech tools that can satisfy regulations, lower costs, and improve the effectiveness of both health administrators and health practitioners. Adding that success or failure of these technologies often depends on financial resources, effective leadership and, perhaps most of all, intent, whether healthcare providers are using them as a means to enhance quality of care, and not just to increase the speed at which it is delivered, is a matter of concern.

According to Haasteren et al. [7], healthcare is increasingly engaging with m-Health) and their accompanying software applications are colloquially referred to as "apps." The push toward m-Health is largely driven by encouraging statistics, showing that up to 58% of United States (US) mobile phone owners had downloaded some form of a health app as of 2015, and also that there were around 325,000 health applications on the market in 2017.

7.3 THINKING OF QUALITY AND PERFORMANCE IN HEALTHCARE FACILITIES

Needs in healthcare facilities are increasing notably due a lot of factors, such as population aging and the development of technologies. Because of this, a good quality/cost ratio is required to improve the healthcare systems.

The health sector includes both public (public hospitals, etc.) and private sectors (clinics, private doctors, etc.). Both sectors contribute (each in its own way) to improving the quality of health. Before going to the design of a managerial tool to help health managers, we need first to know about the quality requirements needed in healthcare facilities to be fulfilled with this tool. With the vast spreading of the quality management principles among the researchers, various educators and practitioners have started to experiment with them in recent years in order to explore how they can also be used for the improvement of services in healthcare. These principles in healthcare focus on the quality management in a general way, but it still works when adapted to the specifications of healthcare sector as shown in Table 7.1 as presented in Pejović et al. [4].

7.4 THE NEED FOR A MANAGERIAL TOOL IN HEALTHCARE FACILITIES

Managers in healthcare have a legal and moral responsibility to ensure a high quality of patient care and to strive to improve care. These managers are in a key position to mandate policy, systems, procedures, and organizational environments [8].

The limitations of resources in developing countries and the need for a managerial solution to provide a better-quality management/patient satisfaction/sustainable facilities represent a big motivation for adapting m-Health.

The World Health Organization defines m-Health as "[t]he provision of health services and information via mobile technologies such as mobile phones and Personal Digital Assistants (PDAs)." There has been a recent expansion of various innovative m-Health solutions in many functionalities due to the increasing use of Internet and mobile devices and apps. Therefore, it is very promising that such technologies could be used in a wide way within management of healthcare facilities, especially in complicated tasks such as quality and performance management.

TABLE 7.1
Quality Management Principles in Healthcare [4]

Customer focus	This principle is a fundamental objective in the development of public and private services as it constitutes one of the main drivers for healthcare services reforms.
Stakeholder involvement	Adequate worth must also be provided to employees, local and global community, investors, and society in general, in terms of both financial and nonfinancial aspects of a company's performance.
Leadership	Leadership is crucial for the management of the healthcare organizations and the quality management system of those organizations that adopted customer-centered approach. Leaders have the role to inspire, promote, and support the organizational culture of quality. (ISO 9001)
People and care vision	Drawing information, consciously or unconsciously, man creates values, beliefs, and attitudes, and, guided by a variety of external influences, makes decisions. This is an exceptional role of employees in the organization that is present in all areas of life and work.
Process orientation	Healthcare services require the implementation of integrated and multidisciplinary processes that unite different functions, clinical specialist activities, as well as the variety of providers of healthcare services.
Guidance through information	Healthcare organizations exchange a great number of different healthcare information and provide a great number of healthcare services, all with the support of modern information technologies.
Partnerships for quality across healthcare services	It is necessary to ensure coordination between several healthcare organizations when providing healthcare services. These may be two or three different healthcare organizations and, sometimes, in a regional context, we can talk about a whole network of healthcare organizations.
Demand-oriented care	It is important to change the treatment paradigm based on the opinion of the doctor (without taking into account the patient's opinion) to the treatment based, particularly, on the needs, demands, and expectations of the customer.
Mutually beneficial supplier relationship	Third-party services such as technical support, information and communication services, business consulting, recruitment services, sanitation, catering, and training have a critical effect on the quality of healthcare organization and its outcomes.
Continual improvement	According to ISO 9001:2015, "[t]he organization shall continually improve the suitability, adequacy and effectiveness of the quality management system."

7.5 IDEA AND OBJECTIVE OF THE TOOL: METRIC MEDIC

The main idea of the application is to provide a space for data collection by different categories of users (doctors, nurses, lab workers, and so on), including a set of metrics to be assessed (KPI's) and tracked in a specified period of time in order to have a clear view about the current situation of the facility's quality management that offers a support to help managers in decision-making and strategies updating in four main perspectives: social, economic, environmental, and internal processes. After the collection of data provided by the staff in a sequential manner, the app presents in dashboards the metrics' scores with the possible positive or negative progress from the previous assessment cycle (e.g., mortality rate: –2%), which gives a major aid to decide whether the managers are keeping the current strategy or making a change in a really specified areas. It also allows the implication of stakeholders and the ideas exchanging in a professional representative way.

7.6 METRICS

The application presents metrics (indicators) to assess the organizational performance in healthcare facilities in four main domains: social, economic, technical, and internal processes.

7.6.1 Social Indicators

The social indicators are presented in Table 7.2.

7.6.2 Economic Indicators

The economic indicators are presented in Table 7.3.

7.6.3 Internal Process Indicators

The internal process indicators are presented in Table 7.4.

7.6.4 Technical Indicators

The technical indicators are presented in Table 7.5.

7.7 FUNCTIONALITY OF THE APP: A MANAGERIAL TOOL

In Figures 7.1–7.3, we took a screenshot of the application while running it to track the indicator: "patient satisfaction" as an example to explain how it works.

Figure 7.1 displays the interface that appears when we run the application with the name and logo in the middle of the page. Then in Figure 7.2, a description of the app with four main domains of key performance indicators (KPIs) – social, economic, internal processes, and technical indicators – is presented. Figure 7.3 presents the set of indicators in each domain to choose and start entering data.

TABLE 7.2
Social Indicators

Indicators	Definition
Patient satisfaction	It is an important indicator for the healthcare performance, and it measures the degrees to which medical service responds to patients' expectations [9].
Average hospital stay	It shows how quickly medical staff are able to diagnose and prescribe treatment that does not require further stay. Also it helps the facility to predict how many patients they can bring into the facility during a specific time frame [9].
Hospital readmission rate	This indicator calculates the rate of patients who come back to the facility shortly after they were seen. If high, it can indicate a lack of staff, experience, or attention during treatment [10].
Patient waiting time	It indicates the time a patient waits in a facility's waiting room before being seen by one of the medical staff. It measures the average length of time patients spend in the hospital per admission category [11].
Patient safety	This indicator displays a healthcare facility's ability of keeping patients safe from contracting infections, complications, and other issues by tracking it in a recorded period that helps to recognize what areas are causing issues that can be improved [9].
Waiting time in the emergency room	It gauges the time that the patient stays waiting in the emergency room until he or she gets a care service in the area [9].
Number of new patients	This indicator measures the number of unique individuals who were first-time patients during the reporting period [9].
Rate of vacant patients in beds	It shows the average rate at which beds in the facility are vacant.
Patient transfer rate to other facilities	It tracks the number of patients being transferred to other healthcare facilities during the reporting period.
Patient's age range (%)	It tracks the range of patient's age: • 0–12 years • 1–20 years • 21–40 years • 41–60 years • 60 years and above
Patient's gender (%)	• Female • Male
Patient complaint rate	It logs the number of complaints filed by patients before, during, or after their period of care.

Source: Authors' own contribution based on a review of the literature.

TABLE 7.3
Economic Indicators

Indicators	Definition
Average care costs	It is an image of the average out-of-pocket cost paid by the patient to the healthcare facility.
Costs per payer	It reflects the averages of the cost that the patients pay for care services.
Average maintenance costs	It measures the direct and indirect costs to maintain equipment throughout the facility.
Current cost per bed	Averages of the cost that the facility incurs for a patient's entire stay.
The cost of drugs and equipment	The cost that the facility pays for the total of drugs, medicines, and medical equipment during the reporting period.
Average hospital expenses	It records the overhead expenses for direct operations of the facility. It affects the pricing of services.
Average care costs of insured patients	Averages of the cost that the facility incurs for a patient's care after the elimination of costs % paid by the insurant.

Source: Authors' own contribution based on a review of the literature.

TABLE 7.4
Indicators of Internal Processes

Indicators	Definition
Medication errors	It can be used to improve the medical process by reporting mistakes made in the medication of inpatient and outpatient services [9].
Bed occupancy rate	It assesses the number of occupied beds in the facility from all the departments divided by the number of actual available beds by a predefined number of days recorded [12].
Mortality rate	A critical indicator that measures the number of deaths by the actual number of patients per the time of measuring the metric [13].
Infection rate	It is an indicator used in healthcare facilities to predict the probability of being infected; it measures the frequency of occurrence of new infection cases among patients during the recorded period [14].
Clinical errors	It measures the frequency of clinical errors in the facility, which indicates the medical staff and equipment's effectiveness [9].
Medical errors	It measures the frequency of making an error of medications or dosage in prescribing medication within the facility [9].
Waiting time for admission to the operating room	It measures the mean time from presentation to the emergency department to the first surgical consultation [15].
Average length of stay in the emergency room	It measures the average time from the patient's arrival at the emergency room until discharge after care service in the facility [16].
Laboratory test time	It measures the average amount of time taken to run a test in the laboratory [9].

Source: Authors' own contribution based on a review of the literature.

TABLE 7.5
Technical Indicators

Indicators	Definition
Natural light penetration	It measures the amount and distribution of natural light needed for the good practices inside the healthcare facility's different spaces [17].
Degree of thermal comfort	It measures the degree of satisfaction with the thermal environment inside the facility; dissatisfaction may be caused by thermal noncomfort of the body expressed by the medical staff or the patients, and could be tracked with the predicted mean vote (PMV) and predicted percentage od dissatisfied (PPD) indices [18]
Distributions of medical devices	This metric assesses the availability and distribution of the medical devices in the facility during the recorded period.
Sufficient air-conditioning	It measures the sufficiency of air out of an HVAC system compared to the standard norm for the room volume and the general well-being of staff and patients in the facility.
Water consumption	It measures the average individual water usage calculated on a daily basis at the facility's level to provide an indication of the water consumption level and set the facility needs and strategies [19].
Artificial lighting	It measures the sufficiency and distribution of the artificial lighting depending on technical metrics: number of units, power per unit, and the type of lamps used for each space to meet the minimum requirements [20].
Energy consumption	It measures the total energy consumption in the facility.
Waste management	It measures the amount of waste collected and/or recycled by the facility, estimated in tones. It takes into account any waste specific to the healthcare activities. "Healthcare waste (HCW) is a by-product of healthcare that includes sharps, non-sharps, blood, body parts, chemicals, pharmaceuticals, medical devices and radioactive materials and toxic materials" [21].
Indoor air quality	Measuring this indicator allows maintaining the optimum indoor air quality using ventilation standards, perceived air quality (PIAQ), by having feedback from people's perceptions of indoor air quality and particles measurements (PM).

Source: Authors' own contribution based on a review of the literature.

After choosing the indicator to make the data entry, a page appears containing a brief definition of the metrics, a calendar, and an option to pick the week, as shown in Figure 7.4. After entering the data, it appears in a form of a chart where we can make a comparison with the previous weeks and have a visual presentation of the tracking process (see Figure 7.5). Finally, sharing the dashboards is possible due to the share option (see Figure 7.6) to a variety of platforms to discuss it with managers or stakeholders.

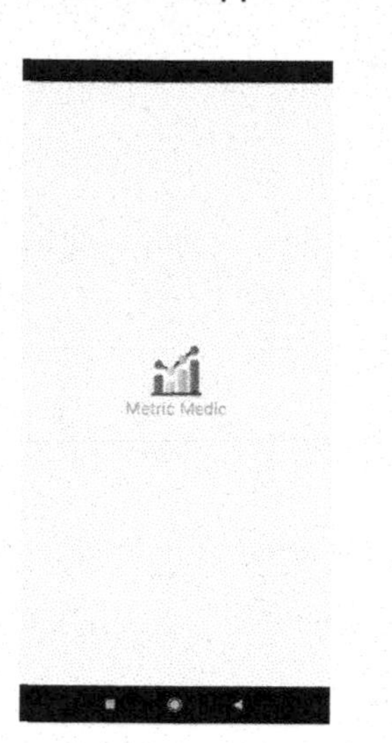

FIGURE 7.1 The interface.

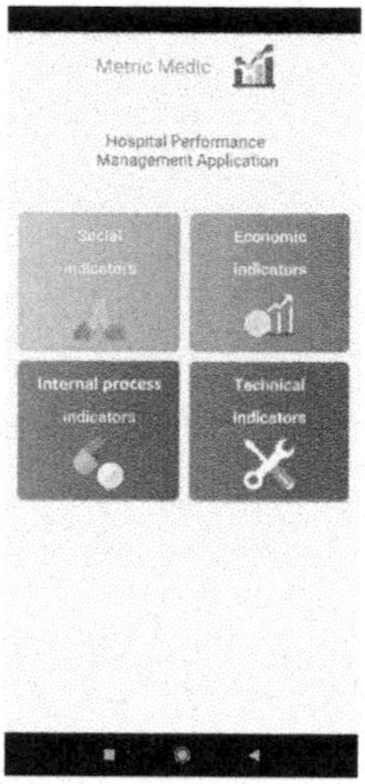

FIGURE 7.2 Description of the app with four main domains of KPIs.

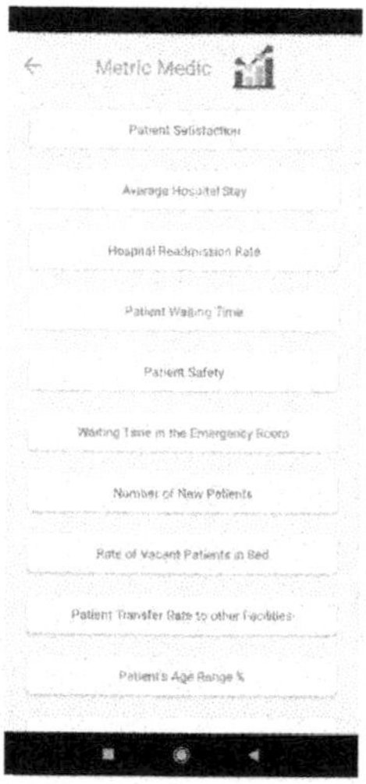

FIGURE 7.3 The set of indicators.

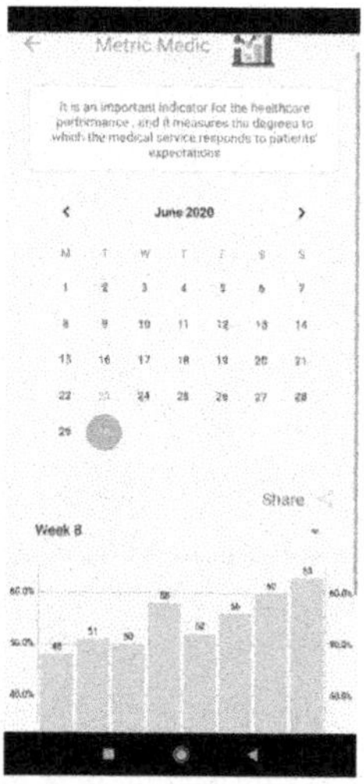

FIGURE 7.4 Brief presentation of the metrics.

7.8 INTEGRATION OF THE MOBILE APPLICATION IN THE HOSPITAL

After integrating the application in a case study hospital in El Taref, Algeria, for a period of time (8 weeks) and studying the collected data and discussing the main

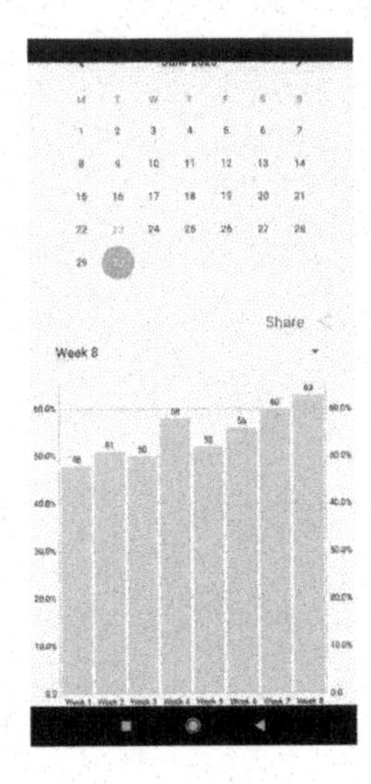

FIGURE 7.5 Metrics of the week.

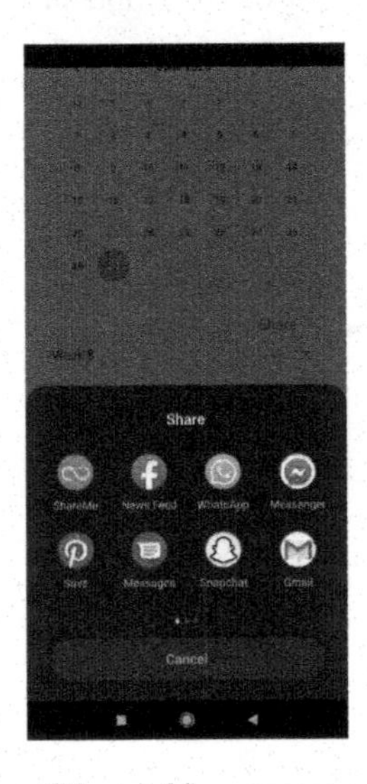

FIGURE 7.6 Visual presentation of the tracking process.

changes in the management of the facility, the impact of the app and its effect in improving the quality of services and performance were assessed.

In this study, we decided to track the following indicators since they are considered as a short-term tracked metrics that affect the facility's management strategy in a direct way. The application Metric Medic was used in the period from April 16 to June 4, 2020 in a public primary hospital to show the following:

TABLE 7.6
Patient Satisfaction % per Week

Week	1	2	3	4	5	6	7	8
%	48	51	50	58	52	56	60	63

1. **Patient satisfaction**
   The method used to collect the data for this indicator is to ask verbally a random group of patients about their satisfaction regarding the services of the facility expressed in a percentage, and then collect it every week and measure the average satisfaction percentage.

Data in Table 7.6 show that there is an observable increase in patient's satisfaction from the first week with 48% to the last one with 63% as recorded in eight successive weeks.

2. **Average hospital stay**
   In this metric, we choose to track the average hospital stay of patients in the mother and child unit from the moment the patient is accepted in the facility till he or she is authorized to go home. This healthcare metric is a very general one and can vary greatly according to the type of stay it measures as we observed while tracking it in the previous 8 weeks because the stay after a surgical operation is not like having a tooth removal, for example.

The data in Table 7.7 show that the average hospital stay varies from 4 days as a minimum to 12 days as a maximum, and there is a direct relationship between the quality of care and the length of hospital stay and of course the nature of the medical situation of the patients. We observe that the numbers start to go down starting from the fifth week, with an average stay of 4 days than 5 days in the sixth and seventh weeks, then back to 6 days in the last week.

3. **Patient waiting time in the emergency room**
   In order to assess the patient waiting time in the emergency room, a chronometer was used to record the time that a patient waits from the moment he or she arrives at the facility until he or she meets a doctor in the emergency room. The situations were different taking into consideration the epic days and hours, and that is the reason why we calculated the average waiting time of all the cases assessed.

From the data shown in Table 7.8, the waiting time is going from a minimum of 29 minutes in the fifth week to a maximum of 51 minutes in the third week, with an observable decreasing from the first 4 weeks to the last 4 weeks.

TABLE 7.7
Average Hospital Stay per Week

Week	1	2	3	4	5	6	7	8
Day	9	10	8	12	4	5	5	6

TABLE 7.8
Patient Waiting Time per Week

Week	1	2	3	4	5	6	7	8
Min	48	52	51	42	29	32	40	37

4. **Mortality rate**
   A standardized mortality ratio is calculated as the observed number of deaths divided by the expected number of deaths [22]. In this metric, we assess the number of death cases every week in the given healthcare facility.

From the data in Table 7.9, it shows that the death cases in the facility go from a minimum of 0 case in weeks 1, 3, 6, and 7 to a maximum of 4 cases in week 5.

5. **Bed occupancy rate**
   To measure the percentage of bed occupancy in the facility, we assessed the number of occupied beds from the total number of beds in every week.

Data in Table 7.10 show that generally the occupancy rate of beds in the facility is high, varying from 62% to 92% of the total beds, as it goes from high percentages in the first 4 weeks to a bit lower percentage in the last 4 weeks during the study period.

6. **Laboratory test time**
   To track this metric, we picked a random set of blood tests (blood cholesterol test, blood glucose, tuberculosis test, full blood count [FBC], etc.) and measured the average time from the sampling moment till the delivery of results to patients in the hospital (see Table 7.11).

In the majority of the weeks (1, 2, 4, 5, and 08), the laboratory test time is fixed as 24 hours, but it can go up to 48 hours as in the week 7. It is needless to say that the average time can vary from a really short amount of hours (4 hours) to a long amount of hour (60 hours) depending on the type of the test and its complexity, as well as the number of the tests needed to be done in the hospital's test laboratory.

TABLE 7.9
Mortality Rate per Week

Week	1	2	3	4	5	6	7	8
Death	0	3	0	1	4	0	0	1

TABLE 7.10
Bed Occupancy Rate per Week

Week	1	2	3	4	5	6	7	8
%	78	65	71	92	64	62	73	69

TABLE 7.11
Laboratory Test Time per Week

Week	1	2	3	4	5	6	7	8
Hour	24	24	36	24	24	30	48	24

7. **Patient transfer rate to other facilities**
   In this metric, we calculated the number of patients being transferred to other healthcare facilities during the reporting period: either specialized facilities in the same *wilaya* or to other facilities in another *wilaya*.

Table 7.12 shows that the facility makes transfers of the patients to other facilities with a minimum of two patients and a maximum of nine patients per week (during the study period). The reason behind this is that, according to the facility's staff, there is either the lack of specialized doctors or the lack of required technical resources to deal with their cases. Overall, we can notice that the number of transferred patients is developing decreasingly in the timeline of the study.

7.9 RELATIONSHIP BETWEEN METRICS AND IMPACT EVALUATION

The results of this study show that integrating Metric Medic as a managerial tool in the healthcare facility had a positive effect on the quality of care services and the organizational performance as shown in Figure 7.7. Also, the metrics have a direct influence on each other. For example, when the patient transfer rate becomes less starting from week 6, the patient satisfaction increases at the same time, which

TABLE 7.12
Patient Transfer Rate per Week

Week	1	2	3	4	5	6	7	8
Patient	8	5	5	9	7	2	3	3

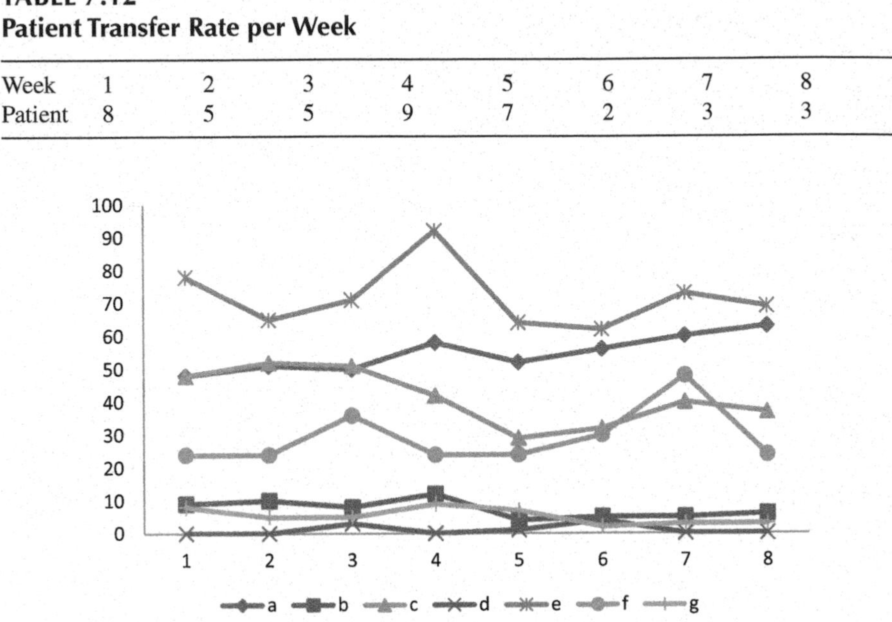

FIGURE 7.7 Metrics evolution during the study.

presents a great interest to health managers to study the possible correlation between indicators to ensure the best decision-making supports for a better performance and care service quality in the healthcare facility. Finally, the application helped the work staff in the facility to have a clearer vision about the existing data and to use it, share it, and discuss it for the good practices.

REFERENCES

1. Imteaj A, Hossain M K. A smartphone based application to improve the health care system of Bangladesh. International Conference on Medical Engineering, Health Informatics and Technology (MediTec), 2016, pp. 1–6.
2. Chuckun V, Coonjan G., Nagowah L. Enabling the disabled using mHealth. *2019 Conference on Next Generation Computing Applications (NextComp)*, 2019, pp. 1–6.
3. Batista MA, Gaglani SM. The future of smartphones in health care. *AMA Journal of Ethics, Virtual Mentor*, 2013; 15(11):947–950. DOI: 10.1001/virtualmentor.2013.15.11.stas1-1311
4. Pejović G, Tosic B, Ruso J. Benchmarking as the quality management tool for the excellence assessment of medicines regulatory authorities in Europe. *International Scientific Symposium SymOrg Conference*, Zlatibor, Serbia, June 7-10 2018.
5. WHO Global Observatory for eHealth. mHealth New horizons for health through mobile technologies: second global survey on eHealth. World Health Organization,

2011. Available online: https://apps.who.int/iris/handle/10665/44607 (Accessed 29 May 2020)
6. Herzlinger RE. Why innovation in health care is so hard. *Harvard Business Review*, 2006. Available online: https://hbr.org/2006/05/why-innovation-in-health-care-is-so-hard (accessed 20 June 2020).
7. Van Haasteren A, Gille F, Fadda M, Vayena E. Development of the mHealth app trustworthiness checklist. *Digital Health*, 2019. DOI: 10.1177/2055207619886463
8. Parand A, Dopson S, Renz A, Vincent C. The role of hospital managers in quality and patient safety: A systematic review. *BMJ Open*. 2014;4(9):e005055. DOI: 10.1136/bmjopen-2014–005055
9. Rosdia A. KPI of the day – Healthcare:% patient satisfaction. *Performance Magazine*, June 8, 2017. www.performancemagazine.org/kpi-day-healthcare-patient-satisfaction/ (Accessed 28 May 2020)
10. Oche MO, Adamu H. Determinants of patient waiting time in the general outpatient department of a tertiary health institution in North Western Nigeria. *Annals of Medical Health Sciences Research*. 2013;3(4):588–592.
11. Collins AS. *Preventing Health Care-Associated Infections.In* Hughes RG, editor. *Patient Safety and Quality: An Evidence-Based Handbook for Nurses*, Rockville, MD: Agency for Healthcare Research and Quality (US). 2008, vol. 1, Chapter 41, Available online: https://www.ncbi.nlm.nih.gov/books/NBK2683/ (Accessed 12 May 2020)
12. World Health Organization (WHO). European health information gateway 2008. Bed occupancy rate (%), acute care hospitals only, 2008. https://gateway.euro.who.int/en/indicators/hfa_542-6210-bed-occupancy-rate-acute-care-hospitals-only/ (Accessed 10 April 2020)
13. Porta M. Mortality Rate, morbidity rate; death rate; cumulative death rate; case fatality rate. *A Dictionary of Epidemiology* (5th edn.). Oxford: Oxford University Press, 2014, p. 60.
14. Utah Department of Health. Calculation of infection rates. 2017. http://health.utah.gov/epi/diseases/HAI/resources/Cal_Inf_Rates.pdf (Accessed 21 February 2020)
15. Acharya S, Dharel D, Upadhyaya S, Khanal N, Dahal S, Dahal S, Aryal K. Study of factors associated with waiting time for patients undergoing emergency surgery in a tertiary care centre in Nepal. *Journal of Society of Anesthesiologists of Nepal,* 2015;1(1):7–12. https://doi.org/10.3126/jsan.v1i1.13582
16. Sreekala P, Arpita D, Varghese ME. Patient waiting time in emergency department. *International Journal of Scientific and Research Publications*, 2015;5(5).
17. Gherri B. Natural light and daylight assessment, a new framework for enclosed space evaluation. 2020. http://thedaylightsite.com/natural-light-and-daylight-assessment/ (Accessed 31 May 2020)
18. Olesen BW, Hagström K. *Industrial Ventilation Design Guidebook*. 2001. www.sciencedirect.com/book/9780122896767/industrial-ventilation-design-guidebook#book-description (Accessed 26 March 2020)
19. World Health Organization (WHO). Domestic Water Quantity, Service, Level and Health, 2003. https://www.who.int/water_sanitation_health/diseases/WSH0302.pdf (Accessed 18 February 2020).
20. Balaras CA, Dascalaki EG, Droutsa KG, Kontoyiannidi S, Guruz R, Gudnason G. Energy and other key performance indicators for buildings – Examples for Hellenic buildings. *Global Journal of Energy Technology Research Updates*, 2014; 1:71–89.

21. Nwachukwu NC, Anayo Orji F, Ugbogu OC, Health care waste management – Public health benefits, and the need for effective environmental regulatory surveillance in Federal Republic of Nigeria, 2012, pp. 150–177.
22. Mausner JS, Bahn AK. *Epidemiology an Introductory Text.* Philadelphia, PA: Saunders, 7, 1974, pp. 146–159.

8 Intelligent Approaches for Developing Knowledge-Based System for Diabetes Diet

Ibrahim M. Ahmed, Marco Alfonse, and Abdel-Badeeh M. Salem

CONTENTS

8.1 INTRODUCTION

Diabetes is a serious health problem today. It is the single most important metabolic disease. It can affect nearly every organ system in the body. Diabetics find difficulty to observe a healthy lifestyle in their diets and eating patterns. Treatment of a diabetic requires a strict regimen that typically includes carefully calculated and controlled diet. Type-2 diabetes is becoming more common due to risk factors such as older age, obesity, lack of exercise, family history of diabetes, and heart diseases. Most of the people are unaware that they are at risk of or may even have type-2 diabetes.

On the other hand, knowledge-based expert systems (KBS) certainly became an essential tool for diagnosis and personalized treatments. They are widely used in domains where knowledge is more prevalent than data and that require heuristics and reasoning logic to derive new knowledge. The knowledge in a KBS is stored in a knowledge base that is separate from both the control and inference programs and can be represented by various formalisms, such as frames, Bayesian networks, and production rules. Recently, expert systems technology provides efficient tools for diagnosing diabetes and hence providing a sufficient treatment. The research in diabetic systems is important for both the medical staff and diabetes patients. An efficient tool for diagnosing diabetes and hence providing a sufficient treatment is urgently needed for helping both specialist doctors and patients.

The expert system went through many stages, starting from requirement specification of the problem, addressing the technical difficulties, knowledge acquisition for the healthy food that helps type-2 diabetic people to monitor and control the proper diet, challenges in the designing phase, implementation constrains, and, finally, testing the developed Sudanese intelligent medical expert system.

Visual Prolog was used for designing the graphical user interface and the implementation of the system. The Visual Programming Interface (VPI) is a high-level application programming interface (API) and is designed to make it easy for Prolog applications to provide sophisticated user interfaces utilizing the graphical capabilities of today's operating systems and display hardware. It makes possible to create portable source code. Rule base is used as knowledge representation and backward chaining is used as inference engine.

Our results showed a meal planner of a recommended five meals a day for every patient. These are breakfast, lunch, snack1, dinner, and snack2. These meals suggest appropriate diet using calorie-based or serving-based planner for Sudanese diabetic people. Therefore, the proposed expert system is a helpful tool that reduces the workload of physicians and provides diabetics with simple and valuable assistance.

8.2 DIABETES MELLITUS

Diabetes mellitus is a disease that causes a rise in blood glucose level (BGL) in the human body. It is known that the normal BGL lies between 70–100 mg/100 mL when fasting and around 140 mg/100 mL otherwise. For a diabetic person, the blood glucose is around 126 mg/100 mL when fasting and 200 mg/100 mL otherwise. The most common symptoms observed in diabetic patients are polyuria, weight loss, excessive thirst, continuous hunger, blurring and changes in vision, and fatigue.

Diabetes mellitus can create many complications [1]: (1) heart disease, (2) stroke, (3) kidney disease, (4) blindness, (5) nerve damage, (6) leg and foot amputations, and (7) death.

There are different types of diabetes: type 1 diabetes or insulin-dependent diabetes mellitus (IDDM), an autoimmune disease in which no insulin is produced, must be treated by insulin injections. Treatment also includes regular exercise and development of a meal plan. Type-2 diabetes, or non-insulin-dependent diabetes mellitus (NIDDM), in which tissues do not respond to insulin, is linked to heredity and obesity and may be controlled by diet; it accounts for 90% of all cases, many of which go undiagnosed for years. During pregnancy, usually around the 24th week, many women develop gestational diabetes [2].

Most medical resources reported that 90%–95% of diabetics are diagnosed as type-2. Furthermore, it can affect not only adults but also young people. Over 80%–90% of type-2 diabetics are overweight, and this in turn contributes to many diabetes symptoms. Therefore, reducing daily carbohydrates and fat intake and adhering to a healthy diet with a simple walking keep your glucose level within normal ranges and help dropping those extra pounds [4].

Recommendations of diabetic diet differ from one person to another based on their nutritional needs, lifestyle, and the action and timing of medications.

In type-2 diabetes, the concern may be more oriented to weight loss in order to improve the body's ability to utilize the insulin that it produces. Thus, learning about the basics of food nutrition will help in adjusting diets to suit the particular condition. Table 8.1 shows the desirable blood sugar level supply by the American Diabetes Association [5]. Table 8.2 shows the recommended daily food portion by the American Diabetes Association.

Fortunately, reducing daily carbohydrates and fat intake and adhering to a healthy diet combined with a simple exercise like walking keep your glucose within normal ranges and help dropping those extra pounds [3]. Diabetes may be diagnosed based

TABLE 8.1
Blood Glucose Goals – Desirable Blood Sugar Levels [5]

Time of Test	Person without Diabetes	Person with Diabetes
Before meals	Less than 115 mg/dl	80–120 mg/dl
Before bedtime	Less than 120 mg/dl	100–140 mg/dl

TABLE 8.2
Recommended Daily Food Portion [4]

Food Portion	Daily Calories Count
Carbohydrates	50%–60%
Protein	12%–20%
Fat	Not more than 30%

on A1C criteria or plasma glucose criteria, either the fasting plasma glucose (FPG) or the 2-h plasma glucose (2-h PG) value after a 75-g oral glucose tolerance test (OGTT) [6].

8.3 INTRODUCTION TO DIABETIC INFORMATICS

8.3.1 Medical Informatics

The field of medical informatics has drawn increasing popularity and attention, and has been growing rapidly over the past two decades due to advances in new molecular, genomic, and biomedical techniques and applications such as genome sequencing, protein identification, medical imaging, and patient medical records. The digitization of critical medical information, such as lab reports, patient records, research papers, and anatomic images, has also resulted in large amounts of patient care data. New computational techniques and information technologies are needed to manage these large repositories of biomedical data and to discover useful patterns and knowledge from them [7].

8.3.1.1 Intelligent Medical Informatics

Intelligent medical informatics consist of five main domains: medical imaging, medical knowledge engineering, robotic surgery, medical education/training, and medical expert systems (Figure 8.1).

8.3.1.1.1 Medical Knowledge Engineering

The term "knowledge engineering" refers to computer-based symbolic reasoning issues such as knowledge representation, acquisition, explanism, and self-awareness or self-modification. The inference engine makes inferences. It decides which rules are satisfied by the facts, prioritizes them, and executes the rule with the highest priority. There are two types of inference: forward chaining and backward chaining. Forward chaining is the reasoning from facts to the conclusion, while backward chaining is from hypothesis to facts that match and check for halt.

Significant clinical problems require large knowledge bases that contain complex interrelationships including time and functional dependences. The knowledge of such domains is inevitably open-ended and incomplete, so the knowledge base must be easily extensible. Not only does this require a flexible representation of knowledge, but it also encourages the development of novel techniques for acquisition and integration of new facts and judgments. Similarly, the inexactness of medical

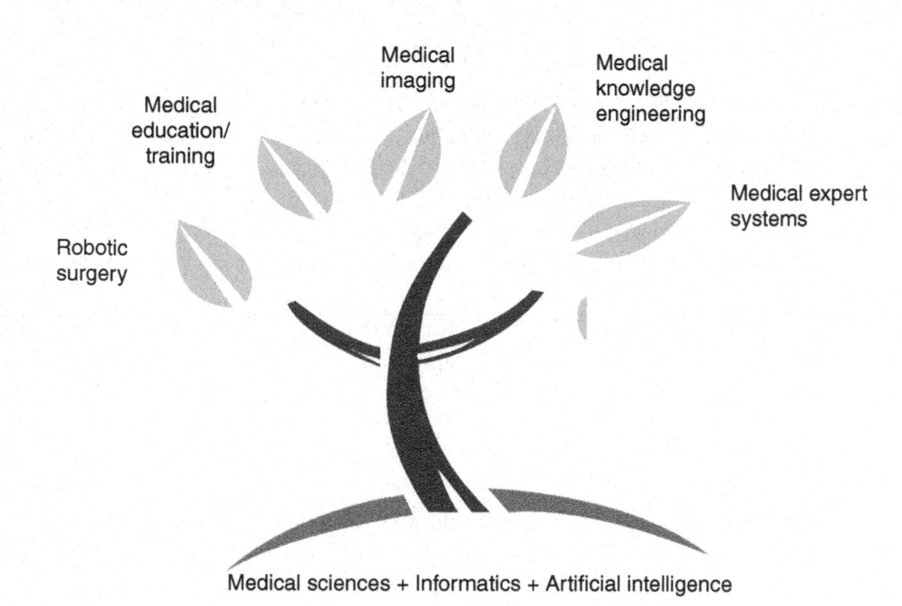

FIGURE 8.1 Intelligent medical informatics tree

inference must somehow be represented and manipulated within effective consultation systems.

The most successful paradigms in medical domain are symbolic reasoning approaches, decision theory approaches, Bayesian analysis approaches, statistical pattern recognition, mathematical models of physical processes, data bank analysis for prognosis and therapy selection, and clinical reasoning [8].

8.3.1.1.2 Evaluation Methodologies

There are several popular methods used for such evaluation, including holdout sampling, cross-validation, leave-one-out, and bootstrap sampling.

In the holdout method, data are divided into a training set and a testing set. Usually two-thirds of the data are assigned to the training set and one-third to the testing set.

In cross-validation, a data set is randomly divided into a number of subsets of roughly equal size. Tenfold cross-validation, in which the data sets are divided into ten subsets, is most commonly used. The system is trained and tested for ten interactions. In each interaction, nine subsets of data are used as training data and the remaining set is used as the testing data. In rotation, each subset of data serves as the testing set in exactly one interaction. The accuracy of the system is the average accuracy over the ten interactions. Leave-one-out is the extreme case of cross-validation, where the original data are split into n subsets, where n is the size of the original data. The system is trained and tested for n interactions, in each of which n–1 instances are used for training and the remaining instance is used for testing.

In the bootstrap method, n independent random samples are taken from the original data set of size n.

8.3.2 Electronic Health Records (EHRs)

EHRs, also known as electronic medical records or computerized patient records, are found in an increasing number of physician offices and hospitals. They provide the ability to manage health information using modern information techniques that are impossible to apply to paper record-keeping.

EHR is processed and stored in electronic healthcare information (EHI) systems. EHR includes patient demographic and clinical health information such as medical histories and problem lists [9].

A diagrammatic example of a simple EHR is shown in Figure 8.2, indicating some areas feeding into the record from units/departments within the institution. There could be others depending on the extent and scope of the system [10].

8.3.3 Diabetic Diet

The diet for a diabetic patient is in principle no different from the diet considered healthy for the population as a whole [11]. Diabetic diet is simply a balanced healthy diet that is vital for diabetes treatment. The regulation of blood sugar in the nondiabetic is automatic, adjusting to whatever foods are eaten. However, for the diabetic, extra caution is needed to balance the food intake with exercise, insulin injections, and any other glucose altering activity. This helps diabetic patients to maintain the desirable weight and control their glucose level in their blood. It also helps to prevent diabetes patients from heart and blood vessel-related diseases [12].

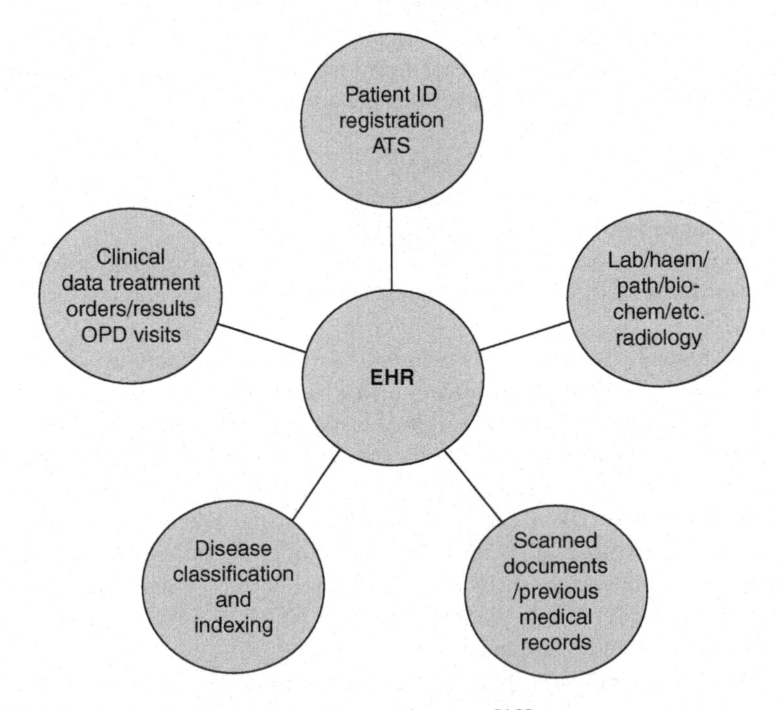

FIGURE 8.2 A simple electronic health record system [10]

Food groups are exchange lists of foods that contain roughly the same mix of carbohydrates, protein, and fat; serving sizes are defined so that each will have the same amount of carbohydrate, fat, and protein as any other. Foods can be "exchanged" with others in a category while still meeting the desired overall nutrition requirements. Food groups can be applied to almost any eating situation and make it easier to follow a prescribed diet [13].

8.4 MEDICAL EXPERT SYSTEMS

8.4.1 Expert System

The expert system is a computer program that represents and reasons with knowledge of some specialist subject with a view to solving problems or giving advice. To solve expert-level problems, expert systems will need efficient access to a substantial domain knowledge base, and a reasoning mechanism to apply the knowledge to the problems they are given. Usually they will also need to be able to explain, to the users who rely on them, how they have reached their decisions. They will generally build upon the ideas of knowledge representation, production rules, search, and so on, that we have already covered [7].

8.4.1.1 The Architecture of Expert Systems

The process of building expert systems is often called knowledge engineering. The knowledge engineer is involved with all components of an expert system. Building expert systems is generally an iterative process. The components and their interaction will be refined over the course of numerous meetings of the knowledge engineer with the experts and users. We will look in turn at the various components shown in Figure 8.3 [14].

8.4.1.1.1 Knowledge Acquisition

The knowledge acquisition process usually comprises three principal stages:

1. Knowledge elicitation is the interaction between the expert and the knowledge engineer/program to elicit the expert knowledge in some systematic way.

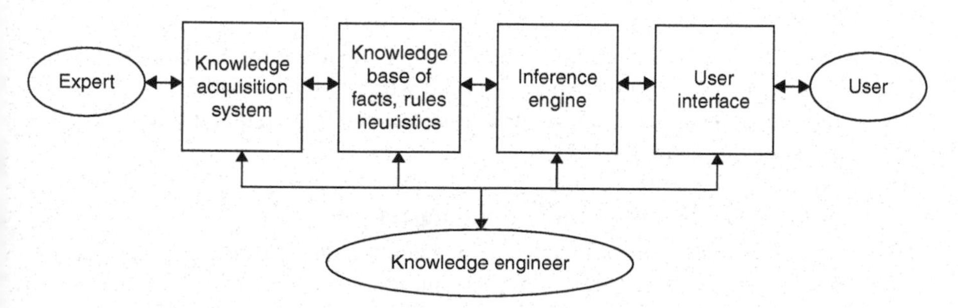

FIGURE 8.3 Architecture of expert systems [29]

2. The knowledge thus obtained is usually stored in some form of human-friendly intermediate representation.
3. The intermediate representation of the knowledge is then compiled into an executable form (e.g., production rules) that the inference engine can process.

8.4.1.1.2 The Inference Engine

We have already looked at production systems, and how they can be used to generate new information and solve problems.

Recall the steps in the basic recognize act cycle:

1. Match the premise patterns of the rules against elements in the working memory. Generally, the rules will be domain knowledge built into the system, and the working memory will contain the case-based facts entered into the system, plus any new facts that have been derived from them.
2. If there is more than one rule that can be applied, use a conflict resolution strategy to choose one to apply. Stop if no further rules are applicable.
3. Activate the chosen rule, which generally means adding/deleting an item to/from working memory. Stop if a terminating condition is reached or return to step 1. Early production systems spent over 90% of their time doing pattern matching, but there is now a solution to this efficiency problem [14].

8.4.1.1.3 The User Interface

The expert system user interface usually comprises two basic components:

1. The interviewer component
   This controls the dialogue with the user and/or allows any measured data to be read into the system. For example, it might ask the user a series of questions, or it might read a file containing a series of test results.
2. The explanation component
   This gives the system's solution, and also makes the system's operation transparent by providing the user with information about its reasoning process [14].

8.4.1.2 Representing the Knowledge

We have already discussed various types of knowledge representation. In general, the knowledge acquired from our expert will be formulated in two ways:

1. Intermediate representation is a structured knowledge representation that the knowledge engineer and expert can both work with efficiently.
2. Production system is a formulation that the expert system's inference engine can process efficiently [14].

8.4.1.3 Knowledge Representation Techniques

Knowledge representation is defined as "[t]he encoding and storage of knowledge in computational models of cognition." Representation of knowledge in computational models is a complex problem. Its complexity makes it difficult to devise good knowledge representation techniques. However, there are criteria for judging their goodness [15]:

- Semantic networks
- Production rules
- Frames

8.4.2 Medical Expert Systems

Medical expert systems will begin to appear, however, as researchers in medical artificial intelligence (AI) continue to make progress in key areas, such as knowledge acquisition. It is accordingly important for physicians to understand the current state of such research and the theoretic and logistic barriers that remain before useful systems can be made available.

8.4.2.1 Expert Systems Tasks of Medical Domains

1. Diagnostic assistance
2. Expert laboratory information systems
3. Therapy critiquing and planning
4. Agents for information retrieval
5. Generating alerts and reminders
6. Image recognition and interpretation [14]

8.4.2.2 Medical Diagnosis Using Machine Learning

Machine intelligence plays a crucial role in the design of expert systems in medical diagnosis. Expert or knowledge-based systems are the most common type of AI systems in routine clinical use. They contain medical knowledge, usually about a very specifically defined task, and are able to reason with data from individual patients to come up with reasoned conclusions.

Although there are many variations, the knowledge within an expert system is typically represented in the form of a set of rules.

Machine learning systems can be used to develop the knowledge bases used by expert systems. Given a set of clinical cases that act as examples, a machine learning system can produce a systematic description of those clinical features that uniquely characterize the clinical conditions. This knowledge can be expressed in the form of simple rules, or often as a decision tree [16].

8.5 STUDY AND REASONING IN DIABETES

Intelligent systems in diabetes focus on the main technical characteristics of four reasoning methodologies that are commonly used in developing diabetic expert systems, namely, reasoning with production rules, fuzzy reasoning, case-based reasoning (CBR), and ontological-case-based reasoning.

8.5.1 Reasoning with Production Rules

Production rules are the most commonly technique used in developing the inference engine of expert system. Forward chaining can be used to produce new facts (hence the term "production" rules), and backward chaining can deduce whether statements are true or not. Rule-based systems were one of the first large-scale commercial successes of AI research [17, 18].

8.5.2 Reasoning with Fuzzy Rules

In the rich history of rule-based reasoning in AI, the inference engines almost without exception were based on Boolean or binary logic. However, in the same way that neural networks have enriched the AI landscape by providing an alternative to symbol processing techniques, fuzzy logic has provided an alternative to Boolean logic-based systems. Unlike Boolean logic, which has only two states (true or false), fuzzy logic deals with truth values that range continuously from 0.0 to 1.0. Thus, something could be half true (0.5) or very likely true (0.9) or probably not true (0.1) [19].

Reasoning with fuzzy rule systems is a forward-chaining procedure. The initial numeric data values are fuzzified, that is, turned into fuzzy values using the membership functions. Instead of a match and conflict resolution phase where we select a triggered rule to fire, in fuzzy systems, all rules are evaluated because all fuzzy rules can be true to some degree (ranging from 0.0 to 1.0). The antecedent clause truth values are combined using fuzzy logic operators (a fuzzy conjunction and/or operation takes the minimum value of the two fuzzy clauses). Next, the fuzzy sets specified in the consequent clauses of all rules are combined, using the rule truth values as scaling factors. The result is a single fuzzy set, which is then defuzzified to return a crisp output value.

8.5.3 Reasoning with Cases

CBR means reasoning from experiences (old cases) in an effort to solve problems, critique solutions, and explain anomalous situations. The CBR approach to problem-solving and learning has drawn significant attention within the AI community over the last few years [20]. The CBR systems' expertise is embodied in a collection (library) of past cases rather than being encoded in classical rules. Each case typically contains a description of the problem plus a solution and/or the outcomes. The knowledge and reasoning process used by an expert to solve the problem is not recorded, but is implicit in the solution [21].

8.5.4 Ontological Case-Based Reasoning Methodology for Diabetes Management

Ontology is a formal and explicit specification of a shared conceptualization. It defines a common vocabulary for researchers who need to share information in a domain. It includes machine-interpret definitions of basic concepts (classes) in the domain, properties of each concept describing various features and attributes of the concept (slots, relationships), and restrictions on slots (facets or role restrictions). Ontology together with a set of individual instances of classes constitutes a knowledge base [22].

8.6 THE PROPOSED SYSTEM

Body mass index (BMI) of the diabetics is divided into six categories [23].

8.6.1 Knowledge Analysis

The structure of the system contains three main steps. First, it calculates the total needs of calories; second, it determines the actual amount of calories of the items; and third, it concludes the proper diet.

8.6.2 Total Calories

A first step to calculate the total calories (TC) is to calculate the BMI using equation (8.1):

$$\text{BMI} = (\text{weight (kg)})/(\text{height (m)})^2 \tag{8.1}$$

Then, using the BMI we determine whether the diabetic patients are classified as slim, obese, or normal according to the World Health Organization (WHO) BMI classification. Furthermore, the activity type of the patient is needed to be specified, where it could be very active, moderately active, or little active, according to Figure 8.4. Then equation (8.2) is used to calculate the TC. Figure 8.4 shows the flow diagram to calculate the TC.

$$\text{TC} = \text{activity type (calorie/kg)} * \text{weight (kg)} \tag{8.2}$$

8.6.3. Amount of Items

The diet recommendations made by the American Diabetes Association contain carbohydrates, proteins, and fats [24]. The diet uses portion control and scheduling to help manage glucose levels throughout the day. From the TC we determine the daily amount of each item.

8.6.4. List of Diet

A proper diabetes diet is balanced and based on healthy foods. We select the contents of the proper diet that satisfy the amount of each item from the exchange list where, for example, 1 g of carbohydrates = 4 cal, 1 g of protein = 4 cal, and 1 g of fats = 9 cal.

Food groups are exchange lists of foods that contain roughly the same mixture of carbohydrates, protein, fat, and calories; serving sizes are defined so that each will have the same amount of carbohydrate, fat, and protein as any other. Actually, we determine the amount of each item in the food groups as shown in Table 8.3.

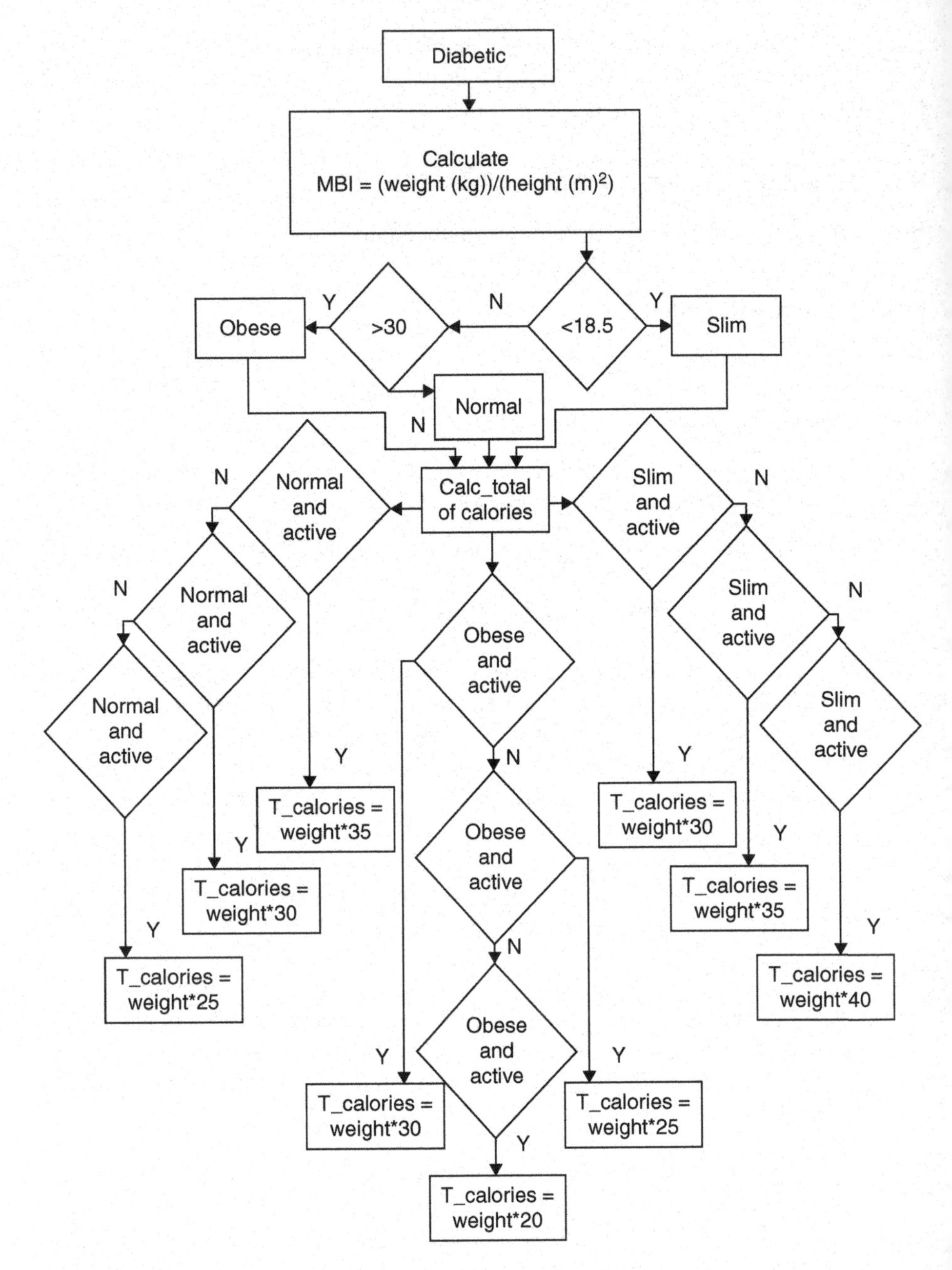

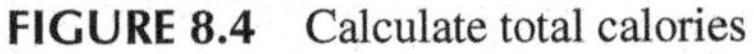
FIGURE 8.4 Calculate total calories

8.6.5 Knowledge Representation

Knowledge representation allows one to specify and emulate systems of a growing complexity. Knowledge representation schemes indeed have known an important evolution, from basic schemes supporting a rather heuristic approach to advanced

TABLE 8.3
Standards of Items [66]

Fat & Milk		Sugar		Proteins	
Name	**Amount**	**Name**	**Amount**	**Name**	**Amount**
Oil	1 spoon (20 g)	Sugar	1 spoon (20 g)	Chicken	1/4 piece (250 g)
Shortening	1 spoon (20 g)	Jam	1 spoon (20 g)	Egg	1 piece
Synths	1 spoon (20 g)	Cake	1 piece	Fish	125 g
Milk	1 cup	Tahnia	1 spoon (20 g)	Meat	Kumsha (100 g)
Yogurt	100 g	Sweet	1 piece	Tamiea	4 pieces (40 g)
Cheese	50 g	S_drinks	75 mL	Bean	Kumsha (100 g)
–	–	Pasta	1 small piece	Lentils	Kumsha (100 g)
				Foul	Kumsha (100 g)

Fruits		Vegetables		Starch	
Name	**Amount**	**Name**	**Amount**	**Name**	**Amount**
Banana	Small piece (100 g)	Salad	Free (open)	Custer	1 cup
Orange	Small piece (100 g)	Molokhia	Kumsha	Kissra	2 pieces (100 g)
Mango	Small piece (100 g)	Bazenjan	Kumsha	Gorasa	1/2 piece (100 g)
Dates	3 pieces (24 g)	Okra	Kumsha	Bread	1 piece (120 g)
Grapes	10 pieces (120 g)	Potatoes	2 Kumsha	Rice	1 cup
W_melon	2 slices (120 g)	Regla	2 Kumsha	Macaroni	1 cup
Apple	1 small piece (100 g)	Taglia	Kumsha	Potato	1 big piece
Guava	1 small piece (100 g)	Roub	2 Kumsha	Noodles	1 cup

schemes involving a deeper consideration of the various dependencies between knowledge elements [25, 26]. There are three types of diabetes: type 1, type 2, and gestational diabetes. We focus on type 2 that can managed by exercise, diagnosis, and diet. We concentrate on diet using serving base and calories base as depicted in Figure 8.5.

8.6.6 Food Groups Servings

Some diseases increase the risk of diabetes disease and affect the number of servings in the food groups. The major diseases we got from our knowledge acquisition

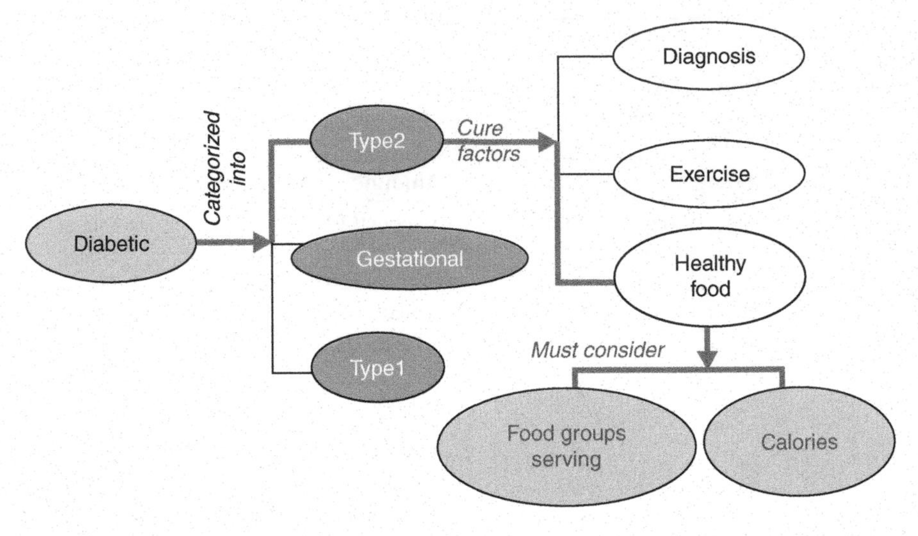

FIGURE 8.5 Types of diabetes

are anorexia, surgery, blood pressure, typhoid, bitter, liver problems, heart disease, and gout. Other factors that affect the serving are the patient activity and weight (see Figure 8.6).

8.6.7 Knowledge Management

Knowledge was managed through the semantic network. The following is the algorithm to specify the number of servings for each patient:

1. Determine whether the patient is slim, moderate, or obese.
2. Determine whether the patient activity is high, moderate, or little.
3. Determine whether the patient is infected with anorexia, surgery, blood pressure, typhoid, bitter, liver problems, heart disease, and gout
4. Calculate the number of servings as follows:
   - Vegetable servings =3
   - If (anorexia=1) or (surgery=1) or (age>65), then fruit servings =4; else fruit servings =2
   - If activity="normal," then crab-servings=6; else if activity="high," then crab servings=8
   - If the patient is underweight, then crab servings=10
   - If ((gout =1) or (heart disease=1) or (bitter=1) or (liver problems=1) or (blood pressure=1) or (typhoid=1)), then protein servings=2; else protein servings=3
   - If ((gout =1) or (heart disease=1) or (bitter=1) or (liver problems=1) or (blood pressure=1) or (typhoid=1)), then milk servings=2; else milk servings=3

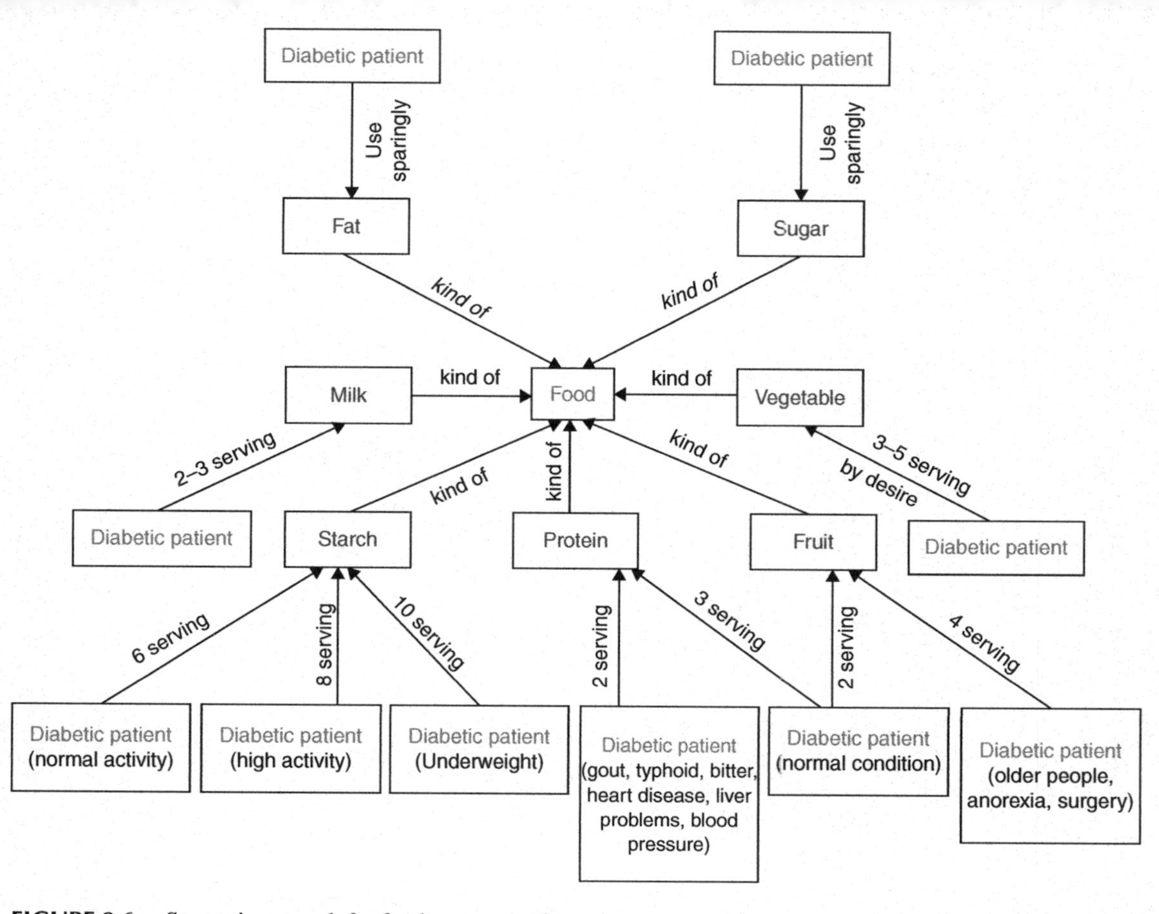

FIGURE 8.6 Semantic network for food groups servings

8.7 DESIGN AND IMPLEMENTATION

The guide pyramid consists of seven main groups: starch, vegetables, fruits, protein, milk, fat, and sugar. Each group has similar amount of calories. Based on the well-defined pyramid, the healthy eating must be high in nutrients, low in fat, and foods that are high in carbohydrates which increase BGLs [23].

Figure 8.7 shows the Sudanese food guide pyramid based on the diabetes food guide pyramid reported in lectures but modified according to the Sudanese food culture. From the pyramid, examples of foods that increase BGLs are grains, beans, starch, and vegetables group, the fruits group, and the milk group. Other foods that raise blood glucose are sweets, found in the top of the pyramid. Starchy foods, sweet foods, fruits, and milk are high in carbohydrate. On the other hand, vegetables group, meat and others group, and fats do not increase the BGL. According to the healthy pyramid, diabetes patients should eat 6–11 servings grains, 2–5 servings vegetable group, 2–4 servings fruit group, 2–3 servings milk group, and 2–3 servings protein group, and sugars group and oils should rarely be eaten [27].

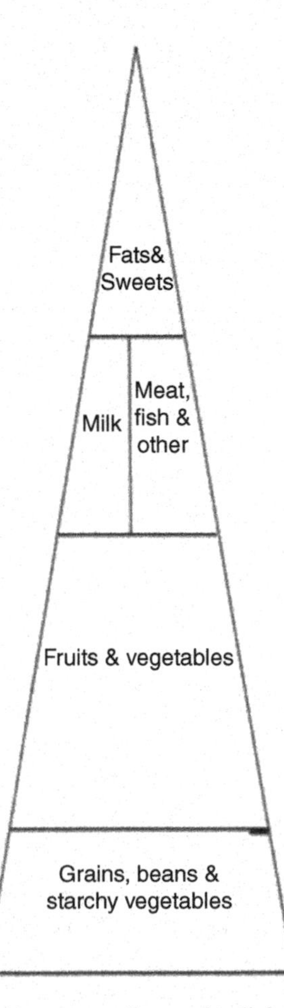

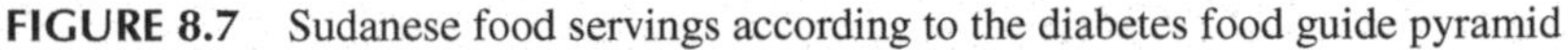

FIGURE 8.7 Sudanese food servings according to the diabetes food guide pyramid

8.7.1 Formalization

The information and knowledge collected were modeled into two forms to facilitate the understanding of how the system will operate and how it arrives at its conclusion:

1. For calculating food servings and the number of calories, rule-based representation is used. Equation 8.1 shows the calculation of the BMI [23].
2. Frame based representation is used to connect food types and subcategories of each class according to diabetics healthy food pyramid, where we find that slots provide us with more information about each Sudanese food category and subcategory, and more description means better reflection of the knowledge.

Figure 8.8 shows the sample of diabetics food frame representation and Figure 8.9 shows the proposed system architecture. As shown in the figure, the system starts asking the user to enter his or her personal information showing the Patient dialog. Based on these information, the number of servings is calculated and hence appears in the next Food groups dialog in which the patient gives permission to select the interested food list from the system food recommendations. Finally, the system connects all gathered information and performs inferences through its knowledge engine process to output a recommended five meals a day for every patient (breakfast, lunch, dinner, and two snacks).

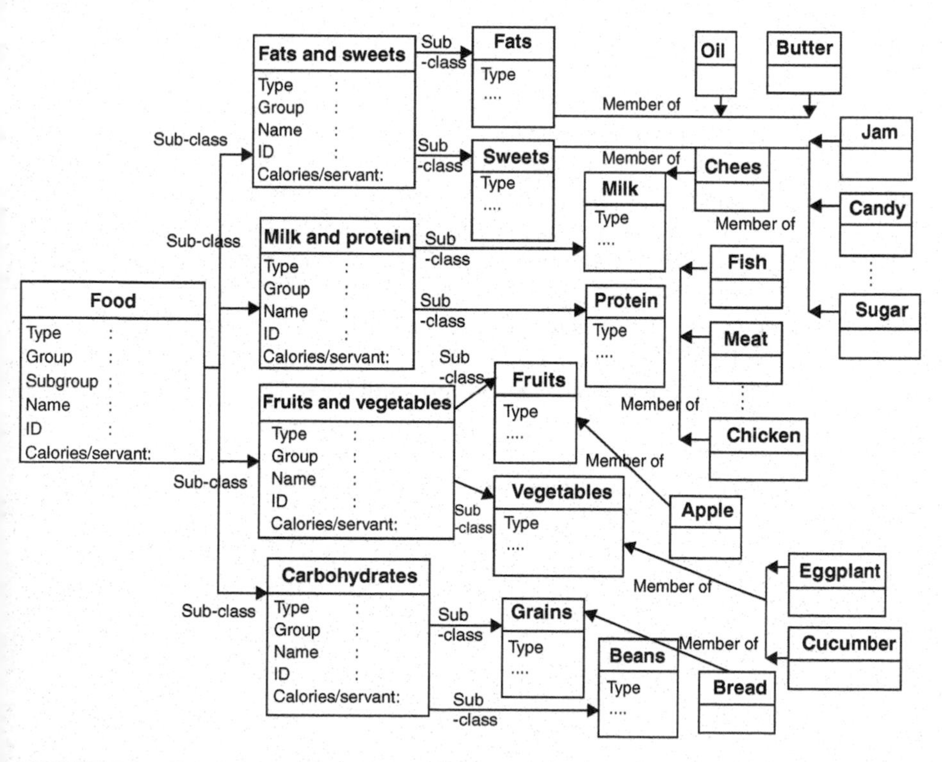

FIGURE 8.8 Sample of diabetics food frame representation

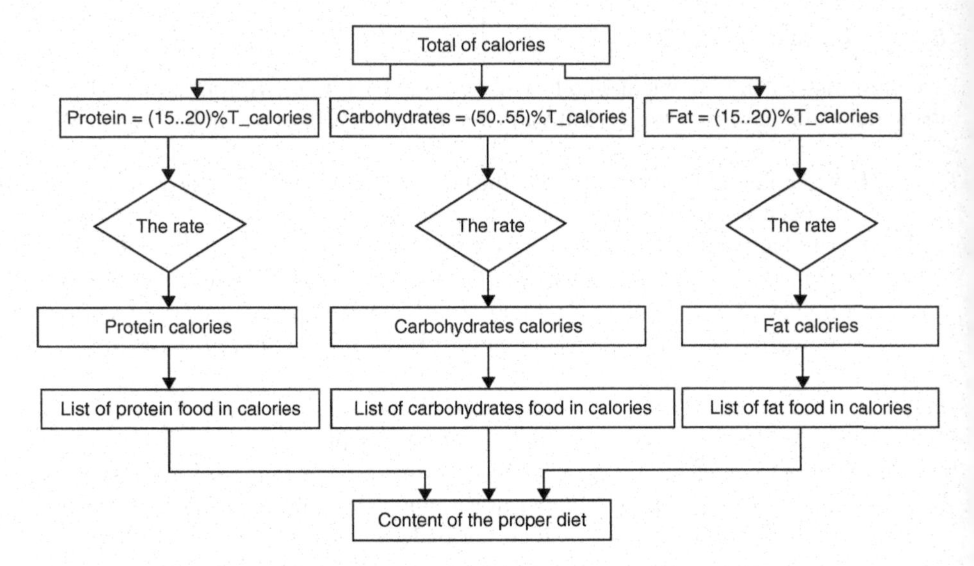

FIGURE 8.9 The structure of the proposed system

Another step is to calculate the TC, which needs to calculate the BMI using equation (8.1).Then using the BMI we determine whether the diabetic patients are classified as slim, obese, or normal according to the WHO BMI classification. Furthermore, the activity type of the patient is needed to be specified where it could be very active, moderately activity, or little active. Then equation (8.2) is used to calculate the TC.

The systems developed so far have used a command-driven, dialog-type user interface. Increasingly windows and menus are being used to make interfaces easier to understand and work with. In the context of the meal plan, age, gender, BMI, BGL, physical activity, and the related diseases with diabetes are the main risk factors to consider. The outcome of each of these factors directly or indirectly depends on one or more of the other(s), and the overall reaction determines the plan outcomes.

The system consists of two main graphical user interface components. The first component is the Patient dialog which consists of name, gender, age, weight, height, activity type, BGL, favorite meals, and additional diseases. The second is the Food groups dialog which consists of items names and items list

The Implementation phase involves the actual coding of the system (writing of the Prolog commands that run the system). The codes were developed and customized in Visual Prolog.

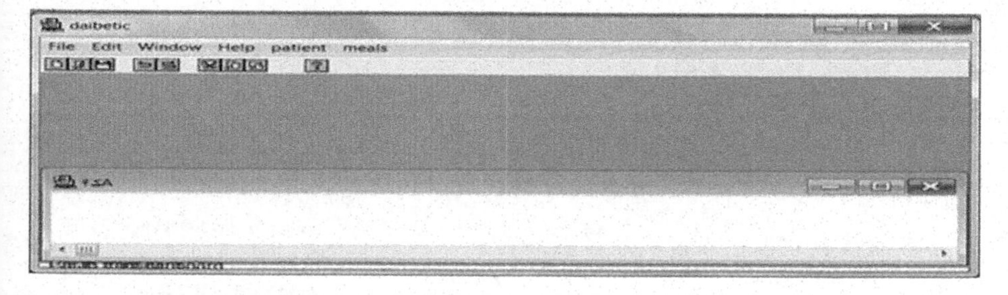

FIGURE 8.10 The main window of the system.

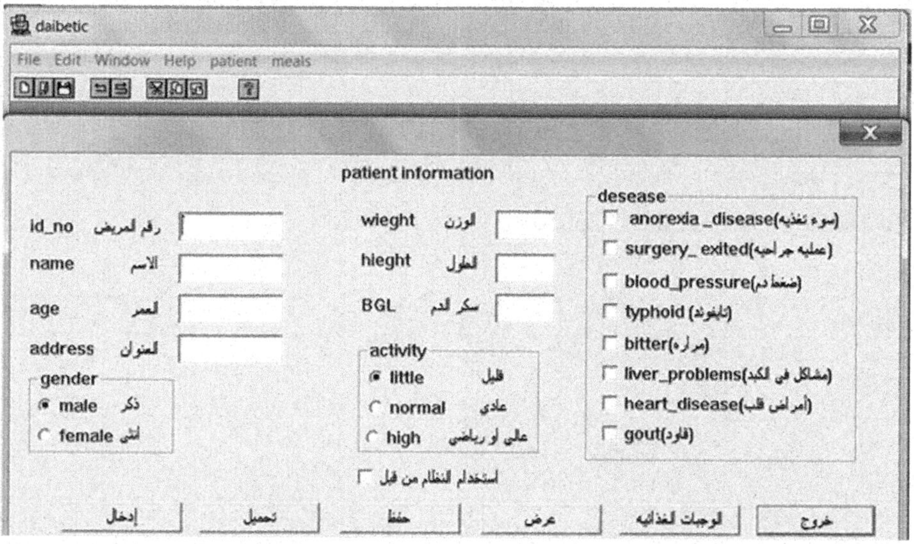

FIGURE 8.11 Submenu patient dialog

8.7.2 How the System Works

The system started from the main menu which consisted of two submenus, Patient menu which led to Patient dialog and Meals menu which led to meals dialog. Figure 8.10 presents the main window of the system.

When the user selects the patient from the main window, the Patient dialog box appears (see Figure 8.11).

Then the user fills his or her personal information including the diseases from the check boxes and then clicks the insert button and saves the knowledge to the database after loaded to the file (see Figure 8.12).

If the user used the meal plan before and his or her BGL is still above 140, the system recommends him or her to visit the doctor through the new dialog (see Figure 8.13).

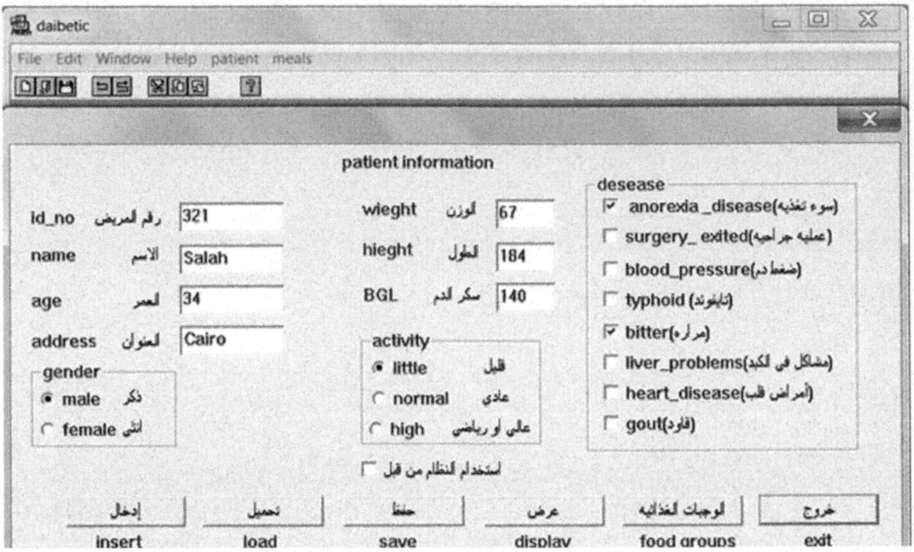

FIGURE 8.12 Filled patient information

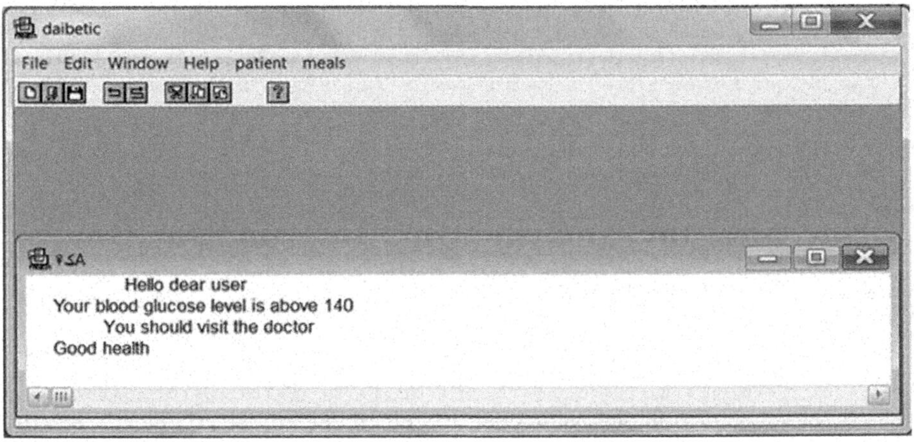

FIGURE 8.13 Recommendation to doctor

In the Food group dialog, the recommended number of servings appears and the patient is allowed to select the different type of any item from the concerning list. After selection of the items from the list, the user (patient) clicks the food group button to appear the report which contains the five recommended meals (see Figure 8.14).

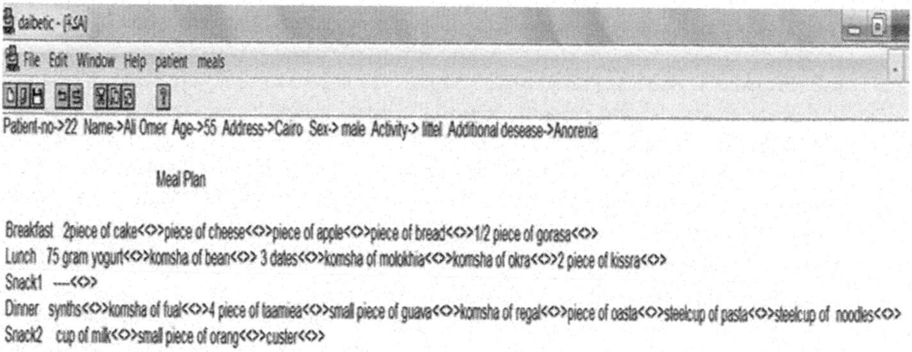

daibetic - [FSA]

File Edit Window Help patient meals

Patient-no->22 Name->Ali Omer Age->55 Address->Cairo Sex-> male Activity-> littel Additional desease->Anorexia

Meal Plan

Breakfast 2piece of cake<<>>piece of cheese<<>>piece of apple<<>>piece of bread<<>>1/2 piece of gorasa<<>>
Lunch 75 gram yogurt<<>>komsha of bean<<>> 3 dates<<>>komsha of molokhia<<>>komsha of okra<<>>2 piece of kissra<<>>
Snack1 ---<<>>
Dinner synths<<>>komsha of fual<<>>4 piece of taamiea<<>>small piece of guava<<>>komsha of regal<<>>piece of oasta<<>>steelcup of pasta<<>>steelcup of noodles<<>>
Snack2 cup of mik<<>>small piece of orang<<>>custer<<>>

FIGURE 8.14 Serving based meal plan report

REFERENCES

1. Shyi-Ming Chen and Yun-hou, "Fuzzy reasoning techniques and domain ontology for anti-diabetic drugs recommendation", *Lecture Notes in Computer Science*, Vol. 7196, pp. 125–135, Taiwan, 2012.
2. F. Ekram, L. Sun, O. Vahidi, E. Kwok, R and B. Gopaluni, "A feedback glucose control strategy for type II diabetes mellitus based on fuzzy logic", *The Canadian Journal of Chemical Engineering*, pp. 1411–1417, 5 Mar 2012.
3. Audrey Mbogho, Joel Dave and Kulani Makhubele, "Diabetes advisor a medical expert system for diabetes management", University of Cape Town, pp. 84–87, 2005.
4. Diabetic Diet Plan and Food Guide. www.diabeticdietfordiabetes.com/foods.htm (Accessed 22 May 2014).
5. Awad M. Ahmed and Nada Hassan Ahmed, "Diabetes mellitus in Sudan: The size of the problem and the possibilities of efficient care", *Practical Diabetes* Int, Vol. 18, No. 9, pp. 324–327, 2001.
6. William T. Cefalu, "Standards of medical care in diabetes", *American Diabetes Association*, Vol. 38, 2015.
7. Hsinchun Chen, Sherrilynne S. Fuller, Carol Friedman and William Hersh, Medical Informatics, Springer Science+Business Media, Inc., 2005.
8. Edward H. Shortliffe, Bruce G. Buchana and Edward A. Feigenbaum, "Knowledge engineering to medical decision making: A review of computer-based clinical decision aids", *Proceedings of the IEEE*, pp. 1207–1224, 1981.
9. Okechukwu Felix Erondu, "Medical imaging", *Janeza Trdine* 9, 51000 Rijeka, Croatia, 2011.
10. Principles_of_Good_Medical_Education. www.gmcuk.org/ (Accessed 30 May 2015).
11. Kumar and Clark, Clinical Medicine Fifth Edition, British Medical Association, www.kumarandclark.com, 2003.
12. "Diet for diabetes patient". www.medmint.com/CONTENT/Diabetics/Diabetics_7.html (Accessed 3 May 2013).
13. World Diabetes Day, "Diabetes education and prevention". www.diabetes-diabetic-diet.com (Accessed July 2012).
14. Amani Al-Ajlan, "*Medical expert systems HDP and PUFF*", King Saud University College of Computer & Information Sciences, Department Of Computer Science, Course CSC 562, 2007.

15. John F. Sowa, "Semantic networks". www.jfsowa.com/pubs/semnet.htm (Accessed December 2015).
16. E.S. Prasadl, N. Krishna Prasad and Y. Sagar, "An approach to develop expert systems in medical diagnosis using machine learning", *International Journal on Soft Computing*, Vol. 2, No. 1, February 2011.
17. Matthew Wiley and Razvan Bunescu, "*Emerging applications for intelligent diabetes management Cindy Marling*", Association for the Advancement of Artificial Intelligence, 2011.
18. Wioletta Szajnar and Galina Setlak, "A concept of building an intelligence system to support diabetes diagnostics", *Studia Informatica*, 2011.
19. P.M. Beulah Devamalar, V. Thulasi Bai and S.K. Srivatsa, "*An architecture for a fully automated real-time web-centric expert system*", World Academy of Science, Engineering and Technology, 2007.
20. Sanjeev Kumar and Bhimrao Babasaheb, "Development of knowledge base expert system for natural treatment of diabetes disease", *International Journal of Advanced Computer Science and Applications*, Vol. 3, No. 3, pp. 44–47,2012.
21. Jaime Cantais, David Dominguez, Valeria Gigante, Loredana Laera and Valentina Tamma, "*An example of food ontology for diabetes control*", International Semantic Web Conference, 2005.
22. M. Cindy, S. Jay and S. Frank, "Toward case based reasoning for diabetes management", *Computational Intelligence Journal*, Vol. 25, No. 3, pp. 165–179, 2009.
23. A. Igbal and M. Nagwa, "Health guide for diabetics", Sudan Federal Ministry of Health, 2010.
24. "The ratio of fats, carbohydrates and protein for diabetics". www.Livestrong.com /article /363268-/ (Accessed May 2011).
25. Stephan Grimm, Pascal Hitzler and Andreas Abecker, "Knowledge representation and ontologies logic, ontologies and SemanticWeb languages", University of Karlsruhe, pp. 37–87, Germany, 2007.
26. Abdullah Al-Malaise Al-Ghamdi, Majda A. Wazzan, Fatimah M. Mujallid and Najwa K. Bakhsh, "An expert system of determining diabetes treatment based on Cloud Computing platforms", *International Journal of Computer Science and Information Technologies*, Vol. 2, No. 5, pp. 1982–1987, 2011.
27. Karen Halderson and Martha Archuleta, "Control your diabetic for life", College of Agriculture and Home Economics, NM State University, pp. 631A1–631A4, 2013.

9 An Approach for Designing of Domain Models in Smart Health Informatics Systems Considering Their Cognitive Characteristics

Olena Chebanyuk, and Olexandr Palahin

CONTENTS

9.1 INTRODUCTION

To design quality model in Smart Health Information System, it is necessary to spend some efforts to design well-structured model. Requirements for the stable and well-designed models are the following:

- Consider peculiarities of human perception.
- Full and strict representation of the system.
- Possibility to analyze the whole system as well as to investigate detailed algorithms or structure of some system components.
- Representation of system functionality or structure in full and noncontradictory way.
- Metamodeling notation for representation of metamodels must provide compact and detailed representation of metamodels in order to design quality models that would satisfy metamodeling notation as well as all stakeholders' needs.

According to peculiarities of human perception, the part of visual perception consists nearly 87%. That is why in order to design a model the visual notation should be involved. Such a notation should allow the representation of systems from different sides and cover different aspects of the Smart Health System. Today one of the most widespread graphical notations for covering all requirements formulated above is unified modeling language – UML (UML, 2017. This modeling language is used by many software development enterprises. Researches devoted to ontologies designing and domain analysis involve UML for representation of both structural and behavioral characteristics of the system. The use of UML for modeling Smart Health Informatics Systems answers the following requirements of the modeling area:

- Representation of different kinds of models, namely, static and dynamic ones. Such models are aimed to represent different scales of the system and consider a system from different points of view.
- Methods of domain engineering techniques and ontology designing use UML diagrams as software development artifacts that contain initial information and resulting information of domain analysis.
- Σ allows to process surface of model structure. Many modeling environments store information about UML diagrams in XMI (XML Metadata Interchange) (OMG, 2015) format. (XMI is a standard for metadata interchange, proposed by Object Management Group (OMG, 2016)). in order to satisfy challenges for well-designed model It supports many tools for software model processing, namely transformation, refinement, merging, and .

- It supports many tools for models transformation, refinement, merging, and comparing; UML diagrams processing (Eclipse Modeling Tools, IBM Rational Products, Microsoft Tools and plugins, online diagram designing tools, and others).
- Presence of well-designed standards (OMG and IEEE) for models and metamodels representation.
- There are business-modeling templates for many problem domains.

Illustration that proves the fact that UML notation is used for representation of system behavior with different levels of details is presented in Figure 9.1.

Figure 9.1 illustrates that more detailed notation allows representing a system by means of drawing more complex diagram for comprehension and analysis. Large number of details allows understanding of the system from the one hand, but making comprehension of model more complex and taking a background for forgetting some details.

After grounding the choice of modeling notation for Smart Health Informatics Systems representation, the next step is to formulate the challenges for good model. The main aspect of models estimation is grounded on human cognitive abilities.

This chapter is organized as follows: Section 9.2 is devoted to considering approaches of domain models designing. Section 9.3 is dealt with the analysis of human cognitive design principles while UML diagrams are comprehended. Section 9.4 provides an introduction to domain analysis, covering aspects of general definitions from domain analysis and explaining terms from cognitive science that are related to mechanisms of human comprehension. Section 9.5 explains the main aspects concerning different types of domain analysis methods. It gives a background for performing comparison of types of domain analysis methods, which is performed in Section 9.6. This section provides a background of theoretical foundation for defining cognitive activities that are performed in different domain analysis activities matching them with theoretical foundations in domain analysis activities performing. Investigated peculiarities of domain analysis allow to formulate tasks and challenges for methods of domain models designing (Section 9.7) and research questions (RQs) (Section 9.8). Then, in Section 9.9, the area of domain models usage is introduced. Section 9.10 is devoted to the investigation of factors that influence domain models' cognitive value. Composition of these factors enables the design analytical models for estimation of domain models' cognitive characteristics. Then rules for estimating cognitive values of UML diagrams are introduced in Section

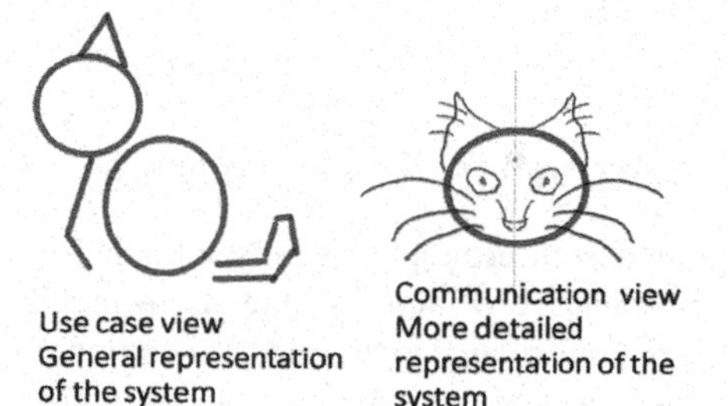

FIGURE 9.1 Analogies between the level of details in different UML diagram notations and possibility to represent details of UML diagram in health information system.

9.11. Researches that are described above become a basis for formulating a proposed approach for domain models designing, which is described in Section 9.12. Section 9.13 explains the sequence of steps performed to design a domain model for deep learning neural networks to investigate brain tumors. The last section (Conclusion) summarizes the performed investigations and illustrates advantages of the proposed approach.

9.2 ANALYSIS OF COGNITIVE MECHANISMS INFLUENCING UML DIAGRAMS PERCEPTION

Cognitive science is concerned with understanding the processes that the brain uses to accomplish complex tasks, including:

- Perceiving
- Learning
- Remembering
- Thinking
- Predicting
- Inference
- Problem solving
- Decision-making
- Planning
- Moving around the environment.

The goal of a cognitive modeling is to design models convenient for human perception according to cognitive processes and laws (Thagard, 1996).

One of the cognitive activities is to design models with the aim of analyzing internal structure of objects (in our case, they are information systems) or system behavior. Another important function of such models is communicative when one can study the system structure and its behavior.

Laws of human comprehension of models' comprehension were studied well. For instance, Mangano et al. (2015) analyzed the role of sketches when pairs of software designers are working on design problems.

At a cognitive level, processing of UML diagrams consists of constructing (generating, transforming, and evaluating) their representations until they became precise and concrete (Allen, 2015). This question was explored by Visser (2006). Effective visualization of complex system is possible when graphical representation of this system allows comprehending a system as a set of components.

9.3 HUMAN COGNITIVE DESIGN PRINCIPLES

Investigation of cognitive design principles is presented in Tversky et al. (2006). The authors underlined two cognitive principles, namely, principles of congruence and apprehension. The idea of *congruence principle* is to compare visual patterns, which are known for person with new ones. Then one can recognize components of some complex structure using the *apprehension principle*. Collaboration of these two principles provides a common cognitive comprehension of visual models.

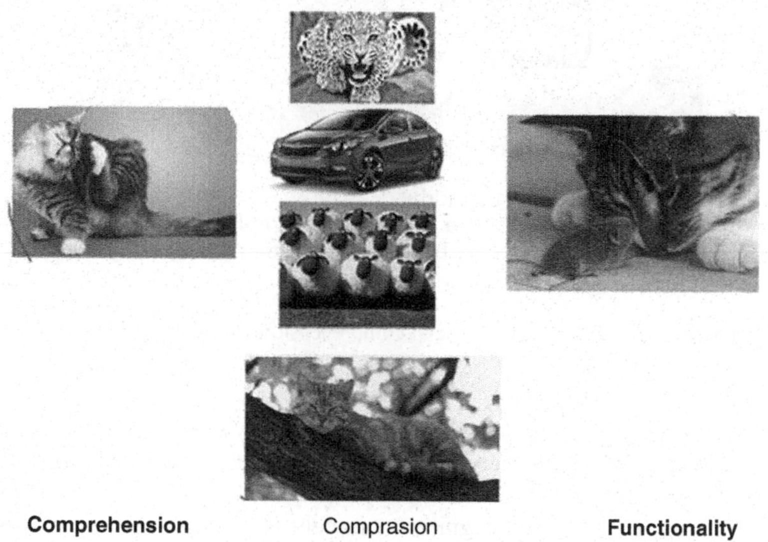

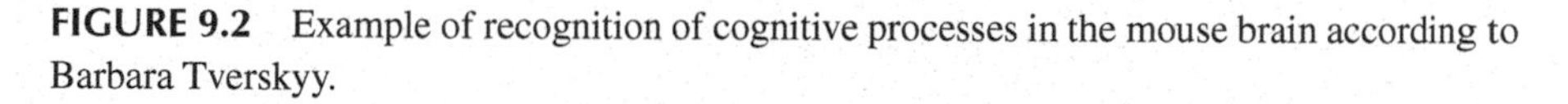

FIGURE 9.2 Example of recognition of cognitive processes in the mouse brain according to Barbara Tverskyy.

Figure 9.2 demonstrates the principles of cognitive comprehension by Barbara Tverskyy.

Figure 9.2 illustrates the process of models comprehension. The essence of the comparison approach is "to load a models into brain" (the first comprehension of visual model). In the comprehension stage, the brain of the mouse fixes the model named "cat." The next stage is comparison. During the comparison stage, the brain of mouse iterates the collection of objects and the comparison procedure is performed by means of matching every object in the collection with the searched model. (According to Figure 9.2, the mouse starts to compare the given object with car, sheep, and cat.) Then every object has an associated behavior with it. According to this behavior, the mouse starts to interact with object (attracting to cat).

Some other examples of different models' visual comprehension are also considered in Tversky et al. (2006). One model is routing maps comprehension and processing. Another model is a representation of a set of sequences goal-oriented actions. In order to represent goal-oriented actions, processes of complex objects assembling are considered. These two examples allow considering that common verbal-oriented approach can facilitate a process of existing visual model modification. Examples of visual models are maps, in the first case, and drawings in the second case (Chebanuyk & Palahin, 2018). It is difficult to estimate the effectiveness of verbal description method reading the paper (Tversky et al., 2006). The authors do not propose alternative methods of visual models comprehension. Also measurement to estimate cognitive characteristics of verbal description method is absent.

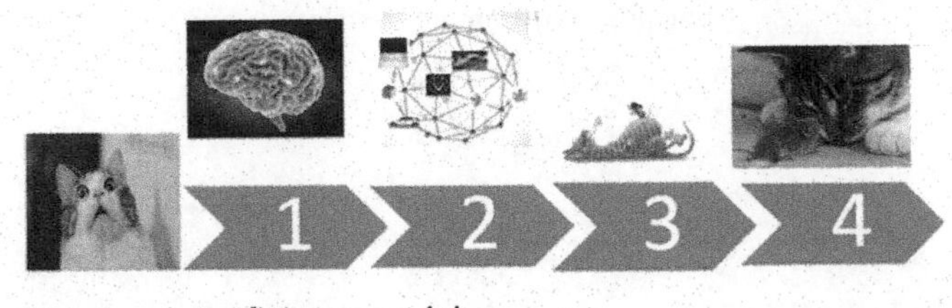

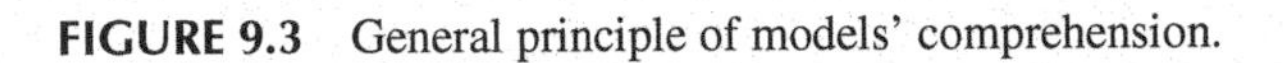

FIGURE 9.3 General principle of models' comprehension.

The general schema of the model by Barbara Tverskyy is presented in Figure 9.3. Usually cognitive behavior depends on the obtained experience and ways of interacting with a model.

Other approaches of human cognitive comprehension of models are proposed by Gureckis and Love (2010).

Gureckis and Love (2010) proposed a definition of two main principles of comprehension, namely, *direct associations* and *internal transformations*.

Using the direct associations principle, one can comprehend a sequence of patterns. The content of a particular pattern from this sequence can be forgotten partially or fully. For example, such a situation occurs when the memory is over. After comprehension of such a sequence in people's memory, just common model is left. Using this model some properties of the investigated object are predicted. Such a principle is used when a sequence of movie or sound frames is comprehended.

Using the internal transformation principle, one can match incoming patterns with those that are already existed in the memory. Existing patterns can be modified by means of adding or removing details. Such a principle is used when structural schemas are refined or new routes are established.

In the next section, an application of these principles while UML diagrams are comprehended for different purposes and situations is considered (Figure 9.4).

9.4 GENERAL DEFINITIONS FROM DOMAIN ANALYSIS AND COGNITIVE SCIENCE AREA

Human cognitive abilities have limits (Green & Blackwell, 1998). For example, Miller (1956) found that a person's short-term memory has limited capacity to remember chunks of information (Endres & Rombach, 2003). Modern psychology has even more sophisticated models of how memory works. Simon (1982) argued that "bounded rationality" is an important aspect of human problem solving, and design activities, in particular.

The goal of a cognitive model is to scientifically explain one or more of these basic cognitive processes, in particular, to understand how these processes interact (Thagart, 1996).

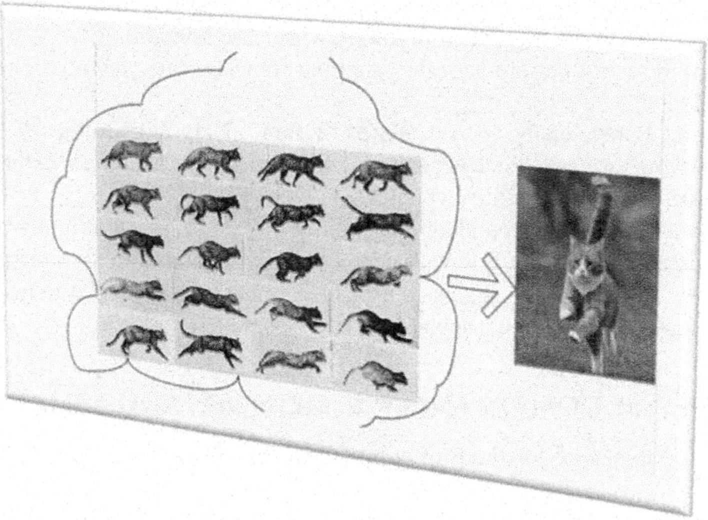

FIGURE 9.4 Illustration of model cognitive recognition process according to Gureckis and Love.

Cognitive modeling is the process of explaining human intelligence behavior by means of designing models that represent different cognitive processes (Olson & Olson, 2015).

In this chapter, we outline an approach for the estimation of different UML diagrams from cognitive science point of view.

The basic notion of this approach is the new term "Software Model Cognitive Value" (UML DIAGRAMCV) (Chebanyuk & Markov, 2015).

Cognitive value is an evaluation of both the convenience of UML diagram comprehension and understanding by humans and its design characteristics' effectiveness.

One of the features of the Agile approach (Allen, 2015; Beck et al., 2001) is that UML DIAGRAMs replace other software artifacts and have both cognitive and communicative functions.

> **Cognitive functions** of Information System models: using software models one can acquaint with algorithms, processes of UML diagram at Health Informatics Systems. The aspect of obtaining new knowledge depends upon UML DIAGRAM notation and purpose of its usage.
>
> **Communicative functions** of Information System models: one can express his understanding about software functionality, structure, or algorithm, to collaborate with other stakeholders. Then these models could be used with cognitive purpose. Using strict notation avoids misunderstanding.

A very important task is to design models of problem domain that correspond to cognitive characteristics.

Domain analysis: This involves the process of identifying, collecting, organizing, and representing the relevant information in a domain based on the study of existing systems and their development histories, knowledge captured from domain experts, underlying theory, and emerging technology within the domain.

Domain model: A definition of the functions, objects, data, and relationships in a domain (Kyo et al., 1990).

The term "domain analysis "was coined by James Neighbors in the 1980s. It is a process by which we are able to exploit commonalities in applications in the domain, capture experiences, and identify variabilities.

Domain analysis is the foundation for reusability. An important improvement of the reuse process happens when we succeed in deriving common architectures, generic models, or specialized languages by using domain analysis that helps the software development process in a specific problem area.

9.5 TYPES OF DOMAIN ANALYSIS METHODS AND APPROACHES

It is proposed to classify methods of domain analysis by the following criteria:

- Approaches aimed to improve processes of domain models designing, namely, family-oriented abstraction, specification, and translation (FAST)
- Approaches aimed to improve domain models features and properties, namely, feature-oriented domain analysis (FODA), feature-oriented reuse method (FORM); component-based product line engineering with UML (KobrA)
- Approaches that are aimed to perform an analysis of initial information sources, namely, domain analysis and reuse environment (DARE), product line UML-based software engineering (PLUS), and Koala (domain engineering approaches for embedment systems).

In order to design a model that represents characteristics of a UML diagram at Health Informatics Systems, let us consider the peculiarities of different domain analysis approaches (Frakes et al., 2005).

9.5.1 APPROACHES CONCENTRATED ON DOMAIN MODELS' DESIGNING

These techniques standards and approaches are concentrated on the designing of domain profiles and the designing of analytical approaches to represent domain models (Chebanyuk, 2013; Gómez-Romero et al., 2011) and constraints (OCL, 2014), or ontologies (Ivanova et al., 2013a; Ivanova et al., 2013b).

Gómez-Romero et al. (2011) devoted to the description of language for formal representation of interconnection between domain entities and their representations. The authors complained that there is no convenient and compact way to propose analytical tools that are compatible with plug-ins for models' transformation operations.

However, the proposed language and architecture do not allow to design models that can be estimated as high-level cognitive models. Many other researchers have proposed the improvement of one of the steps in domain models designing. While some researchers have proposed improved techniques of considering domain constraints, others are devoted to the spreading of existing graphical notation models representation (e.g., UML) for more exact representation of domain models (Ivanova, 2013a; Ivanova, 2013b).

There are works that are concentrated on new or improved methods of initial information gathering about problem domain. In other words, such papers are devoted to the development of new methods of gathering knowledge about domain and establishing relationships between them.

All methods show that the information about initial information gathering and performing domain processes analyses is performed in the mind. Initial information for gathering constrains designed manually. Then methods allowing matching domain entities with components of the model are performed.

Approaches to domain models' improvement are usually performed in the minds of domain experts after finishing the processes of domain model designing.

9.5.2 Approaches Concentrated on Improvement of Existing Techniques of Domain Models' Designing

These works are concentrated on the improvement of process gathering of information about domain models' concepts.

For example, some works have proposed decomposition of knowledges about domain into several layers. On one layer, the domain expert can systemize the knowledge about problem domain. Others have proposed the schema of knowledge systematization in the level of interface.

Asnina (2006) focused on the representation of problem domain processes with given level of precision. Every domain entity is associated with some priority. Then these priorities are arraigned. As use cases are high-level models, they represent only high-level entities. Thus, the selection procedure for defining actors and precedents are proposed. The analytical foundation of entities ranging is grounded on graph theory.

It is proposed to represent processes as graphs considering edges as entities and some actions between them as graph edges. Analyzing edges and vertexes according to priority diagrams illustrating domain processes designed.

9.5.3 Approaches of Reusing Knowledge about Domain

One approach to design knowledge for convenient reuse is storing them into databases. For knowledge database structure, it is possible to prepare different requests to obtain data for different purposes. In this area, there is a set of papers related to the improvement of mechanical UML diagrams of storing domain models into memory.

Such approaches are based on using new techniques, namely, sequentially storing of software model parts into memory, giving links to the next portion of information. Among scientific papers in this regard, the next works known are Ivanova et al. (2013 a) and Ivanova et al. (2013 b).

9.6 COLLABORATION OF DOMAIN ANALYSIS AND COGNITIVE SCIENCES AREA

Table 9.1 illustrates the activities that are performed in domain analysis corresponding to some action in the area of cognitive science.

TABLE 9.1
Matching Cognitive Activities with Domain Analysis Processes

Domain Analysis Processes	Cognitive Activities	Analytical Foundation for Providing of Mentioned Activity
Gathering information about domain	Searching and matching patterns	Graph theory
Ordering domain artifacts according to their value	Extracting knowledge from text or models	Non-strict sets
Composing domain models	Ordering domain knowledge	Predicate logic, Graph theory
Verifying domain models	Designing or refining of cognitive models	Predicate logic, Set theory
Renewing domain models	Extracting knowledge from other text or models Obtaining new domain knowledge refining of cognitive models	Second-order logics Set theory

9.7 TASK AND CHALLENGES

9.7.1 Task

In this section, we propose the domain analysis method that considers cognitive characteristics of the model. Challenges of the proposed method are the following:

- Considering cognitive characteristics of domain model
- Allowing to process initial information for domain models designing of different types (text, software models of different types, etc.)
- Considering the procedure of domain model partially renewing
- Realizing the procedure of tracing initial artifacts
- Designed domain models should satisfy the model-driven development requirements, namely, represent full and noncontradictory information about domain processes.

9.8 RESEARCH QUESTIONS NEEDED TO BE SOLVED FOR DESIGNING OF DOMAIN MODELS FOR SMART HEALTH INFORMATION SYSTEMS

RQ1: Define the aims of using domain models in Smart Health Information Systems.
RQ2: Estimate factors influencing domain models' cognitive value.

RQ3: Propose analytical foundation for domain models' cognitive value estimation.
RQ4: Define rules of domain model cognitive estimation, namely, how to explain values obtained while using mathematical apparatus.
RQ5: Propose new approaches for domain models designing that allow to update initial information about the domain.
RQ6: Make a comparative analysis of two domain models that are designed according to classical domain analysis methods and the proposed approach.

9.9 AREA AND AIMS OF DOMAIN MODELS USAGE IN SMART HEALTH INFORMATION SYSTEMS

As the aim of domain analysis is to prepare reusable knowledge or artifacts about problem domain for further usage, the domain models in Smart Health Information Systems can serve for the next purposes:

Explanation to new specialist interconnections between problem domain entities: This aim can be achieved through the following:

- New doctors involve in specialty.
- Specialists from different areas define information about the diagnosis of patient or search treatment methods.
- Specialists from neighboring areas (engineers about medical equipment, pharmacists, and others) perform actions in Smart Health Information Systems.
- Squinting of patients with information about their disease.
- Systematization of information about problem domains in scientific research.

9.10 FACTORS THAT INFLUENCE DOMAIN MODELS' COGNITIVE VALUE

Different processes of designing models for Smart Health Informatics Systems need different types of models to represent considering aspects of a system with the given level of details. The general cognitive value of a model is characterized by a set of cognitive parameters and designing characteristics, which are different for various reasons. These parameters should be integrated into a common mathematical model and this way the model may be estimated. The main cognitive parameters of software models are outlined below.

The cognitive value of a model depends on the *complexity of its notation* for its representation. Every UML diagram has its own notation. The complexity of notation depends on the number of elements and their combination that can represent some software process or structure. The more difficult model requires more efforts to comprehend it. That is why the cognitive value of a model decreases when the model is expressed by means of complex notation. It requires more time to comprehend all details and more effort to memorize it. Denote the complexity of a notation by *comp*.

The parameter *prec* depends on the *level of representation precision* of software process (behavioral UML diagrams) or structure (static UML diagrams). More precise models contain more information about process details. When a domain expert acquaints himself/herself with the model that allows precise representation of a

TABLE 9.2
Influence of Base Parameters on General Cognitive Value of Model

Parameter	Estimation of General Cognitive Value When the Considered Parameter Is	
	Increased	**Decreased**
Complexity of notation	Reduced	Raised
Precision of process (structure) representation	Raised	Reduced
Scale of domain processes	Raised	Reduced
UML diagram creation time	Reduced	Raised
The resulting: general cognitive value of model	Raised	Reduced

process or structure, he/she can get more concrete knowledge about algorithm or architectural solution. However, precise models usually represent a large amount of software features.

Also for estimating the UML DIAGRAMCV, it is necessary to consider the *time of model designing*. When this parameter is increased, the complexity of the model is increased too.

Analyze the influence of every introduced parameter on the general cognitive value of the model. Table 9.2 presents information about the influence of every parameter on common UML diagram (Chebanyuk & Markov, 2015).

9.11 ANALYTICAL FOUNDATION FOR DOMAIN MODELS' COGNITIVE VALUE ESTIMATION

From the analysis of Table 9.2, define the general cognitive value of the model:

$$CV_{type} = \frac{prec \cdot scale}{comp \cdot time} \quad (9.1)$$

where:

CV_{type} is the cognitive value of a given type UML diagram (examples are collaboration, state, class, and others according to the UML standard).

prec is the level of precision for representation of software process or structure. This parameter is measured by means of coefficient. Matching this coefficient for every type of UML diagram is based on subjective decision. This parameter varies from 0.1 to 1.

scale is the number of features from software requirement specification that are covered by UML diagram. This parameter is measured by the following way:

$$scale = \frac{repr}{total} \quad (9.2)$$

where:

repr is the number of software requirements represented in UML diagram.
total is the number of all software functional requirements for the project.
Coefficient scale is defined for concrete UML diagram, considering its tasks. This parameter also varies from 0.1 to 1.
comp is the complexity of the UML diagram notation. This parameter is defined by the number of elementary components in the specific UML diagram notation and the quantity of combinations created from them. The range for this parameter also varies from 0.1 to 1.
time is the time needed for one software model creation. This parameter sets for concrete specialist.

Such parameters as *prec* and *comp* are general. Values of the time and scale parameters are defined for every UML diagram.

Denote an amount of UML diagrams that are necessary to cover all functionality of all domain processes by C_{type}. That is why the common cognitive value of all UML diagrams of specific type is defined as follows:

$$C_{type} = CV_{type} \cdot n \tag{9.3}$$

where n is the number of UML diagrams that are necessary to represent all domain entities (processes).

When the parameter C_{type} is defined, it is very important to prove that every UML diagram has a unique content that describes the domain structure of processes.

9.12 RULES FOR ESTIMATING COGNITIVE VALUES OF DOMAIN MODELS

Expressions (9.1)–(9.3) define the UML diagram's cognitive value from the software engineering point of view. However, cognitive aspects of the UML diagram's effective processing and human perceptional abilities should be considered (Endres & Rombach, 2003; Green & Blackwell, 1998; Miller, 1956).

In order to make precise the proposed approach, rules of estimating UML diagram's cognitive value, which is designed with different aims (to represent domain processes or structure), are proposed in the following:

- The best UML diagram has the highest cognitive value.
- Every UML diagram from the set of C_{type} must have unique contents, namely, nonrepeatable elements.
- The number of UML diagram elements must be nearly to the number suggested by Miller (1956), that is, 7 (more or less two).

Both the rules for estimating general cognitive value of UML diagram and mathematical apparatus (equations 9.1–9.3) allow the estimation of general cognitive value of the UML diagram by the following way:

TABLE 9.3
Recommended Values of Miller and Unique Coefficients

Diapason (Range)	Considered Coefficient
Miller	
$elem < 9$	miller = 1.0
$10 < elem < 13$	miller = 0.6
$13 < elem < 15$	miller = 0.2
$elem > 15$	miller = 0.1
Unique	
$\lvert elem_1 - elem_2 \rvert < 3$	unique = 1.0
$3 < \lvert elem_1 - elem_2 \rvert < 5$	unique = 0.5
$5 < \lvert elem_1 - elem_2 \rvert < 7$	unique = 0.25
$\lvert elem_1 - elem_2 \rvert > 7$	unique = 0.15

$$CV_{type} = \frac{prec \cdot miller \cdot unique}{total \cdot comp \cdot time}$$

where *unique* is a coefficient defining the correspondence of general cognitive value of the UML diagram to the second rule, and *miller* is the coefficient considering the correspondence of general cognitive value of the UML diagram to the third rule. Measurements of both these coefficients are proposed in Table 9.3.

To introduce the recommended values of miller and unique coefficients (Table 9.3), an additional parameter *elem* is used. It defines the number of UML diagram's elements.

9.13 PROPOSED APPROACH OF DOMAIN ANALYSIS CONSIDERING COGNITIVE CHARACTERISTICS OF DOMAIN MODELS

The general schema of the method is presented in Figure 9.5. The proposed method integrates the model-driven software development approaches and domain analysis (Chebanyuk & Palahin, 2019).

The proposed method of domain analysis consists of the following operations:

1. Artifacts that contain information about the problem domain are gathered.
2. Between all types of artifacts, trace links are established. These links indicate how the problem domain semantic is linked with different parts of software models.
3. The transformation of behavioral UML diagram into static ones is performed by the proposed methods of transformation of models (Chebanyuk 2014a; Chebanyuk 2014b).
4. Domain models that contain both class diagrams and restrictions inherent in a particular domain are designed using a combination of known methods.

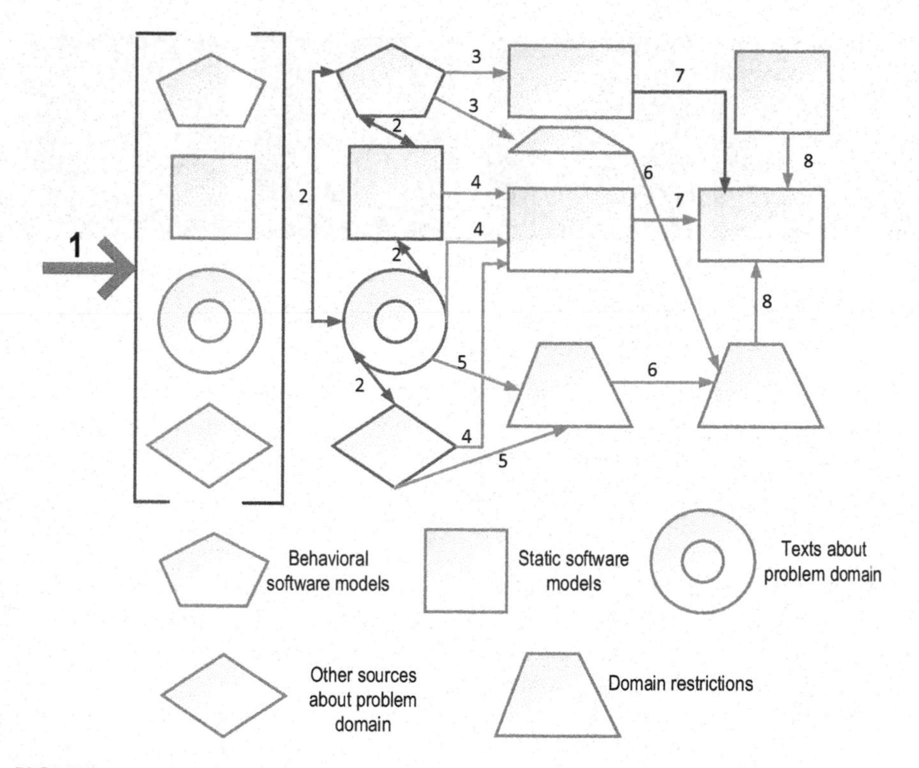

FIGURE 9.5 General schema of domain method analysis.

5. The restrictions (mostly Object Constraint Language (OCL) restrictions) are generated by means of the analysis of different sources of information about the application domain (any sources that are not static or behavioral software models).
6. The existing problem domain restrictions are complemented by newly obtained ones.
7. Newly generated software models are verified in accordance with the cognitive properties of models.
8. A trace link of the domain models and restrictions and other artifacts containing the information about the domain is conducted.

9.14 DESIGNING DOMAIN MODEL TO PERFORM DEEP LEARNING NEURAL NETWORKS TO INVESTIGATE BRAIN TUMORS

Let us consider the proposed approach by means of designing a domain model of problem domain "deep learning in the investigation of brain tumors."

The first task is to gather artifacts that contain information about the problem domain.

Gathered artifacts contain information about principles of processing images showing different brain diseases, and pictures showing photos of the brain with different diseases.

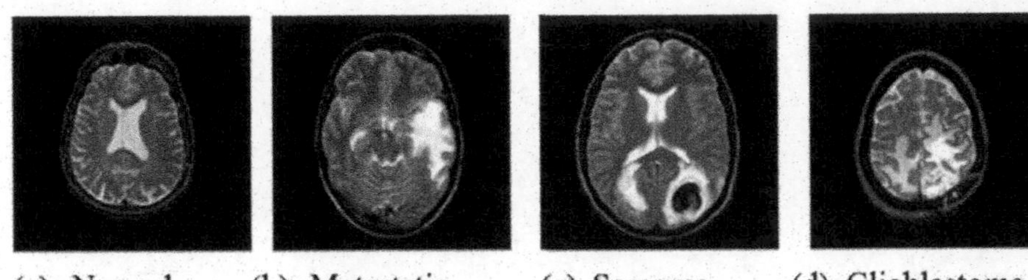

(a) Normal (b) Metastatic bronchogenic carcinoma (c) Sarcoma (d) Glioblastoma

FIGURE 9.6 Pictures of brain diseases. (From Heba et al., 2018. www.researchgate.net/profile/El-Sayed_El-Dahshan/publication/322038024_Classification_using_Deep_Learning_Neural_Networks_for_Brain_Tumors/links/5b1f9909458515270fc4e7b5/Classification-using-Deep-Learning-Neural-Networks-for-Brain-Tumors.pdf.)

Pictures showing diseases are templates for comparing a healthy and a weak brain. They are given in Figure 9.6. Information extracted from these pictures represents names of the brain diseases that are entities of problem domain: metastatic bronchogenic carcinoma, sarcoma, and glioblastoma.

Let us analyze the methodology of deep learning. The method involved in feature-oriented domain analysis defines aspects that can be treated as problem domain entities.

The proposed methodology for classifying the brain tumors in brain MRIs is as follows:

Step 1: Brain MRIs data set acquisition
Step 2: Image segmentation using Fuzzy C-means
Step 3: Feature extraction using discrete wavelet transform (DWT) and reduction using the principal component analysis (PCA) technique
Step 4: Classification using deep neural networks (Mohsen et al., 2018).

Other available information includes the principle of image segmentation when information about brain diseases is processed.

Figure 9.7 shows a two-level DWT decomposition of an image where the functions $h(n)$ and $g(n)$ represent the coefficients of the high-pass and low-pass filters, respectively. As a result, there are four subband images (LL, LH, HH, HL) at each level. The LL subband can be regarded as the approximation component of the image, while the LH, HL, and HH subbands can be regarded as the detailed components of the image (Mohsen et al., 2018).

The second step of the domain analysis is to establish links between entities. Table 9.4 summarize the results of investigation. Figure 9.8 represents the First vision of Domain model for problem domain “Deep learning system for brain tumors recognition”.

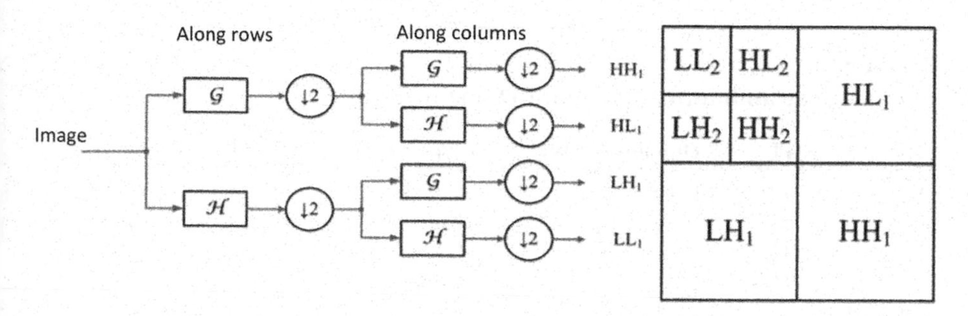

FIGURE 9.7 Principles of image processing implement discrete cosine transformation. (From Heba et al., 2018. https://www.researchgate.net/profile/El-Sayed_El-Dahshan/publication/322038024_Classification_using_Deep_Learning_Neural_Networks_for_Brain_Tumors/links/5b1f9909458515270fc4e7b5/Classification-using-Deep-Learning-Neural-Networks-for-Brain-Tumors.pdf.)

Let us demonstrate the process of domain model cognitive value estimation. An attempt is made to estimate this model according to cognitive value. The cognitive characteristics of the designed model are presented in Table 9.5.

Table 9.5 shows that the obtained cognitive value for the UML diagram is 0.77. Thus, such a model needs structural optimizations while designing (see Figures 9.9 and 9.10).

Involving an approach of changing elements into collection of objects provides an optimization of some UML diagram fragments.

The next step is to consider the proposed optimizations to design a new domain model that could satisfy the requirements of domain model cognitive values.

Let us estimate the characteristics of a domain model that is designed in Figure 9.11.

9.15 CONCLUSION

The approach for designing of domain models represented as UML diagrams considering their cognitive characteristics is proposed in this chapter. It consists of two main steps, namely, designing of domain model, and its next optimization by means of re-designing the model structure with the aim to improve its cognitive characteristics.

The proposed method of domain analysis has the following features:

- It allows to use different sources of information.
- Tracing helps to systematize different sources of information as well as avoiding its duplication.
- Constraints allow to process the model from semantic point of view.
- Possibility to trace OCL constraints with domain model parts allows to match its structural and semantic properties.
- Procedure of domain model correctness, improving its cognitive values, allows to raise its structural characteristics saving the value of semantic.

TABLE 9.4
Summarizing an Information about Domain Entities

Domain Entity1	Domain Entity2	Type of link	Reason
Part of image (LH2)	Image	Composition	LH2 is a part of image
Part of image (LH1)	Image	Composition	LH1 is a part of image
Part of image (HL1)	Image	Composition	HL1 is a part of image
Part of image (HL2)	Image	Composition	HL2 is a part of image
DWT decomposition	Image	Aggregation	DWT process images
Part of image (LH2)	DWT decomposition	Association	Algorithm that gets part of image
Part of image (LH1)	DWT decomposition	Association	Algorithm that gets part of image
Part of image (HL1)	DWT decomposition	Association	Algorithm that gets part of image
Part of image (HL2)	DWT decomposition	Association	Algorithm that gets part of image
Image segmentation	DWT decomposition	Association	One of the algorithms allowing to obtain part of image that is obtained by some rules
Brain MRIs Data set	Image	Aggregation	Images can be added or removed from databases
Metastatic bronchogenic carcinoma	Image	Composition	Image contains information about disease
Sarcoma	Image	Composition	Image contains information about disease
Glioblastoma	Image	Composition	Image contains information about disease
Metastatic bronchogenic carcinoma	Brain	Composition	Disease cannot be separated from the brain
Sarcoma	Brain	Composition	Disease cannot be separated from the brain
Glioblastoma	Brain	Composition	Disease cannot be separated from the brain

The basics for estimation cognitive characteristics of software model, related to comprehension, are introduces un paper (Tverskyy et al., 2006) and Gureckis and Love (2009), as well as on the analytical foundation of cognitive principles (the number of Miller factors that influence the choosing of notations for representation model, and foundations of cognitive principles). Investigation of interconnections between factors, which influenced the forming of domain models' total cognitive value, is presented. Then mathematical apparatus for estimation of cognitive characteristics of domain models is outlined.

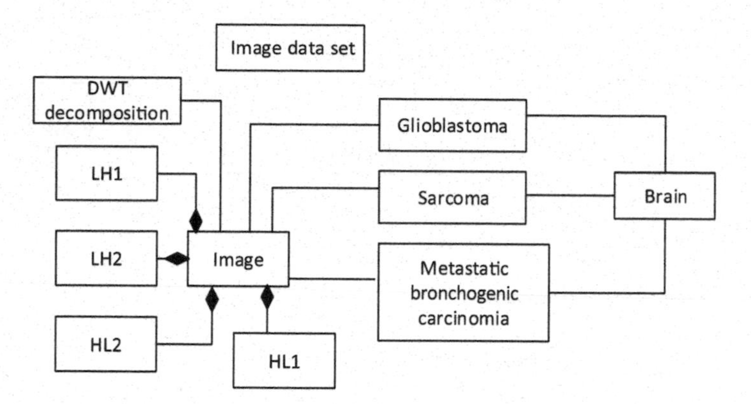

FIGURE 9.8 First vision of domain model of problem domain "deep learning system for brain tumors recognition."

TABLE 9.5
Estimation of Domain Model Cognitive Characteristics (First Approximation)

Parameter	Value	Explanation
Comp	0.3	Notation is not complex, it contains five elements (classes, interfaces, association, aggregation, and composition)
Prec	0.8	Very precise notation for understanding
Time	1 hour	Analysis of big and complex models of problem domain takes an hour
CV_{type}	$CV_{type} \frac{prec * repr * miller * unique}{total * comp * time} = \frac{0.8 * 5 * 0,6 * 1}{0,3 * 11 * 1} = \frac{2,11}{3,11} = 0,77$	The more the better
Scale	1	All problem domain entities are covered
Repr	5	
Total	1	Number of entities in diagram
Unique	1	Model contains nonrepeatable information
Miller	0.6 (10<elem<13)	Meaning is taken from Table 9.2
Elem	11	Number of elements in diagram

The proposed approach is illustrated using problem domain "deep learning neural networks for brain tumors." Designing of the problem domain model is performed in two steps, namely gathering of initial information for the model of problem domain designing, and its further structural optimization.

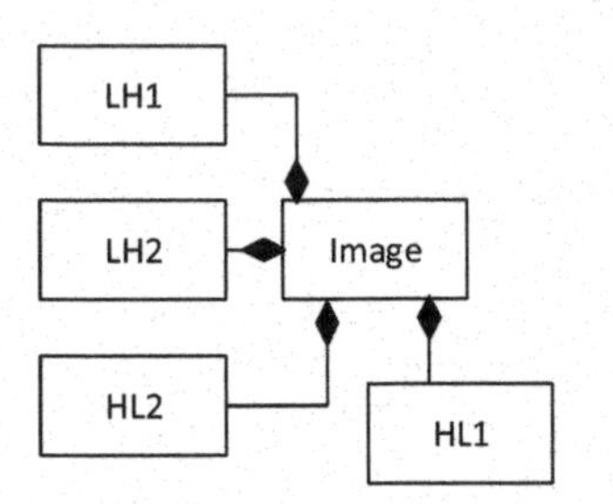

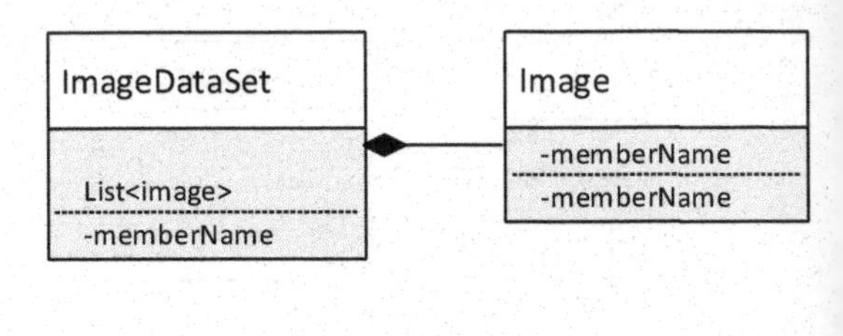

a) Image segmentation parts

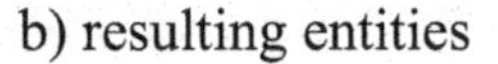

FIGURE 9.9 Representing a collection of images.

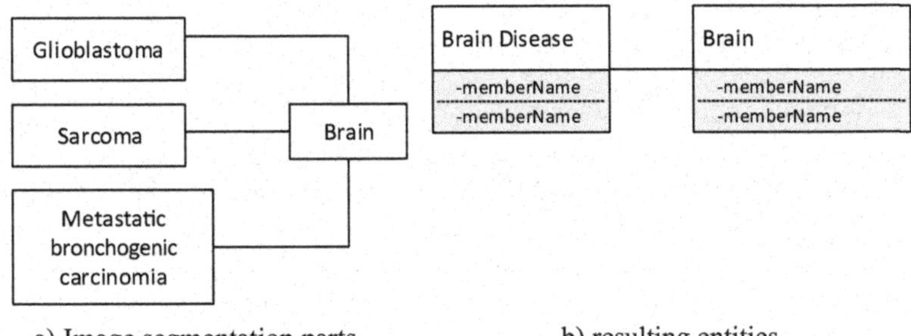

FIGURE 9.10 Representing a collection images.

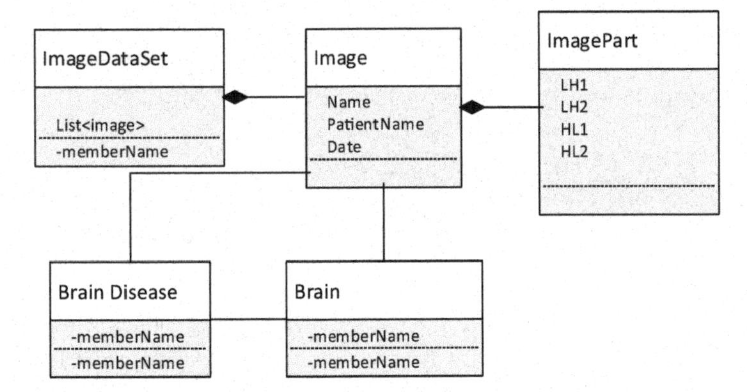

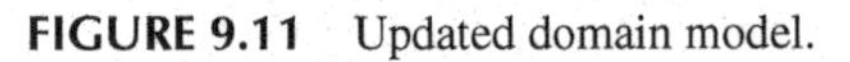
FIGURE 9.11 Updated domain model.

Great values of initial information lead to creation of great Table 9, showing interconnection between entities (Table 9.5). Estimation of model cognitive characteristics (Table 9.6) proves the necessity to perform optimization operations as composing whole objects and their parts (Figures 9.9 and 9.10).

Domain model optimization aimed to optimize the structure of model implementing collections of images and linking the entity "brain disease" with the

TABLE 9.6
Estimation of Domain Model Cognitive Characteristics after Improvement of Its Structural Characteristics

Parameter	Value	Explanation
Comp	0.3	Notation is not complex, it contains five elements (classes, interfaces, association, aggregation, and composition)
Prec	0.8	Very precise notation for understanding
Time	0.5 hour was 1 hour	Analysis of big and complex models of problem domain takes an hour
CV_{type}	$CV_{type}\frac{prec * repr * miller * unique}{total * comp * time}$ $= \frac{0.8 * 5 * 1 * 1}{0,3 * 5 * 0,5} = \frac{4}{0,75} = 5,33$	The more the better
Scale	1	All problem domain entities are covered
Repr	5	
Total	1	Scale of system representation
Unique	1	Model contains nonrepeatable information
Miller	miller = 1.0 (*elem*<9) was 0.6 (10<elem<13)	Meaning is taken from Table 9.2
Elem	5	Number of elements in diagram

entity "brain" allows to design a model whose general characteristics correspond to cognitive values. Another optimization is to represent parts of images as a collection of segments (Figure 9.9).

After modernizing the model structure (Figures 9.8 and 9.11), its cognitive value is increased by $5.33 / 0.77 = 6.922$ times.

9.16 FURTHER RESEARCH

It is planned to use the new method of domain analysis for quick updating of actual information about domain considering newly appeared domain artifacts. To achieve this goal, it is necessary to do the following things:

1. Propose a method for estimation of cognitive value of newly appeared artifacts that contain information about the problem domain (Figure 9.5). This estimation will play the role of a filter allowing exclude not valuable parts of information under the analysis.

2. Design an approach for merging domain models. It will allow considering structural interconnections between problem domain entities when borders of problem domains are merged.
3. Propose a method for domain models comparison. As a comparison operation is a basic for further refinement, merging, and many other activities, comparison methods allow to estimate the degree of two problem domain models' similarities and take a conclusion about expediency of their processing together.

REFERENCES

Allen, E.B. "Design artifacts are central: Foundations for a theory of software engineering", Technical Report MSU-20150420. Mississippi State University, Mississippi, April 2015.

Asnina, E. "The formal approach to problem domain modelling within model driven architecture", *Proceedings of the 9th International Conference on "Information Systems Implementation and Modelling"(ISIM'06)*, Přerov, Czech Republic, April 25-27, 2006.

Beck, K., Beedle, M., van Bennekum, A., Cockburn, A., Cunningham, W., Fowler, M., Grenning, J., J.High UML Diagramith, Hunt, A., Jeffries, R., Kern, J., Marick, B., Martin, R.C., Mellor, S., Schwaber, K., Sutherland, J., Thomas, D. *Agile Manifesto* Copyright 2001.

Chebanyuk, O., Palahin O. "A multi-layer approach of view models designing", *International journal "Informational Content and Processing"*, 5(3), 2018, 203–216.

Chebanyuk, O., Palahin O. "Domain analysis approach", *International Journal "Informational Content and Processing"*, 6(2): 3–20, 2019.

Chebanyuk E., Markov K., "Software model cognitive value", *International Journal "Information Theories and Applications"*, 22(4):338–355, 2015.

Chebanyuk E. "Algebra describing software static models", *International Journal "Information Technologies and Knowledge"*, 7(1):83–93, 2013.

Chebanyuk, E. "An approach to class diagram design", *Proceedings of the 2nd International Conference on Model-Driven Engineering and Software Development*, 2014a, pp.448–453.

Chebanyuk, E. "Method of behavioural software models synchronization", *International Journal Informational Models and Analysis,* 2:147–163, 2014b.

Endres A., Rombach, D. *A Handbook of Software and Systems Engineering*: *Empirical Observations, Laws and Theories*. Pearson – Addison Wesley, Harlow, England, 2003. 327 pp.

Frakes, W.B., Kang, K. "Software reuse research: Status and future", *IEEE Transactions on Software Engineering.*

Frakes, W.B., Kang, K. "Software reuse research: Status and future", *IEEE Transactions on Software Engineering* 31(7):529– 536, 2005.

Gómez-Romero, J., Patricio, M. A., García, J., & Molina, J. M. (2011). Ontology-based context representation and reasoning for object tracking and scene interpretation in video. *Expert Systems with Applications*, *38*(6), 7494–7510.

Green T., Blackwell, A. *Cognitive Dimensions of Information Artefacts: A tutorial.* October 1998.

Gureckis, T.M., Love, B.C. "Direct associations or internal transformations? Exploring the MechaniUML diagrams underlying sequential learning behavior", *Cognitive Science* 34, pp. 10–50, 2010.

Ivanova, K.B., Vanhoof, K., Markov, Kr., Velychko, V. "Storing ontologies by NL-addressing", *IVth All–Russian Conference "Knowledge-Ontology-Theory" (KONT-13)*, Novosibirsk, Russia, 2013a, pp. 175–184.

Ivanova, K.B., Vanhoof, K., Markov, K., Velychko, V. "Introduction to storing graphs by NL-addressing", *International Journal "Information Theories and Applications"*, 20(3):263–284, 2013b.

Kang, K.C., Cohen, S.G., Hess, J.A., Novak, W.E., Peterson, A.S. "Feature-Oriented Domain Analysis (FODA) Feasibility Study", Technical Report CMU/SEI-90-TR-21 ESD-90-TR-222, Software Engineering Institute, Carnegie Mellon University, Pittsburgh, PA, 1990, pp. 1–148.

Mangano, N., LaToza, T.D., Petre, M., van der Hoek, A. "How software designers interact with sketches at the whiteboard", *IEEE Transactions on Software Engineering*, 41(2):135–156, Feb. 2015.

Miller, G.A., "The magical number seven plus or minus two: Some limits on our capacity for processing information", *Psychological Review*, 63(2):81–97, March 1956.

Mohsen, H., El-Dahshan, E.-S.A., El-Sayed, M., El-Horbaty, Abdel-Badeeh. M. Salem., "Classification using deep learning neural networks for brain tumors", *ScienceDirect, Future Computing and Informatics Journal*, 3:68–71, 2018.

OCL. "About the object constraint language specification version 2.4", OCL, 2014. https://www.omg.org/spec/OCL/About-OCL/.

Olson J.R., Olson, G. M. "The growth of cognitive modeling in human computer interaction since GOMS", University of Michigan, 2015.

Simon, H.A. *Models of Bounded Rationality*. MIT Press, Cambridge, MA, 1982, 392 pp.

Thagard, P. *Mind: Introduction to Cognitive Science*. MIT Press, Cambridge, MA, 1996.

Tversky, B., Agrawala, M., Heiser, J., Lee, P., Hanrahan, P., Phan, D., Stolte, C., Daniel, M.-P. "cognitive design principles: From cognitive models to computer models", In: L. Magnani, editor, *Model-Based Reasoning in Science and Engineering*, College Publications, pp. 1–20. 2006.

Willemien, V., *The Cognitive Artifacts of Designing*. Lawrence Erlbaum Associates, Mahwah, NJ, 2006, 280 pp.

UML. "About the unified modeling language specification version 2.5", UML 2017. www.omg.org/spec/UML/2.5/.

10 Medical Images of Breast Tumors

Classification with Application of Hybrid CNN–FNN Network

Yuriy Zaychenko and Galib Hamidov

CONTENTS

10.1 INTRODUCTION: STATE-OF-THE-ART PROBLEM ANALYSIS

Nowadays at every stage of medical diagnostics information technology is widely utilized. The main goal of medically automated systems is to extend spheres of practical tasks that may be solved with the aid of computers, raising the level of intellectual decision support of doctors, particularly in the process of express diagnostics based on processing and analyzing medical images of human tissue obtained by different sources (e.g., magneto-resonance tomography (MRT), computer tomography [CT]).

The advantages of medical diagnostics systems include speed, automation-tomography and stability of work, which make these systems as efficient tools for express medical diagnostics. Despite the young age of medical informatics, which does not exceed 30 years, information technology as a whole is quickly penetrating various spheres of medicine and health defense (e.g., family medicine, insurance medicine, and integration into European medical space).

The latest achievements in image processing technology and machine learning have enabled to construct systems of automatic detection and diagnostics that may help pathologists and anatomists to make faster and more accurate diagnosis and accelerate their work. Classification of histopathology images on different patterns, which correspond to cancerous and noncancerous states of tissue), is often the primary goal of image analysis systems for automatic cancer diagnostics. Among the different types of cancers, breast cancer takes the second place by its occurrence in women. Besides, breast cancer mortality is very high compared with other cancer diseases (Boyle & Levin, 2012).

Up to date, several models and methods have been developed for breast cancer detection using various machine learning algorithms. Using methods and technologies such as artificial intelligence (AI) as neural networks and support vector machine (SVM) (Lakhani Schnitt, Tan, & van de Vijver, 2012; Zhang, Zhang, Coenen, & Lu, 2013), the accuracy of diagnostics was attained from 76% to 94% with a data set of 92 images.

The most part of last papers referring to the field of breast cancer classification were oriented on integer image (Doyle et al., 2008; Singh et al., 2015; Zhang et al., 2013; Zhang, Zhang, Coenen, Xiau, & Lu, 2014). Widespread implementation of breast image classification (BIC) and other forms of digital pathology, however, face barriers such as high cost of implementation, insufficient productivity compared to the amount of clinic procedures, interior technological problems, and opposition from pathologists and anatomists. Until now, most of the works based on histology breast cancer analysis were performed on small data sets. Some improvement in medical images data sets presented data set with 7,909 breast images obtained from 82 patients (Spanhol Oliveira, Petitjean, & Heutte, 2016). In this research, the authors estimated various texture descriptors and various classifiers and carried out their experiments with 82%–85% accuracy. The alternative to this approach is the application of convolutional neural network (CNN) for medical images processing and diagnostics, which is considered and developed in the present research.

It was shown that CNNs are able to overcome the conventional texture descriptors (Le Cun, Bengio, & Hinton, 2015; Krizhevsky, Sutskever, & Hinton, 2012). Moreover, the traditional approach to detection of features based on descriptors demands great effort and high-level knowledge of experts and usually is specific for every task, which prevents its direct application for other similar tasks.

Therefore, in this research, the authors suggested and developed hybrid fuzzy CNN for a medical image classification system. In the suggested hybrid system, CNN is utilized to extract informative features of images and fuzzy neural network (FNN) NEFClass is applied for the classification of detected breast tumors on images in two classes: benign and malignant.

The main goal of this chapter is to develop and investigate algorithmic and software tools for fast analysis of breast tissue images, detection of tumors, and their classification into two classes: benign or malignant. These tools will enable specialists to provide express analysis of images and raise the quality of medical diagnostics.

10.2 DATA SET DESCRIPTION

For this investigation BreaKHis data set was used, which was especially created for estimating the efficiency of different approaches and methods for medical images of breast tumor diagnostics. The data set BreaKHis (Spanhol et al., 2016) contains microscopic biopsies from benign and malignant tumors of the breast. The images were obtained in clinical research from January 2014 through December 2014. BreaKHis consists of 7,909 clinically representative microscopic images of breast tumors received from 82 patients with different scale augmentation (40X, 100X, 200X, and 400X).

During this period, the researchers investigated all patients in the Research & Development (R&D) medical lab. They invited all patients who were diagnosed with breast cancer to take part in this investigation. All data were anonymized. The researchers collected the patterns by surgery biopsy and prepared them for histologic research. The main goal of this procedure was to preserve the original structure of tissue and molecular composition, which allows researchers to observe it with optical microscope.

For the investigation, all images were split into slides of size 3 mkm (micrometer = 10^{-6} m). Experienced pathologist-anatomists made the final conclusion for each case, and the researchers confirmed the conclusions through an additional investigation, such as immune histology-chemistry (IHC).

The researchers used the microscope system Olympus BX-50 with augmentation 3.3 connected with a digital camera, Samsung SCC- 131AN, to obtain digitized images of breast tissues. The images were obtained in a three-channel color space (24 bits value, 8 bits color channels of red, green, and blue) with magnification coefficients 40X, 100X, 200X, and 400X.

In Figures 10.1–10.4, four images are presented with four magnification coefficients: (a) 40 ×, (b) 100 ×, (c) 200 ×, and (d) 400 ×. The researchers obtained these images from one slide of breast tumor that contains malignant tumor (breast cancer). In Figure 10.5, the slide of breast is presented with benign tumor. The pathologist-anatomist chose a separated rectangular region of interest (ROI). Up to this date, the BreakHis data set consists of 7,909 images, divided into benign and malignant tumors. Table 10.1 presents the distribution of images (Spanhol et al., 2016).

10.3 CONVOLUTIONAL NEURAL NETWORKS: A BRIEF DESCRIPTION

A CNN model is a state-of-the-art method that has been widely utilized for image processing. A CNN model has the ability to extract global features in a hierarchical manner that ensures local connectivity as well as the weight-sharing property. CNN consists of the following layers (Le Cun et al., 2015, Krizhevsky et al., 2012).

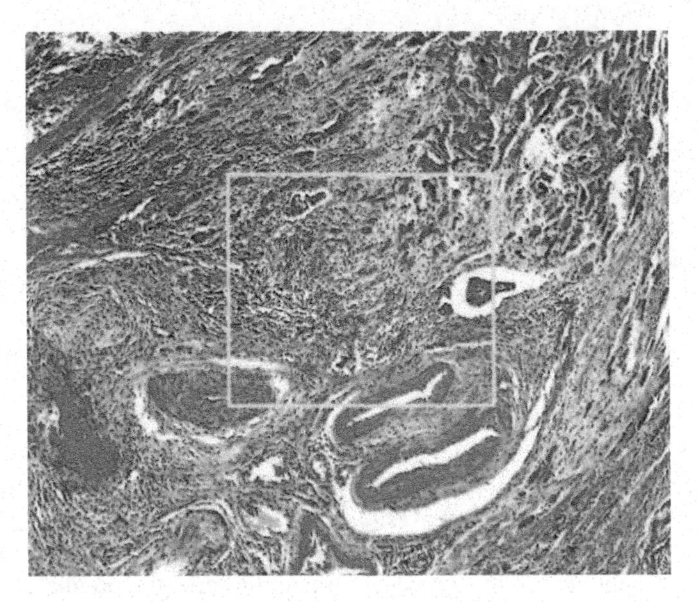

FIGURE 10.1 Slide of malignant tumor with magnification 40×.

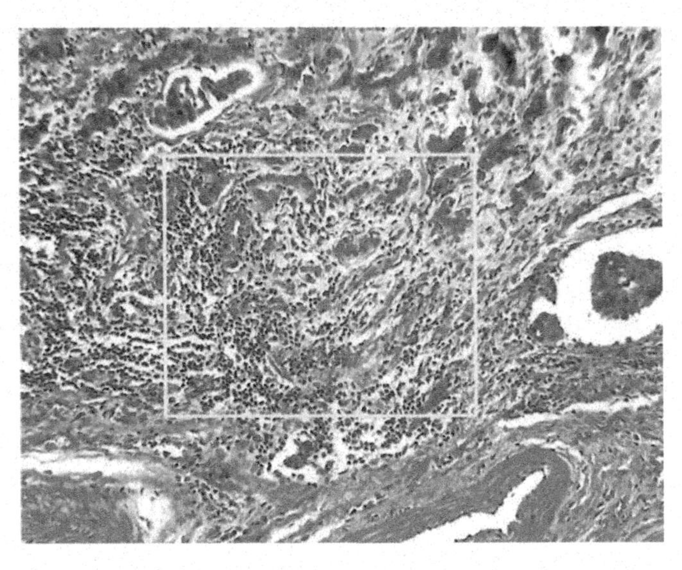

FIGURE 10.2 Slide of malignant tumor with magnification 100×.

10.3.1 Convolutional Layer

The convolutional layer is considered to be the main working ingredient in CNN model, and it plays a vital role in this model. A kernel (filter), which is basically an $n \times n$ matrix, successively goes through all the pixels and extracts the information.

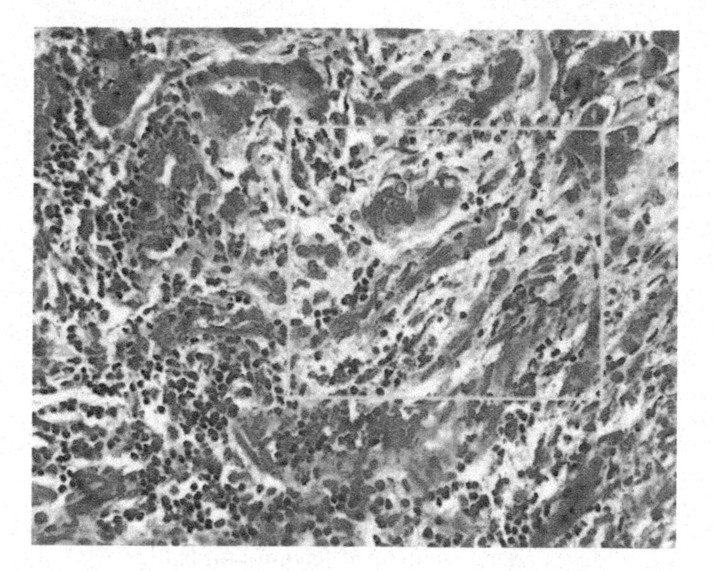

FIGURE 10.3 Slide of malignant tumor with magnification 200×.

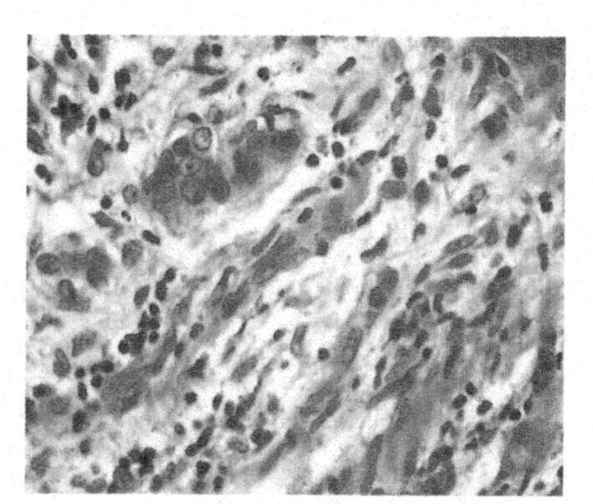

FIGURE 10.4 Slide of malignant tumor with magnification 400×.

TABLE 10.1
Distribution of Images by Magnification Coefficients and Class

Magnification	Benign	Malignant	Total
40×	625	1,370	1,995
100×	644	1,437	2,081
200×	623	1,390	2,013
400×	588	1,232	1,820
Total	2,480	5,429	7,909
Number of patients	24	58	82

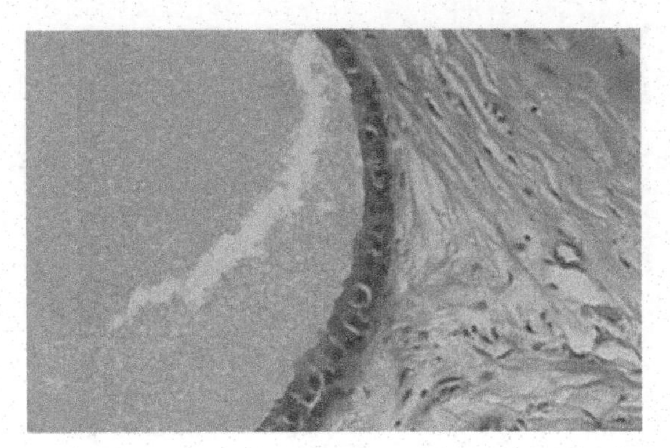

FIGURE 10.5 Slide of benign tumor with magnification 100×.

10.3.2 Pooling Operation

A CNN model produces a large amount of feature information. To reduce the feature dimensionality, researchers have performed a downsampling method named a pooling operation. A few pooling operation methods are well known, such as Max Pooling and Average Pooling.

For this research, Max Pooling operation was utilized. This method selects the maximum values within a particular patch of data.

10.3.3 Nonlinear Performance

Each layer of the neural network (NN) produces linear output and, by definition, adds two linear functions that will also produce a linear output. Due to the linear nature of the output, adding more NN layers will show the same behavior as a single NN layer. To overcome this issue, a rectifier function, such as Rectified Linear Unit (ReLU), Leaky ReLU, Tanh, and Sigmoid, has been introduced to make the output nonlinear.

10.3.4 Dropout

The model shows very poor performance on the test data set due to its overtraining, which is also known as overfitting. Researchers have controlled overfitting by a technique known as Dropout, which removes some of the neurons from the network.

10.3.5 Decision Layer

For the classification decision at the end of a CNN model, researchers introduce a decision layer (usually multi-layered perceptron [MLP]). Normally, a Softmax layer or SVM layer is introduced for this purpose. This layer contains a normalized exponential function and calculates the loss function for the data classification.

10.3.5.1 CNN Model for Image Classification

In Figure 10.6, the architecture of VGG-16 is presented. The authors used VGG-16 in this study as a detector of informative features. VGG-16 was trained by different algorithms, including stochastic gradient descent (SGD), differential evolution (Zaychenko, Petrosyuk, & Jaroshenko, 2009; Zgurovsky & Zaychenko, 2016), and basin hopping (Olson, Hashmi, Molloy, & Shehu, 2012).

10.4 FUZZY NEURAL NETWORK NEFCLASS

As classifier of obtained features in this research, various sources suggested using FNN NEFClass. FNN NEFClass was first suggested by Nauck and Kruse (1997). It was modified and developed in future studies (the so-called FNN NEFClass M) (Zaychenko, Fatma, & Matsak, 2004; Zaychenko, Petrosyuk, & Jaroshenko, 2009).

Zaychenko et al. (2009) developed and investigated the learning algorithms for FNN NEFClass: stochastic gradient (SG), conjugate gradient descent (CGD), and genetic algorithm for the optical images pattern recognition.

In the work (Zaychenko et al., 2015), FNN NEFCLASS was successfully applied for analysis of medical images of cervix tissue obtained with the use of colposcope and diagnostics.

The main advantages of FNN NEFClass as a classifier are the possibility to work with incomplete and fuzzy input data, performing fuzzy classification of input patterns (images) using the so-called membership functions, speed, and high accuracy (Zaychenko et al., 2004; Zaychenko et al., 2009; Zgurovsky & Zaychenko, 2016).

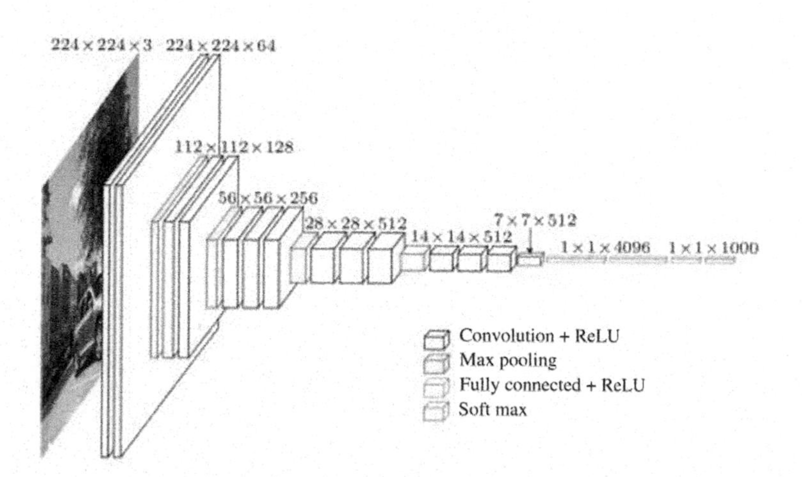

FIGURE 10.6 Convolutional neural network VGG-16.

10.4.1 Architecture of FNN NEFClass

The authors use the NEFClass model for the definition of class or category of an input sample (the so-called patterns). Patterns are feature vectors $X = (x_1, x_2, \ldots, x_n) \in R^n$ of a certain object, and a class is some set in R^n.

A feature of a pattern (sample) is represented by a fuzzy set, and classification is performed by a set of linguistic rules. For each input feature x_i, there are q_i fuzzy sets described by membership functions (MF) $\mu_1^i, \ldots, \mu_{q_i}^i$.

Also there is a rule base which contains k fuzzy linguistic rules, such as $R_1, \ldots, R_k$. Fuzzy rules that describe data have the following form (Zaychenko et al., 2004):

If x_1 *is* μ_1 *and* x_2 *is* μ_2 *and … and* x_n *is* μ_n, *then the sample* $(x_1, x_2, \ldots, x_n)$ *belongs to a class i, where* $\mu_1, \ldots, x_n$ *are fuzzy sets.*

The main tasks of NEFClass are defining these rules and providing a type of membership functions for fuzzy sets. The NEFClass system, which classifies input samples with two features and two separate classes using five linguistic rules, is presented in Figure 10.7.

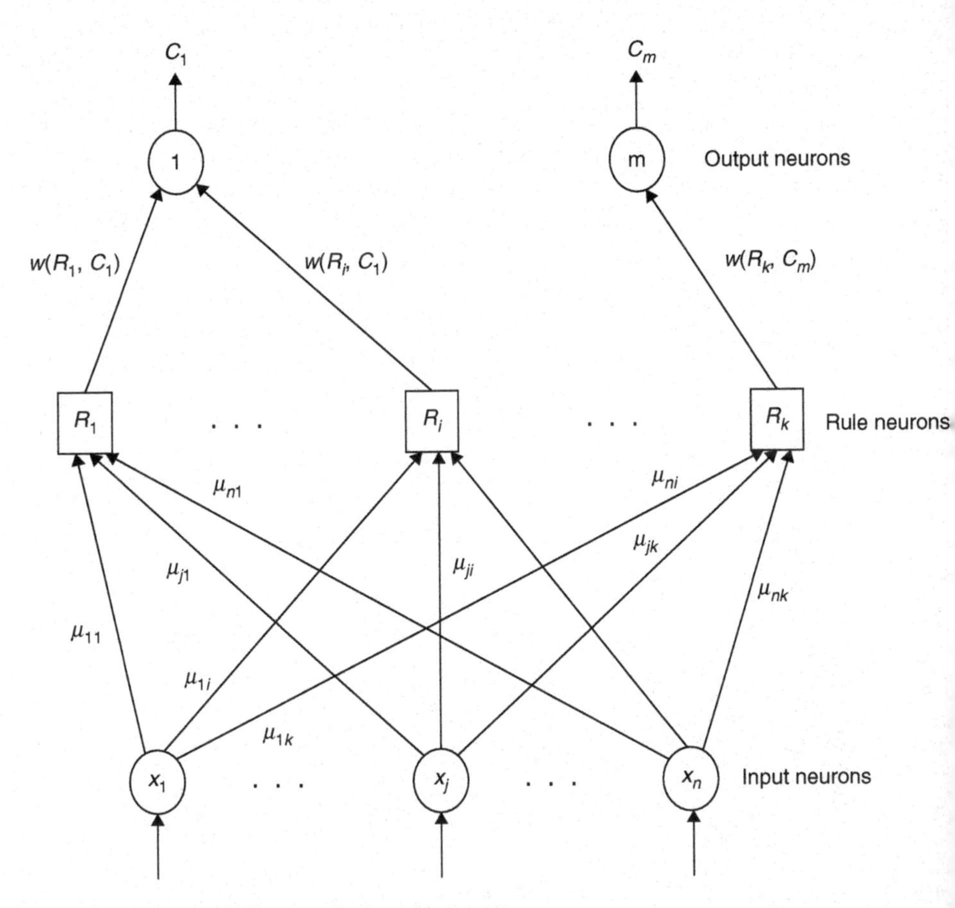

FIGURE 10.7 NEFClass network architecture.

FNN NEFClass has a three-layer architecture (Figure 10.7). The first layer is a layer of input neurons that contain the input samples. Activation of the neurons in this layer does not change the input value. The hidden layer contains fuzzy rules neurons $R_{1,} R_{2,}...,R$, and the third layer consists of output neurons of each class $\left(C_1,...,C_m\right)$.

Training algorithm of FNN NEFClass consists of two stages. In the first stage, fuzzy rules base is generated using a training sample.

There are three algorithms of rules generation:

1. Simple rules base training
2. Best rules training
3. Best for each class training.

After generating a rules base, the authors proceeded to the *second training stage* at which the parameters of fuzzy sets MF are trained. For this stage, the authors developed the goal of several training algorithms, including SGD, CGD, genetic algorithm, differential evolution, and the so-called basin hopping algorithm.

10.4.2 Stochastic Gradient Algorithm for FNN NEFClass

The following criterion of training FNN NEFClass was used:

$$e = \sum_{i=1}^{M} \left(t_i - NET_i\left(W\right)\right)^2 \to \min, \tag{10.1}$$

wheret t_i is the desirable output value of a neural network and $NET_i(W)$ is the actual value of the ith output of a neural network for a weight matrix. $W = \left[W^I, W^O\right]$.

$$W^I = W\left(x, R\right) = \mu_j\left(x\right),\ W^O = W\left(R, C\right).$$

The criterion of $e(W)$ is a mean squared error of approximation.

Let the function of activation for neurons of the hidden layer (neurons of rules) be:

$$O_R = \prod_{i=1}^{n} \mu_{j_i}^{(i)}\left(x_i\right),\quad j = 1,\ldots,q_i, \tag{10.2}$$

where $\mu_{j_i}^{(i)}$ is the membership function that has the following form:

$$\mu_{j_i}^{(i)}\left(x\right) = e^{-\frac{\left(x - a_{ji}\right)^2}{b_{ji}^2}} \tag{10.3}$$

and the activation function of output neuron layer is:

$$NET_c = \max_{R \in U_2} W\left(R, C\right) O_R \tag{10.4}$$

Consider the gradient learning algorithm of fuzzy perceptron.

1. Let $W(n)$ be the current value of the weights matrix. Then the algorithm has the following form:

$$W(n+1) = W(n) - \gamma_{n+1} \nabla_w e(W(n)), \tag{10.5}$$

where γ_n is the step size at nth iteration and
$\nabla_w e(W(n))$ is the gradient (direction), which reduces the criterion (10.1).

2. At each iteration, first the input weight W are trained, which depend on the parameters a and b (see the expression (10.3).

$$a_{ji}(n+1) = a_{ji}(n) - \gamma_{n+1} \frac{\partial e(W)}{\partial a_{ji}}, \tag{10.6}$$

$$b_{ji}(n+1) = b_{ji}(n) - \gamma'_{n+1} \frac{\partial e(W)}{\partial b_{ji}}, \tag{10.7}$$

where γ'_{n+1} is the step size for parameter b.

$$\frac{\partial e(W)}{\partial a_{ji}} = -2\sum_{k=1}^{M} ((t_k - NET_k(w)) \cdot W(R,C)) O_R \cdot \frac{(x - a_{ji})}{b_{ji}^2}, \tag{10.8}$$

$$\frac{\partial e(W)}{\partial b_{ji}} = -2\sum_{k=1}^{M} ((t_k - NET_k(w)) \cdot W(R,C)) \cdot O_R \cdot \frac{(x - a_{ji})^2}{b_{ji}^3}. \tag{10.9}$$

3. Then output weight are trained:

$$\frac{\partial e(W^o)}{\partial W(R,C_k)} = -(t_k - NET_k(W^o)) O_R, \tag{10.10}$$

$$W_k^o(n+1) = W_k^o(n) - \gamma''_{n+1} \frac{\partial e(W^o)}{\partial W(R,C_k)}. \tag{10.11}$$

4. $n := n + 1$ and go to the next iteration.

The gradient method is the first proposed learning algorithm. It is easy to implement, but it has the following disadvantages:

1. The gradient method converges slowly.
2. The gradient method only finds a local extremum.

Therefore, in this research, the authors also applied the conjugate gradient method and the basin hopping algorithm.

10.5 EXPERIMENTAL INVESTIGATIONS AND ANALYSIS

As mentioned earlier, in this investigation, the authors used the pretrained CNN VGG-16. The authors applied this method of training transfer. There are two main training scenarios:

1. **Features extraction**: In this case, the last full-connected layer is deleted, and the rest part of CNN is used as an extractor for new data sets.
2. **Fine tuning**: In this case, a new data set is used for fine training the previously pretrained neural network.

In this research, the authors used CNN VGG-16 for features extraction in medical images of breast tumors. Then they fed the features found as input data to FNN NEFClass. As algorithms of training FNN, three algorithms were used: basin hopping (Olson et al., 2012), SGD, and differential evolution (Zgurovsky & Zaychenko, 2016).

10.5.1 Description of Experiments

The authors carried out a series of experiments and compared the results with previous works. In Tables 10.2 and 10.3, the results of classification (accuracy, %) with different parameters are presented. The authors divided all samples into training and testing subsamples with a ratio of 80% to 20%.

In the first experiment, the authors varied the number of linguistic variables (terms) and rules to determine the best parameter values (Table 10.2).

From the table, one can easily see that beginning from six fuzzy sets per variable and six rules, the accuracy does not increase, but the complexity of training increases.

It can be inferred from Table 10.2 that for two classes, the best values of parameters for FNN NEFClass in this problem are four fuzzy sets per variable and six rules. To estimate the efficiency of the hybrid CNN network, the authors compared the results obtained with the results of previous work (Singh et al., 2015), using different classifiers for the same problem (Table 10.3).

As shown in Table 10.3, FNN NEFClass shows better results than the previous classifiers SVM machine and random forest suggested by Singh et al.

In this study, to train FNN NEFClass, three algorithms were applied, namely, basin hopping, SGD, and differential evolution. Using basin hopping and SGD algorithms, approximately equal results with high accuracy were obtained, while the training results of differential evolution appeared to be much worse.

It is worth noting that in this problem, the number of features extracted by CNN VGG16 was very large: 4,096 features.

Therefore, the authors decided to cut the number of features and reduce the dimensionality of classification problem. For this aim, they applied principal components method (PCM) (Jindal, 2013). In Table 10.4, the results of such reduction are presented.

TABLE 10.2
Classification Results of FNN NEFClass

Initial Number of Fuzzy Sets (Linguistic Terms)/ Number of Rules	40× (%)	100× (%)	200× (%)	400× (%)
2/2	73	74	74.2	73.5
4/2	75.3	74.8	75.7	75.4
6/2	78.2	79	78.4	78
8/2	76	75.4	76.5	75.8
2/4	75	74	73.8	73
4/4	78.3	76.3	75.7	75.4
6/4	82	83	82.4	83.2
8/4	82.2	81.5	81.5	83.8
2/6	75.4	73.8	74.4	73.2
4/6	**90**	**91**	**90.5**	**90**
6/6	89	89.7	90.2	89.5
8/6	90.3	90.5	92	91.2
4/8	89.3	89.8	89.7	89.3
6/8	89.2	88	89.4	88.4
8/8	88	87.2	87.2	87

TABLE 10.3
Comparison of Different Classifiers' Accuracy

Classifier/Magnification Coefficient	40× (%)	100× (%)	200× (%)	400× (%)
Linear SVM	89	89	88	88
Polynomial SVM	88	90	89	85
Random forest	89.18	88	87.74	80
FNN NEFClass	90	91	90.5	90

From Table 10.4, it follows that the results of reduction with 250 principal components are most acceptable as the complexity of training increases approximately proportional to the dimension of input data. Due to the lack of time, the next experiments were performed using data with magnificence factor 100× (2,081 images). In Table 10.5, the accuracy of classification using 250 features is presented with various NEFClass parameters.

In Table 10.6, the dependence of classification accuracy versus the number of features is presented. One can see from the table that the accuracy dropped only by 4%–7% due to features reduction, but at the same time, the training time was substantially reduced.

TABLE 10.4
The Dependence of Total Variance on Number of Components and Approximate Training Time

Number of Principal Components	Variation	Approximate Training Time (in hr)
100	0.84058	~2 hr
200	0.89736	~3 hr
250	0.91232	~4 hr
500	0.95486	~9 hr

TABLE 10.5
Classification Accuracy with 250 Features

Number of Fuzzy Sets/Number of Rules	100× (%)
4/4	80.64
4/6	87.24
4/8	88.18

TABLE 10.6
Classification Accuracy with Different Number of Features

Number of linguistic terms, number of rules/ number of features	100	250	4096
4,4	75.23%	80.64%	86.3%
4,6	83.34%	87.24%	91%
4,8	84.21%	88.18%	89.8%

From Table 10.6, one can easily see that the accuracy drops with a decrease of features number, but this decrease of 3%–5% is insignificant if one compares the results with 100 and 250 features. The authors compared the classification with the full set of features (4,096 features) and found that with decreased features in 20 times the accuracy falls, on average, only by 3%–6%. This conclusion supports the efficiency of PCM method application for the reduction of dimension of medical images classification problems.

10.6 CONCLUSION

- In this chapter, the authors considered the problem of analysis of breast tumor medical images and classification of detected tumors into two classes: benign and malignant.

- For pattern recognition of breast tumors, the authors suggested the new hybrid CNN–FNN network in which the CNN VGG-16 is used for informative features extraction, while FNN NEFClass is used for classification of detected tumors.
- For training FNN NEFClass, the authors suggested basin hopping, SGD, and differential evolution algorithms and investigated their efficiency.
- The authors carried out experimental investigations of suggested hybrid CNN–FNN network in the problem of classification of real images of breast tumors using the BreakHis data set.
- They compared the classification of accuracy of the suggested hybrid CNN–FNN network with known results based on the use of classification algorithms SVM and random forest, which confirmed the efficiency of the suggested approach.
- The authors investigated the problem of reducing the number of features in medical images classification problem using PCM and explored its efficiency.

REFERENCES

Aditi Singh, A., Mansourifar, H., Bilgrami, H., Makkar, N., & Shah, T. (2015). Classifying biological images using pre-trained CNNs. Retrieved from https://docs.google.com/document/d/1H7xVK7nwXcv11CYh7hl5F6pM0m218FQloAXQODP-Hsg/edit?usp=sharing

Bernard W. Stewart & Christopher P. (Eds.). World Cancer Report 2014. Published by the International Agency for Research on Cancer, 150 cours Albert Thomas, 69372 Lyon Cedex 08, France, 2014. ISBN 978-92-832-0443-5.Doyle, S., Agner, S., Madabhushi, A., Feldman, M., & Tomaszewski, J. (2008). Automated grading of breast cancer histopathology using spectral clustering with textural and architectural image features. *Nano to Macro, 61,* 496–499.

Jindal, N. (2013). Enhanced face recognition algorithm using PCA with artificial neural networks. *International Journal of Advanced Research in Computer Science and Software Engineering, 3*, 864–872.

Krizhevsky, A., Sutskever, I., & Hinton, G. E. (2012). Imagenet classification with deep convolutional neural networks. *Advances in Neural Information Processing Systems, 25*, 1097–1105.

Lakhani, S. R., Schnitt, S., Tan, P., & van de Vijver, M. (2012). *WHO Classification of Tumours of the Breast* (4th edn.). Lyon: WHO Press.

Le Cun, Y., Bengio, Y., & Hinton, G. (2015). Deep learning. *Nature, 521*, 436–444.

Nauck, D., & Kruse, R. (1997). New learning strategies for NEFCLASS. *Proceedings of the Seventh International Fuzzy Systems Association World Congress IFSA'97, IV*, 50–55.

Olson, B., Hashmi, I., Molloy, K., & Shehu, A. (2012). Basin hopping as a general and versatile optimization framework for the characterization of biological macromolecules. *Advances in Artificial Intelligence, 3,* 115–122.

Spanhol, F., Oliveira, L. S., Petitjean, C., & Heutte, L. (2016). A dataset for breast cancer histopathological image classification. *IEEE Transactions on Biomedical Engineering, 63*(7), 1455–1462.

Zaychenko Y., Fatma, S., & Matsak, A.. (2004). Fuzzy neural networks for economic data classification. *Vestnik of National Technical University of Ukraine "KPI", section "Informatics, Control and Computer Engineering*, 42, 121–133.

Zaychenko, Y., & Huskova, V. (2015). Recognition of objects on optical images in medical diagnostics using fuzzy neural network NEF class. *International Journal "Information Models and Analysis", 4*(1), 13–22.

Zaychenko Yu, P., Petrosyuk, I. M., & Jaroshenko M. S. (2009). The investigations of fuzzy neural networks in the problems of electro-optical images recognition. *System Research and Information Technologies, 4*, 61–76.

Zgurovsky, M., & Zaychenko, Y. (2016). *The Fundamentals of Computational Intelligence: System Approach*. Switzerland: Springer International Publishing, 308p.

Zhang, Y., Zhang, B., Coenen, F., & Lu, W. (2013). Breast cancer diagnosis from biopsy images with highly reliable random subspace classifier ensembles. *Machine Vision and Applications, 24*(7), 1405–1420.

Zhang, Y., Zhang, B., Coenen, F., Xiau J., & Lu, W. (2014). One-class kernel subspace ensemble for medical image classification. *EURASIP Journal on Advances in Signal Processing, 2014*(17), 1–13.

11 Artificial Intelligence-Empowered Mobile Healthcare

A Wireless Access Perspective

S. Lenty Stuwart and El-Sayed A. El-Dahshan

CONTENTS

11.1 INTRODUCTION

Intelligent computing is viewed as a great conqueror of next-generation wireless systems. In wireless systems, the form factor of fixed wireless devices is reduced to ease the difficulty of handling them, which emerge as mobile devices. The way mobile communication proliferates into every nook and corner of human presence is really astonishing. The present-day mobile technology is supporting and allowing one to invent new allied technologies to which the technology at our hand is considered to be a backbone. Although the use of mobile technology in healthcare is increasing in moderate pace, the real face of the technology boom is expected to be seen in the upcoming days with the advent of new features in the 5G-and-beyond technologies.

In the beginning of mobile networks era, the primary objective was to increase the data rate because the mobile network was considered to be a homogeneous network. The demand for the data rate is slowly diminished by new mobile elements such as wearable healthcare devices, smart hand-held devices, mobile ad hoc devices, and sensors. The presence of these elements changed the status of network from homogeneous to heterogeneous mix of mobile devices. The demand is also migrated from high data rate to low latency, security, ultra-reliability, interoperability, and adaptive nature to the change in environment and network characteristics.

An interesting paradigm shift observed in heterogeneous mix network is traffic congestion rise in the uplink on par with downlink, in some cases uplink congestion surpassing its downlink counterpart. This network behavioral change is due to the fact that a massive real-time data collection from autonomous and semiautonomous devices is deployed to observe the environmental changes. For instance, in healthcare system, in order to collect health-related data from patients, huge numbers of wearable and non-wearable mobile devices are utilized, which periodically populate uncountable data in real time to the host for monitoring and subsequent follow-up. Due to some of the reasons stated above and more, reliability requirements, quality of service (QoS), and health-related applications insist on revolution in design, analysis, modeling, and optimization. Some of the ingredients mandated in the next-generation mobile system are millimeter wave communication, device-to-device communication (D2D), ultra-reliability and low-latency communications, dense small cell deployment, etc. Even though these are favorable choices for mobile healthcare, these systems require intelligent functions to optimize network function by adaptive exploitation of collected data and resources. This kind of intelligent function can be realized by artificial neural network(ANN)-based machine learning technique. Hence, the use of intelligent computing is not going to be optional anymore; rather it would become an integral part of next-generation wireless systems.

This chapter primarily intends to focus on how the existing physical layer techniques aid the development and practice of healthcare system, and then focuses on the salient features being incorporated in the next-generation wireless system to promote the healthcare. This discussion on mobile healthcare (m-healthcare) brings forward different progressive modules needed, on the one hand, and briefs the lead role of intelligent learning, on the other hand. Furthermore, this chapter travels along physical layer problems in m-healthcare network, and new possibilities and solutions are offered with incorporation of intelligent technology.

11.2 M-HEALTHCARE SERVICES AND CHALLENGES

The health condition of a patient must be available anywhere anytime for timely advice and treatment from medical practitioners. Where, when, and how to access health-related information are serious issues in distributed and highly dynamic healthcare enterprises. The operating cost of such healthcare organizations could be minimized when effective methods are employed to improve the efficiency, and to decrease medical errors. The present-day wireless technology plays a pivotal role in providing medical solutions to these underlying problems. M-healthcare services concentrate on exploiting the salient features of mobile technology. There is a common belief that mobile technology is aimed at connecting people. However, it can also provide connectivity among devices, from which these devices can reap the benefits out of network access. Delivery of the services from end to end using mobile network is closely associated with acquiring, analyzing, manipulating, and transmitting data from wearable and non-wearable biomedical devices.

Various scenarios associated with m-healthcare applications are tele-surgery, real-time patient monitoring, remote medication, tracking and management of healthcare organization assets, mobile-assisted living, seamless biomedical device connectivity and self-sustainability, and enhanced information privacy. As shown in Figure 11.1,

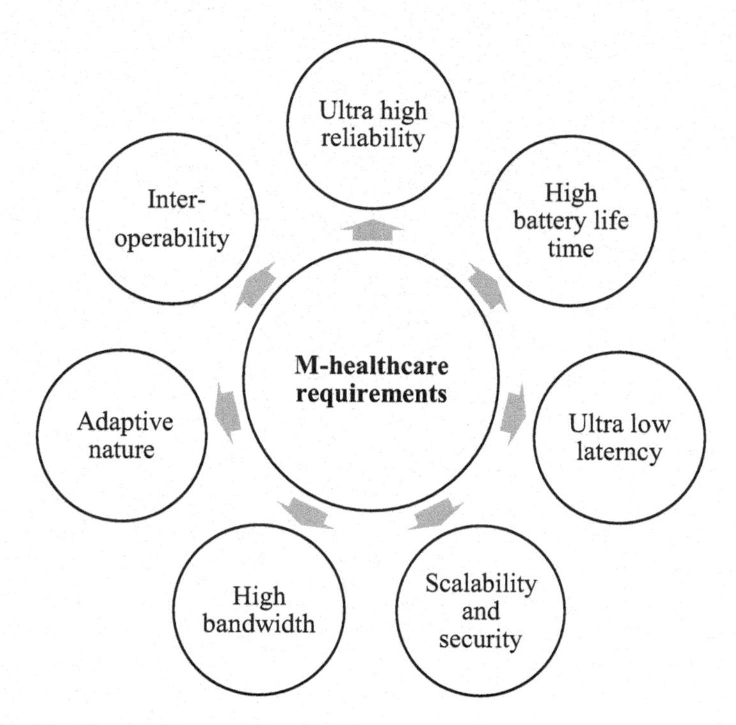

FIGURE 11.1 Required features in m-healthcare network.

although the m-healthcare services provided by the present-day technology consider these aspects, the full-fledged network functionality is not realized due to nonavailability of some features in the existing wireless standards. For instance, tele-surgery is a recommended alternate for a critical patient when the surgery specialist is far away from the hospital where performing the surgery is urgent. The robotic assisted tele-surgery should tackle many hurdles, out of which latency is a crucial factor because it has direct impact on the survival of the patient.

Real-time patient monitoring in m-healthcare faces a different problem. Massive deployments of biomedical devices are subjected to continuous monitoring and transmission of environmental changes. Due to bandwidth limit in existing m-healthcare network, transfer of such huge health-related information in real time is restricted. This reduces clarity on the diagnosis of certain medical conditions of patients by physicians, while remotely accessing low-resolution images received from high-quality biomedical equipment. Similarly, new connection request by a device and the number of simultaneous accesses from multiple sources create scalability problems, which put a cap on seamless connectivity. That is, massive deployment of biomedical devices affects m-healthcare network operation. In the same way, self-sustainability of the devices, especially when implanted, relies on the life time of the battery attached, which is not fully guaranteed in the present wireless technology. A new technology supporting the biomedical device with a tiny and low-power battery can extend the life time of the device. This can make the device self-sustainable for the entire duration of medical care or treatment without battery replacement or recharge.

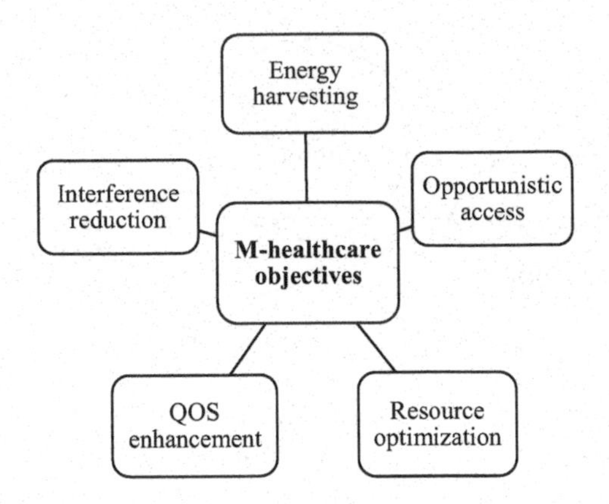

FIGURE 11.2 Major objectives of m-healthcare network.

Finally, m-healthcare network is vulnerable to breach by unauthorized users due to heterogeneous mix network access by different kinds of devices and new business models promoted. Improvement in network privacy and patient health information protection is highly expected in the upcoming wireless standards. Some of the features that can remove hurdles and eradicate the problems faced by the existing m-healthcare network, with the objectives presented in Figure 11.2), are mobile edge computing, software-defined radio, network function virtualization, intelligent radio, cognitive radio, massive multi-input multi-output (MIMO), D2D communication, machine-to-machine (M2M) communication, massive machine-type communication (mMTC), ultra-reliable low-latency communication (uRLLC) or critical machine-type communication (cMTC), and enhanced mobile broadband (eMBB). On top of this, artificial intelligence (AI)-empowered mobile technology is a suitable candidate for next-generation m-healthcare services because the success of m-healthcare is closely interrelated to the development of intelligent capabilities that can boost both energy and spectrum efficiencies.

11.2.1 Interoperability, Scalability, and Security Challenges

The service rendered by healthcare system becomes challenging due to interoperability, scaling, and security problems. That is, next-generation wireless standards aim at integrating devices belonging to networks with different characteristics into a heterogeneous healthcare system. Data exchange among such devices triggers the interoperability problem in the absence of potential AI approach.

Similarly, the deployment in time-varying channel exposes the healthcare devices to vulnerable situations. Network with healthcare devices of different traffic patterns must have a dynamically scalable capability. AI-enabled dynamic network can allow seamless addition/removal of devices in the network. Finally, forecasting the network vulnerability in the hostile environment is a challenging task in a heterogeneous healthcare network. Privacy-aware data transfer and cloud-based data integrity are some of the essential features that can be implemented with the help of AI. The following section further discusses the physical layer issues in the conventional biomedical devices, and AI approach to resolve them.

11.3 WIRELESS CHANNEL AND SUITABLE MACHINE LEARNING APPROACHES

Deployment of massive biomedical devices in wireless channel places fundamental limits on the characteristics of m-healthcare network. The communication channel is nonstationary and random in nature, which makes the channel parameters unpredictable and offers highly complex analysis. The transmitted signal carrying sensitive medical information undergoes scattering, reflection, and diffraction due to severe obstructions, and mobility of devices and obstacles, which distort the information when a strong line-of-sight (LOS) component is unavailable. As a result, large-scale variation in the average received signal strength, and rapid fluctuation in the received signal strength over short time/distance, can be noticed. The large-scale variation is observed in very large transmission distance, like remote medical assistant application via mobile network, which generally leads to loss in the form of log-distance path loss and log-normal shadowing.

On the other hand, multiple biomedical devices deployed in a closed environment, like healthcare clinics, encounter rapid fluctuation in the received signal strength, which leads to small-scale fading. Mobility of biomedical devices, movement of surrounding objects, reception of multiple copies of a transmitted signal also known as multipath propagation, and communication bandwidth are four key physical factors influencing small-scale fading or simply fading. Mobility of devices or relative motion between devices and fixed infrastructure like base station result in Doppler shift, which is nothing but a shift in received signal frequency with respect to its transmitter counterpart. In the same way, in wearable biomedical device communication, every movement by object/person in the channel environment offers a time-varying Doppler shift. *Frequency dispersion* or *time-varying nature* is a characteristic of channel with simple or time-varying Doppler shift. On the other hand, signal distortion also takes place in multipath propagation due to random amplitude and phase of multipath received components. In this case, if a transmitted signal bandwidth is narrower than the channel bandwidth, the information distortion is tolerable because there is no signal dispersion in time; conversely, wider signal bandwidth attracts inter-symbol interference that leads to dispersion in time, thereby distorting the information. *Time dispersion* or *time invariant nature* is another important characteristic of channel with bandwidth constraint. As a final point, frequency dispersion and time dispersion are used to define slow/fast fading and frequency selective/non-selective fading, respectively. A time and frequency selective channel is generally termed as doubly selective channel.

"Channel state information" (CSI) is a term associated with the fading coefficient which specifies the number of taps in the multipath channel, and phase, amplitude, and

Doppler shift of each path. In a closed-loop m-healthcare network, CSI enables the system to adapt to instantaneous channel conditions so as to achieve improved receiver performance, and consequently detecting the information with relatively small errors. Some of the transceiver parameters adapted based on CSI are modulation type, transmit power, coding, antenna, precoding, equalizer, etc. In m-healthcare scenario, the rapid channel variation caused by mobility of biomedical devices and environment influences the accuracy of channel estimation. Nowadays the popularity of AI grows among technicians, academicians, and researchers as a potential candidate to solve various issues related to wireless communication. By interacting with wireless channel, AI can learn the channel variation, classify the issues related to such variations, forecast challenges, and provide possible solutions. In other words, AI algorithms can recommend various solutions to enhance the response of m-healthcare network by means of sensing, mining, prediction, and reasoning.

The broad classification of multidisciplinary AI technique and issues related to wireless communication considered by machine learning are shown in Figure 11.3. Furthermore, various algorithms supporting machine learning approach are listed in Figure 11.4. Machine learning is an algorithm operated in intelligent machines to learn time-varying environment, and to adapt to such environments with learning experience. Huge volume of data originated from uncountable sources demand the use of machine learning algorithms for intelligent processing in many sectors. Machine learning is regarded as a suitable tool for intelligent computing to solve physical layer problems. Based on signal available to learn, and the corresponding nature of learning object, machine learning is generally classified into supervised learning,

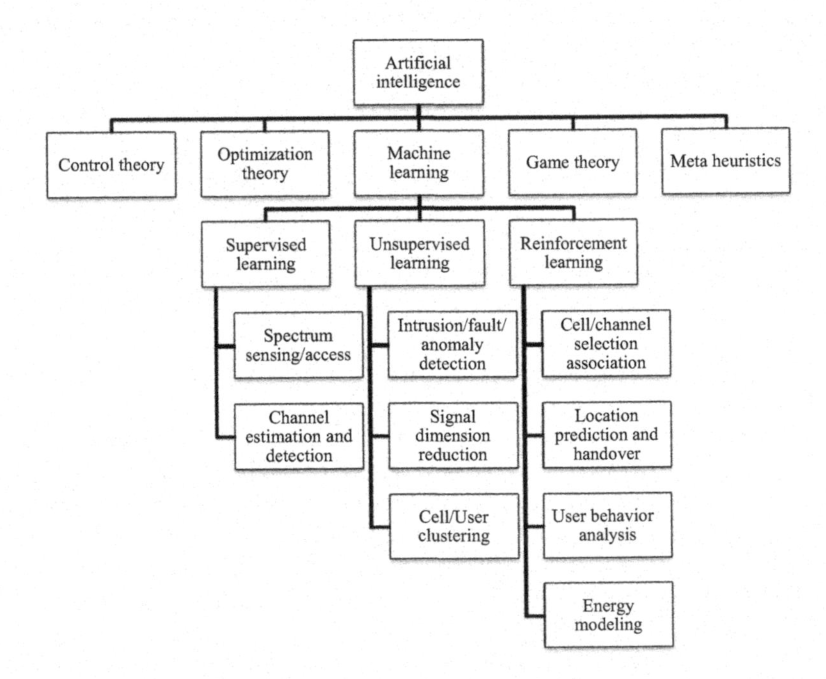

FIGURE 11.3 Classification of artificial intelligence techniques, and wireless access issues handled by machine learning.

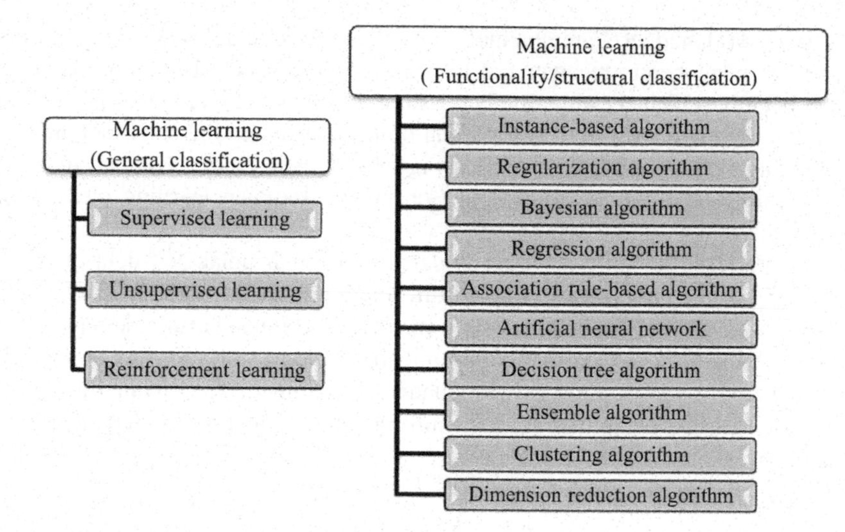

FIGURE 11.4 Machine learning algorithms.

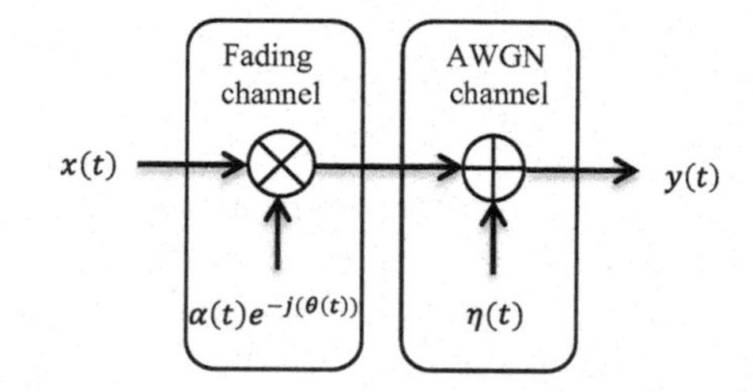

FIGURE 11.5 A basic communication channel.

unsupervised learning, and reinforcement learning. Intelligent data analytics (DA) is the ability of m-healthcare network to gather, analyze, and predict the status of wireless environment using supervised and unsupervised learning.

Supervised learning is a suitable technique to train using labeled data or historical data. A general rule to map input to output is established with past inputs and their corresponding outputs. Therefore, application of supervised learning to deal with channel estimation is accepted as a suitable method.

Consider a frequency nonselective and slow-fading communication channel in an m-healthcare network as shown in Figure 11.5. The medical data collected by a biomedical device are transmitted in the form of signal $x(t)$. The transmitted signal undergoes fading in which magnitude variation and phase shift are constant over at least symbol duration. Hence, the received signal $y(t)$ in faded additive white Gaussian noise (AWGN) channel can be expressed as

$$y(t) = \alpha(t)e^{-j(\theta(t))}x(t) + \eta(t) \tag{11.1}$$

where $\alpha(t)$, $\theta(t)$, and $\eta(t)$ are channel gain, phase shift, and AWGN, respectively. Coherent or noncoherent receiver can be opted to detect the information based on whether accurate channel estimation is possible. In supervised learning, the receiver can exploit the known signal $x(t)$ for some point of time and the corresponding received signal $y(t)$ to estimate the CSI using probabilistic model. Kalman filtering, Bayes learning, and particle filter approach are well-known learning methods in wireless networks.

In unsupervised learning, training is carried out with unlabeled data in which the available data do not possess a priori information. It explores the unlabeled data available and retrieves hidden structure in the data, and finds its suitable representation in the available data. Consider communication among multi-antenna biomedical devices where a time-invariant MIMO channel is assumed. The channel matrix of this generic MIMO system with N_t transmitting antennas and N_r receiving antennas is denotes by:

$$\boldsymbol{H} = \begin{bmatrix} h_{11} & h_{12} & \cdots & h_{1N_t} \\ h_{21} & h_{22} & \cdots & h_{2N_t} \\ \vdots & \vdots & \cdots & \vdots \\ h_{N_r1} & h_{N_r2} & \cdots & h_{N_rN_t} \end{bmatrix} \tag{11.2}$$

where h_{ij} is the transfer function or channel gain corresponding from ith transmitting antenna to jth receiving antenna. A stream of encoded data from a biomedical device is passed to N_t transmitting antennas from which the signal propagates over a frequency-flat quasi-static wireless channel. In this case, the channel gain is not a random but just a scalar value. Let $\boldsymbol{x}$ and · denote the transmitted signal vector and channel noise vector, respectively. The vector representation of the received signal is of the following form:

$$\boldsymbol{y} = \boldsymbol{Hx} + \boldsymbol{\eta} \tag{11.3}$$

Singular-value decomposition (SVD) is a prominent method used in MIMO detection, which can convert the MIMO channel into a parallel channel as shown in Figure 11.6. Unlike the eigenvalue decomposition, SVD supports square and rectangular matrices. In general, SVD decomposes a given matrix into a combination of three matrices. That is, the SVD of channel matrix $\boldsymbol{H}$ is written as:

$$\boldsymbol{H} = \boldsymbol{W} \Sigma \boldsymbol{U}^T \tag{11.4}$$

where $\boldsymbol{W}$ is the unitary matrix describing the row space with left singular vectors, Σ is the diagonal matrix with singular values corresponding to the strength of different eigenmodes, and $\boldsymbol{U}$ is the unitary matrix corresponding to the column space containing right singular vectors. The received signal vector is rewritten as follows:

$$\boldsymbol{y} = \boldsymbol{W} \Sigma \boldsymbol{U}^T \boldsymbol{x} + \boldsymbol{\eta} \tag{11.5}$$

Now, $\boldsymbol{W}^T$ is multiplied with $\boldsymbol{y}$, and yields:

$$\begin{aligned} \boldsymbol{W}^T \boldsymbol{y} &= \boldsymbol{W}^T \boldsymbol{W} \Sigma \boldsymbol{U}^T \boldsymbol{x} + \boldsymbol{W}^T \eta \\ &= \Sigma \boldsymbol{U}^T \boldsymbol{x} + \boldsymbol{W}^T \eta \end{aligned} \tag{11.6}$$

In order to diagonalize the channel $\boldsymbol{H}$, the transmitted signal vector is modified from $\boldsymbol{x}$ to $\boldsymbol{Ux}$. The new received signal vector is then:

$$\tilde{\boldsymbol{y}} = \boldsymbol{HUx} + \eta \tag{11.7}$$

As stated before, the multiplication of $\boldsymbol{W}^T$ diagonalizes the channel which is described as:

$$\begin{aligned} \boldsymbol{y} &= \boldsymbol{W}^T \tilde{\boldsymbol{y}} = \boldsymbol{W}^T \boldsymbol{HUx} + \boldsymbol{W}^T \eta \\ &= \boldsymbol{W}^T \boldsymbol{W} \Sigma \boldsymbol{U}^T \boldsymbol{Ux} + \boldsymbol{W}^T \eta \\ &= \Sigma \boldsymbol{x} + \boldsymbol{W}^T \eta \end{aligned} \tag{11.8}$$

where the matrix Σ contains the number of nonzero diagonal elements equal to the number of eigenmodes or transmitting antennas in each biomedical device. The number of nonzero elements is also equal to the rank of the channel matrix $\boldsymbol{H}$. The squared singular diagonal elements are the eigenvalues of the $\boldsymbol{H}$ matrix. From the above procedure, it is very clear that biomedical signal vector is $\boldsymbol{x}$. The precoded biomedical signal vector $\boldsymbol{Ux}$ is transmitted, which undergoes fading, and the corresponding received signal vector is $\tilde{\boldsymbol{y}}$. Furthermore, $\tilde{\boldsymbol{y}}$ is manipulated with the aid of SVD, which yields $\Sigma \boldsymbol{x}$ in the absence of AWGN component, and eventually, the

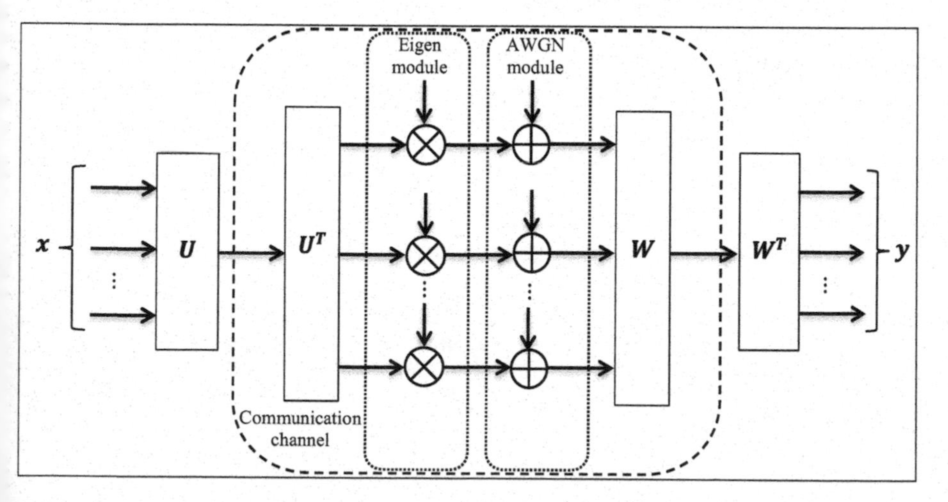

FIGURE 11.6 MIMO channel decomposition.

decoded signal vector $\boldsymbol{x}$ is obtained. In this unsupervised learning, the hidden pattern or structure in the received signal is explored with the help of characterization of channel matrix $\boldsymbol{H}$ using SVD to identify the exact transmitted data.

Machine learning, without proper optimization algorithms, lacks the ability to interacting with environment in solving configuration, uncertainty, and self-healing problems in mobile network. AI can enhance key performances of mobile devices with the network functions, such as sensing, mining, prediction, and reasoning. Therefore, intelligent aware network can support alternative options to the time-varying behavior of the network. The appropriate AI algorithms that are not in place would leave the intelligent computing at stake. The following section explores various AI modules and potential algorithms required to evolve the future m-healthcare applications and services.

11.4 ARTIFICIAL NEURAL NETWORK ALGORITHM IN MACHINE LEARNING

Machine learning is a prominent method of nonlinear computation that is easily implemented with the aid of ANN. Moreover, ANN-based machine learning (ANN-ML) can make use of unsupervised, supervised, and reinforcement learning methods in different m-healthcare services. ANN is a suitable candidate to investigate and predict patient or m-healthcare network behavior. Deep neural network (DNN), spiking neural network (SNN), and recurrent neural network (RNN) are vital ANN techniques recommended for solving wireless physical layer problems, which is presented in Table 11.1. Especially, Deep learning-based algorithms are in use to render a response to combat virus-creating pandemic situation. ANN-ML supports intelligent function in various levels of m-health networks, which include system level, user-centric, and physical layer services.

In system level, in the user context, intelligent monitoring of patients is carried out by learning from the collected data and it predicts the nature of problem that one faces. Apart from this, traffic congestion, behavior of wireless channel, and composition of m-healthcare network are also some of the parameters learned by ANN-ML in system level. This kind of intelligent learning is useful to achieve the predefined objectives, such as low latency and QoS, of the m-healthcare network. Intelligent

TABLE 11.1
ANN-ML Techniques Recommended for Physical Layer Problems

Issues	Intelligent Tool		
	DNN	RNN	SNN
Channel modeling and estimation	DA		DA
Antenna tilting	DA &RL		DA &RL
Resource allocation	RL	RL	
LOS detection	DA		DA
Wireless user behavior estimation	DA	DA	

learning from collected data opens the opportunity for data-driven network operation, decision, and optimization.

Another system-level intelligent function is ANN-ML-based intelligent resource management. From wireless communication point of view, resource handling problems related to spectrum allocation, power control, multiple radio access, cell assignment, diversity, and beamforming are needed to be addressed for improving the efficiency of the m-healthcare network. Conventional methods adopted to resolve such issues involve distributed optimization technique, which is executed either in offline or semi-offline mode. In contrast, the ANN-ML-based intelligent resource management tool is designed with fully online mode of learning. Also, it is a suitable choice for resolving such problems, which extends self-organization and optimization solutions for m-healthcare network decision-making. The ANN-ML- driven network decision-making candidature for next-generation wireless system is going to be a big boom for the m-healthcare services in near future.

The range of user-centric applications of ANN-ML in m-healthcare system varies from device to network level. Consider an example of providing emergency health services to a person from a distant destination who needs an urgent intensive care. In this case ,the intelligent tool at the base station can be used to analyze and study the behavior of the ambulance service. In a short period of time, the mobility pattern of the ambulance is predicted, which allows the optimization of m-healthcare network resources. From the real-time traffic information, the base station takes the intelligent aware decision to reroute the ambulance through the shortest route with least traffic intensity.

The physical layer intelligent function supported by ANN-ML considers selection and implementation of modulation and coding techniques. This tool ensures achieving target bit error rate (BER) to increase the reliability of data collected through implantable, injectable, ingestible, and wearable healthcare mobile devices. In addition, it improves the robustness to impediments caused by multipath wireless channel. Hence, intelligent prediction capable ANN is necessary to harvest its full potential with machine learning to combat the problem of inaccuracy in CSI estimation.

11.5 DEEP LEARNING FOR A DOUBLY SELECTIVE CHANNEL IN M-HEALTHCARE NETWORK

In m-healthcare scenario, signals transmitted from biomedical devices undergo a doubly selective fading. The accuracy of detected data relies on the channel estimation algorithm employed in the m-healthcare network. Basis expansion model (BEM) is a widely accepted method to characterize the doubly selective channel. Least square (LS), recursive LS, minimum mean square error (MMSE), and linear MMSE are examples of BEM-based estimators. Consider that the transmitted signal undergoes rich scattering with A_v, φ_v, and θ_v, respectively, amplitude, angle of arrival, and random phase of the vth propagation path. For a maximum Doppler shift of f_{max}, the doubly selective fading channel, partially characterized by Jakes model, is represented as:

$$h(t,\tau)=\sum_{m=0}^{M}\sum_{v=1}^{V}A_{m,v}e^{\left[j\left(\varphi_{m,v}+2\pi f_{max}\cos\left(\theta_{m,v}t\right)\right)\right]}\delta\left(\tau-\tau_m\right) \tag{11.9}$$

where $A_{m,v}$, $\varphi_{m,v}$, $\theta_{m,v}$, and τ_m are multipath-dependent amplitude, angle of arrival, random phase, and time delay, respectively. Let $h(i,m)$ denote the discrete time equivalent of the above channel, and $\eta(i)$ denote the AWGN component, then the linear time-varying convolution between ith transmitted symbol $x(i)$ and $h(i,m)$ yields the received symbol $y(i)$, which is in the form:

$$y(i)=\sum_{m=1}^{M}h(i,m)x(i-m)+\eta(i) \tag{11.10}$$

The classical estimators support only linear, mathematically modeled channel. The time-varying and time dispersive nature of doubly selective channel presented above leads to nonlinearity in the channel response. The imperfection caused by this nonlinear behavior degrades the performance of the network when classical channel estimation algorithms are employed. The powerful learning capability of DNN for nonlinear channel is greatly supported by its more number of neurons and hidden layers. The DNN approach is recognized for solving issues such as CSI feedback, modulation, channel encoding and decoding, beamforming, etc. Moreover, the data-driven approach of DNN makes the deep learning-based algorithms highly robust to channel imperfection due to doubly selectivity. Their proved superior performance in physical layer design and low computational complexity attract deep learning algorithms in channel estimation.

Let us discuss the role of fully connected feed-forward DNN in channel estimation. DNN-based online deep learning algorithm takes advantages of classical estimator and makes use of previous estimate to exploit the variation in the channel. In addition, more features are extracted from received signal and pilot transmission. DNN is trained in offline during pretraining to initialize the process, and then trained with simulated data in training stage. Next, in testing stage, without prior knowledge of the channel statistics, the DNN is trained using pilot in online to track the dynamic channel. This approach is highly suitable for high-mobility scenarios where the channel is assumed to be nonstationary due to frequent movement of wearable devices.

Consider a frame of biomedical symbol transmission which contains several blocks of data. Each information block, denoted by $\boldsymbol{x}(n)$, consists of pilot symbols, information symbols, and zero padding to tackle multipath fading.

The received symbols in vector form are written as:

$$\boldsymbol{y}(n)=\boldsymbol{H}(n)\boldsymbol{x}_{sp}(n)+\eta(n) \tag{11.11}$$

where $\boldsymbol{H}(n)$, $\boldsymbol{x}_{sp}(n)$, and $\eta(n)$, respectively, are channel transfer function, pilot cum information term, and AWGN component. The deep learning algorithm is aimed at

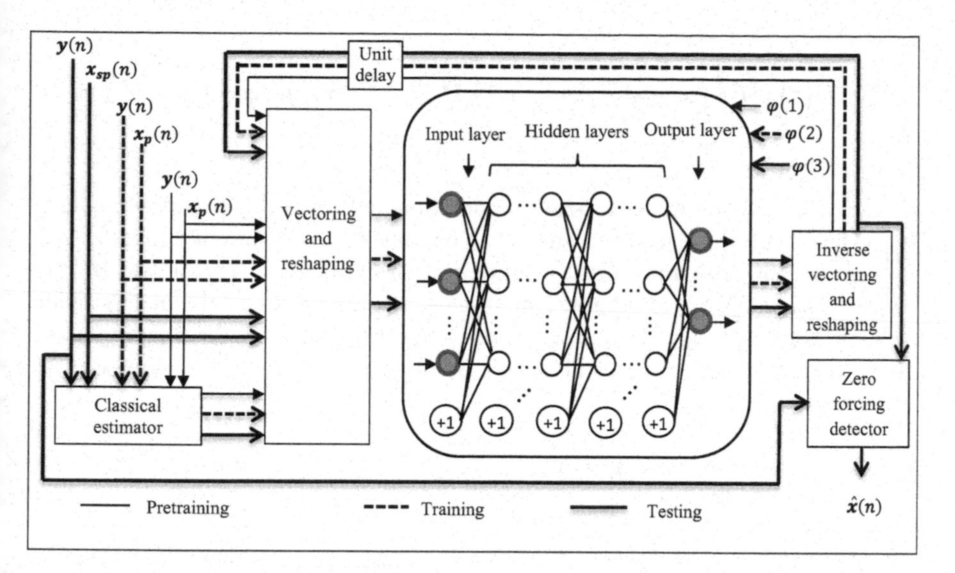

FIGURE 11.7 Deep learning stages in channel estimation.

estimating the channel parameter $\boldsymbol{H}(n)$, which is depicted in Figure 11.7. The DNN structure includes several hidden layers, one input layer, and one output layer. More number of neurons and one bias unit are present in each layer.

DNN with random initialization limits the performance due to poor functioning of optimization algorithm. Therefore, the desirable weight initialization for the DNN training is achieved in pretraining stage. Let $z_1(n)$ and $\boldsymbol{e}_1(n)$ are the input and labels belonging to the DNN. The output/estimate of the DNN is given by:

$$\hat{e}_1(n) = p_{J-1}\left(\dots p_1\left(z_1(n);\varphi_1\right);\varphi_{J-1}\right) \tag{11.12}$$

where $p_1\left(z_1(n);\varphi_1\right)$ is the output and φ_j denotes the parameters of the jth layer. The corresponding loss function using L_1norm is represented as follows:

$$Loss(\varphi) = \frac{1}{VL_e}\sum_{v=0}^{V-1}\hat{z}_1(n) - z_1(n)_1 \tag{11.13}$$

where V is the size of the batch of data processed by deep learning algorithm and L_e is the length of the DNN label vector $\boldsymbol{e}_1(n)$. The optimal $\varphi \triangleq \left\{\varphi_j\right\}_{j=1}^{J-1}$ can be obtained by minimizing the loss function $Loss(\varphi)$ through offline training. Adaptive moment estimation, stochastic gradient descent, and root mean square propagation are some of the optimization algorithms suitable to minimize $Loss(\varphi)$. The input data given to the DNN during pretraining can be written as follows:

$$z_1(n) = f_R\left(\left[x_{sp}(n)^T, y(n)^T, vec\left(\hat{H}_{ce}^{sp}(n)\right)^T, vec\left(\hat{H}_1(n-1)\right)^T\right]^T\right) \tag{11.14}$$

where vec and f_R are the vectorization operation and reshaping function, respectively. Here the input data are reshaped to operate the DNN in real domain. Also it is assumed that the transmitted pilot cum information $x_{sp}(n)$ is known. $\hat{H}_{ce}^{sp}(n)$ is the classical estimator output, and $\hat{H}_1(n-1)$ is the previous channel estimate in the pretraining stage. Using the inverse of vectroization and reshaping operations, the estimated channel from the DNN output $\hat{e}_1(n)$ can be expressed as follows:

$$\hat{H}_1(n) = vec^{-1}\left(f_R^{-1}\left(\hat{e}_1(n)\right)\right) \tag{11.15}$$

In this pretraining stage, the initial parameters $\varphi(1)$ are applied to the DNN, and by adaptive moment estimation algorithm $Loss(\varphi)$ is minimized; therefore, converged parameters $\varphi(2)$ are obtained at the end of pretraining.

The second stage is DNN training with initial parameters $\varphi(2)$. The input data given to DNN in the training stage can be written as follows:

$$z_2(n) = f_R\left(\left[x_p(n)^T, y(n)^T, vec\left(\hat{H}_{ce}^{p}(n)\right)^T, vec\left(\hat{H}_2(n-1)\right)^T\right]^T\right) \tag{11.16}$$

It is assumed that the transmitted pilot $x_p(n)$ is known, but the information is unknown. $\hat{H}_{ce}^{p}(n)$ is the classical estimator output, and $\hat{H}_2(n-1)$ is the previous channel estimate in the training stage. The estimated channel $\hat{H}_2(n)$ from the DNN output $\hat{e}_2(n)$ is $vec^{-1}\left(f_R^{-1}\left(\hat{e}_2(n)\right)\right)$. The time correlation of the nonstationary channel is learned by the previous estimated channel in DNN training; furthermore, this detail is merged with the present data to increase the accuracy of $\hat{H}_2(n)$. The optimization algorithm runs until the DNN converges, and the parameters $\varphi(3)$ are obtained at the end of training.

In the third stage, the trained DNN is loaded with the parameter $\varphi(3)$ obtained from the previous stage. The transmitted pilot $x_p(n)$, the received vector $y(n)$, the classical estimator output $\hat{H}_{ce}^{p}(n)$, and the previous channel estimate $\hat{H}(n-1)$ are given as input to the DNN, which is mathematically expressed as follows:

$$z_3(n) = f_R\left(\left[x_p(n)^T, y(n)^T, vec\left(\hat{H}_{ce}^{p}(n)\right)^T, vec\left(\hat{H}(n-1)\right)^T\right]^T\right) \tag{11.17}$$

The estimated channel $\hat{H}(n)$ from the DNN output $\hat{e}_3(n)$ is $vec^{-1}\left(f_R^{-1}\left(\hat{e}_3(n)\right)\right)$. The estimate of transmitted information, denoted by $\hat{x}(n)$, is obtained from a linear detector. The BER evaluation and robustness test of deep learning-based algorithm can be performed, respectively, by considering the same channel statistics and different channel statistics. A notable performance improvement is recorded by deep learning compared with classical estimators, and the traditional channel estimators built on shallow RNN. Therefore, deep learning-based AI-empowered m-healthcare network will successfully act as the center of digital world in the near future.

11.6 CONCLUSION

The health monitoring devices became modernized after the development of 4G wireless standardization. The mobile device entry in the household list of the present society has taken another leap in the health monitoring. Devices in the form of wearable, implantable, ingestible, injectable, etc., devices remind us about specific needs of mobile health among people in both developed and developing countries. The radio technology is being developed for m-healthcare services, and they are aimed at meeting various system-level requirements involving the technologies, such as power amplifiers, wearable antennas with MIMO and reconfigurable beam arrays, and narrow beams with the support of millimeter wave band.

This chapter detailed a spectrum of AI healthcare on wireless access aspect. Firstly, a discussion on m-healthcare services and challenges associated with them is presented to understand the necessity of AI in the device and network level. Secondly, nonlinear characteristics of the wireless channel, challenges in the upcoming wireless access technology, and contribution of machine learning to solve the issues arising from the fading effect of the channel are elaborated. Next, the role of ANN-based machine learning in m-healthcare network is briefed. Finally, unresolved problems in the existing doubly selective channel estimation methods are discussed, and a deep learning-based solution for such problems is presented for further discussion. It is assured that a humble attempt made in this chapter to explore the widespread use of healthcare system with AI assistance would successfully ignite the minds of academicians, researchers, and practitioners.

BIBLIOGRAPHY

1. A. Ahad, M. Tahir and K. A. Yau, "5G-Based Smart Healthcare Network: Architecture, Taxonomy, Challenges and Future Research Directions," *IEEE Access*, vol. 7, pp. 100747–100762, 2019, doi: 10.1109/ACCESS.2019.2930628.
2. N. F. M. Aun, P. J. Soh, A. A. Al-Hadi, M. F. Jamlos, G. A. E. Vandenbosch and D. Schreurs, "Revolutionizing Wearables for 5G: 5G Technologies: Recent Developments and Future Perspectives for Wearable Devices and Antennas," *IEEE Microwave Magazine*, vol. 18, no. 3, pp. 108–124, May 2017, doi: 10.1109/MMM.2017.2664019.
3. M. Chen, U. Challita, W. Saad, C. Yin and M. Debbah, "Artificial Neural Networks-Based Machine Learning for Wireless Networks: A Tutorial," *IEEE Communications Surveys & Tutorials*, vol. 21, no. 4, pp. 3039–3071, 2019, doi: 10.1109/COMST.2019.2926625.
4. Y. Chong, W. Ismail, K. Ko and C. Lee, "Energy Harvesting for Wearable Devices: A Review," *IEEE Sensors Journal*, vol. 19, no. 20, pp. 9047–9062, 15 October 2019, doi: 10.1109/JSEN.2019.2925638.

5. M. B. Jamshidi, A. Lalbakhsh, J. Talla, Z. Peroutka et al., "Artificial Intelligence and COVID-19: Deep Learning Approaches for Diagnosis and Treatment," *IEEE Access*, doi: 10.1109/ACCESS.2020.3001973.
6. Z. Jia, W. Cheng and H. Zhang, "A Partial Learning-Based Detection Scheme for Massive MIMO," *IEEE Wireless Communications Letters*, vol. 8, no. 4, pp. 1137–1140, August 2019, doi: 10.1109/LWC.2019.2909019.
7. G. Jia, Z. Yang, H. Lam, J. Shi and M. Shikh-Bahaei, "Channel Assignment in Uplink Wireless Communication Using Machine Learning Approach," *IEEE Communications Letters*, vol. 24, no. 4, pp. 787–791, April 2020, doi: 10.1109/LCOMM.2020.2968902.
8. W. Jiang and H. D. Schotten, "Deep Learning for Fading Channel Prediction," *IEEE Open Journal of the Communications Society*, vol. 1, pp. 320–332, 2020, doi: 10.1109/OJCOMS.2020.2982513.
9. G. Karageorgos et al., "The Promise of Mobile Technologies for the Health Care System in the Developing World: A Systematic Review," *IEEE Reviews in Biomedical Engineering*, vol. 12, pp. 100–122, 2019, doi: 10.1109/RBME.2018.2868896.
10. M. G. Kibria, K. Nguyen, G. P. Villardi, O. Zhao, K. Ishizu and F. Kojima, "Big Data Analytics, Machine Learning, and Artificial Intelligence in Next-Generation Wireless Networks," *IEEE Access*, vol. 6, pp. 32328–32338, 2018, doi: 10.1109/ACCESS.2018.2837692.
11. K. B. Letaief, W. Chen, Y. Shi, J. Zhang and Y. A. Zhang, "The Roadmap to 6G: AI Empowered Wireless Networks," *IEEE Communications Magazine*, vol. 57, no. 8, pp. 84–90, August 2019, doi: 10.1109/MCOM.2019.1900271.
12. R. Li et al., "Intelligent 5G: When Cellular Networks Meet Artificial Intelligence," *IEEE Wireless Communications*, vol. 24, no. 5, pp. 175–183, October 2017, doi: 10.1109/MWC.2017.1600304WC.
13. L. Liang, H. Ye, G. Yu and G. Y. Li, "Deep-Learning-Based Wireless Resource Allocation with Application to Vehicular Networks," *Proceedings of the IEEE*, vol. 108, no. 2, pp. 341–356, February 2020, doi: 10.1109/JPROC.2019.2957798.
14. T. Maksymyuk, J. Gazda, M. Ružička, E. Slapak, G. Bugar and L. Han, "Deep Learning Based Mobile Network Management for 5G and Beyond," *2020 IEEE 15th International Conference on Advanced Trends in Radioelectronics, Telecommunications and Computer Engineering (TCSET)*, Lviv-Slavske, Ukraine, 2020, pp. 890–893, doi: 10.1109/TCSET49122.2020.235565.
15. M. Mehrabi, M. Mohammadkarimi, M. Ardakani and Y. Jing, "Deep Adaptive Transmission for Internet of Vehicles (IoV)," *2020 International Conference on Computing, Networking and Communications (ICNC),* Big Island, HI, USA, 2020, pp. 363–367, doi: 10.1109/ICNC47757.2020.9049784.
16. M. Mehrabi, M. Mohammadkarimi, M. Ardakani and Y. Jing, "Decision Directed Channel Estimation Based on Deep Neural Network k -Step Predictor for MIMO Communications in 5G," *IEEE Journal on Selected Areas in Communications*, vol. 37, no. 11, pp. 2443–2456, November 2019, doi: 10.1109/JSAC.2019.2934004.
17. B. Mohanta, P. Das and S. Patnaik, "Healthcare 5.0: A Paradigm Shift in Digital Healthcare System Using Artificial Intelligence, IOT and 5G Communication," *2019 International Conference on Applied Machine Learning (ICAML)*, Bhubaneswar, India, 2019, pp. 191–196, doi: 10.1109/ICAML48257.2019.00044.
18. A. F. Molisch, *Wireless Communications*. New York: Wiley, 2005.
19. T. S. Rappaport, *Wireless Communications*. Upper Saddle River, NJ: Prentice Hall PTR, 2001.

20. F. Tang, Y. Kawamoto, N. Kato and J. Liu, "Future Intelligent and Secure Vehicular Network Toward 6G: Machine-Learning Approaches," *Proceedings of the IEEE*, vol. 108, no. 2, pp. 292–307, February 2020, doi: 10.1109/JPROC.2019.2954595.
21. H. Viswanathan and P. E. Mogensen, "Communications in the 6G Era," *IEEE Access*, vol. 8, pp. 57063–57074, 2020, doi: 10.1109/ACCESS.2020.2981745.
22. T. Wang, L. Zhang and S. C. Liew, "Deep Learning for Joint MIMO Detection and Channel Decoding," *2019 IEEE 30th Annual International Symposium on Personal, Indoor and Mobile Radio Communications (PIMRC),* Istanbul, Turkey, 2019, pp. 1–7, doi: 10.1109/PIMRC.2019.8904390.
23. S. Xia and Y. Shi, "Intelligent Reflecting Surface for Massive Device Connectivity: Joint Activity Detection and Channel Estimation," *ICASSP 2020 – 2020 IEEE International Conference on Acoustics, Speech and Signal Processing (ICASSP)*, Barcelona, Spain, 2020, pp. 5175–5179, doi: 10.1109/ICASSP40776.2020.9054415.
24. Y. Yang, F. Gao, X. Ma and S. Zhang, "Deep Learning-Based Channel Estimation for Doubly Selective Fading Channels," *IEEE Access*, vol. 7, pp. 36579–36589, 2019, doi: 10.1109/ACCESS.2019.2901066.

12 Computational Intelligence in the Identification of COVID-19 Patients

Shaymaa Adnan Abdulrahman and Abdel-Badeeh M. Salem

CONTENTS

12.1 INTRODUCTION

The testing of coronavirus disease 2019 (COVID-19) is currently a difficult task because of the unavailability of diagnosis systems everywhere, which is causing panic. Because of the limited availability of COVID-19 testing kits, we need to rely on other diagnosis measures. As COVID-19 attacks the epithelial cells that line our respiratory tract, we can use medical X-rays to analyze the health of a patient's lung. Medical practitioners frequently use medical X-ray images to diagnose pneumonia, lung inflammation, abscesses, and/or enlarged lymph nodes [1, 2]. Coronavirus refers to a family of viruses that cause respiratory tract diseases and infections, which can be fatal such as COVID-19. Usually there are some kinds of coronaviruses that can also affect animals. In addition, jumps from animal species to humans

Ozturka et al. [3] proposed DarkCovidNet models to provide accurate diagnostics for the classification approach when applied a COVID-19 X-ray image as data set. This data set comprised 43 female and 82 male COVID-19 positive patients. Neural networks (NN) approach was used for extracts features. DarkCovidNet models achieved 87.02% of accuracy. Mohamed et al. [4] analyzed seven deep learning models and studied the performance for each model by applying many of categories of classification such as binary and multiclass. The types of classification are support vector machine (SVM), artificial neural network (ANN), Naive Bayes and random forests. In machine learning approaches, NN model gives the highest detection rate when used (CSE-CIC-IDS2018) as data set. Data mining model used for the prediction of COVID-19-infected patients of South Korea was proposed by Muhammad et al. [5]. In their work, six algorithms (KNN, SVM, logistic regression, Naive Bayes, random forest, and DT) were applied directly on the COVID data set. The authors found that decision tree data mining algorithm is more efficient to predict the infected patients, with an accuracy of 99.85%. Wang et al. [6] used 1,065 computed tomography (CT) images of COVID-19 cases. In that study, accuracy, sensitivity, PPV.NPV, specificity, and area under curve (AUC) were used as markers of the classification process.

Artificial intelligence (AI) has been shown to be an effective tool in the diagnosis of diseases, particularly in emerging corona disease. After the histogram of gradients (HOG) was used as a feature extraction technique, principal component analysis (PCA) was applied in this study to reduce the dimensionality of the data set and to reduce the number of dimensions. Two classifiers (SVM and K-nearest neighbor [KNN]) were applied and compared with each other to find which type of classifier is better in terms of accuracy.

The rest of this chapter is organized as follows: the topics in Section 12.2 include computational intelligence (CI) paradigms and techniques, ANN, SVM, genetic algorithms (GAs), deoxyribo nucleic acid (DNA) computing, evolutionary computing (EC), analogical computing (AC), rough sets computing, fuzzy logic computing, deep learning, and pervasive computing system. Section 12.3 covers materials and methods, data set, feature extraction, and classification methods, while Section 12.4 deals with the study results and analysis. Finally, Section 10.5 concludes the chapter.

12.2 COMPUTATIONAL INTELLIGENCE PARADIGMS AND TECHNIQUES

CI aims to enable computers to learn from data and make improvements without any dependence on commands in a program. This learning could eventually help

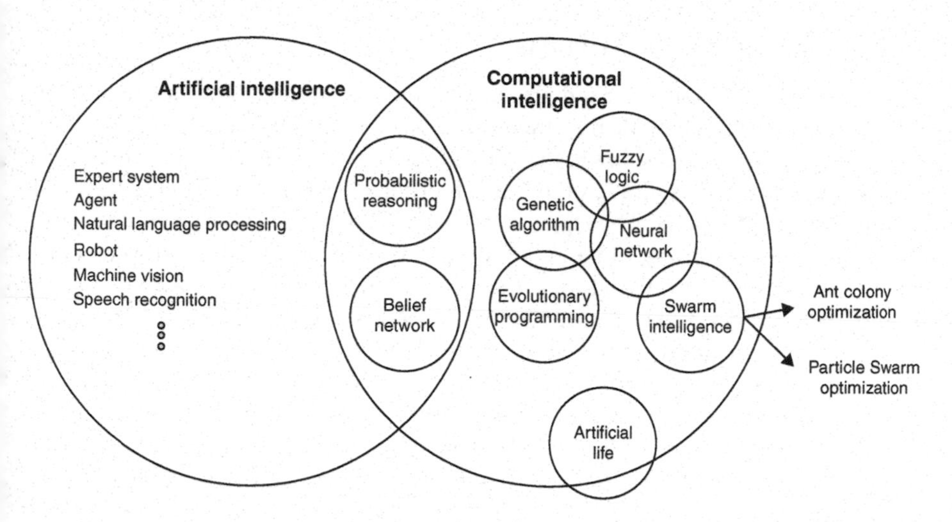

FIGURE 12.1 Computational intelligence techniques.

computers in building models such as those used in the prediction of weather. This section presents a brief account of the well-known CI techniques (see Figure 12.1).

12.2.1 Artificial Neural Networks

ANN is a class of learning algorithms consisting of multiple nodes that communicate through their connecting synapses. NNs imitate the structure of biological systems. ANNs are inspired by biological models of brain functioning [15]. They are capable of learning by examples and generalizing the acquired knowledge. Because of these abilities, NNs are widely used to find out nonlinear relationships that otherwise could not be unveiled due to analytical constraints. The learned knowledge is hidden in their structure and thus it is not possible to be easily extracted and interpreted. The structure of the multilayered perception, that is, the number of hidden layers and the number of neurons, determines its capacity, while the knowledge about the relationship between input and output data is stored in the weights of connections between neurons. The values of weights are updated in the supervised training process with a set of known and representative values of input–output data samples. ANN can be used for the following medical purposes:

- **Modelling:** simulating and modeling the functions of the brain and neurosenory organs.
- **Signal processing:** bioelectric signal filtering and evaluation.
- **System control and checking:** intelligent artificial machine control and checking based on responses of biological or technical systems given to any signals.
- **Classification tasks:** interpretation of physical and instrumental findings to achieve more accurate diagnosis.
- **Prediction:** provides prognostic information based on retrospective parameter analysis

12.2.2 Support Vector Machines

SVMs are new learning by example paradigms for classification and regression problems [16]. SVMs have demonstrated significant efficiency when compared with NNs. Their main advantage lies in the structure of the learning algorithm which consists of a constrained quadratic optimization problem (QP), thus avoiding the local minima drawback of NN. This approach has its roots in statistical learning theory (SLT) and provides a way to build "optimum classifiers" according to some optimality criterion that is referred to as the maximal margin criterion. An interesting development in SLT is the introduction of the Vapnik–Chervonenkis (VC) dimension, which is a measure of the complexity of the model. Equipped with a sound mathematical background, SVMs treat both the problem of how to minimize complexity in the course of learning and how a high generalization might be attained. This trade-off between complexity and accuracy led to a range of principles to find the optimal compromise. Vapnik and coauthors' work has shown the generalization to be bounded by the sum of the training errors and a term depending on the VC dimension of the learning machine, leading to the formulation of the structural risk minimization (SRM) principle. By minimizing this upper bound, which typically depends on the margin of the classifier, the resulting algorithms lead to high generalization in the learning process.

12.2.3 Genetic Algorithms

GA follows the lead of genetics, reproduction, evolution, and the "survival of the fittest" theory by Darwin. GA is a class of machine learning algorithms that is based on the theory of evolution [17]. GAs provide an approach to learning that is based loosely on simulated evolution. The GA methodology hinges on a population of potential solutions, and as such exploits the mechanisms of natural selection well known in evolution. Rather than searching from general to specific hypothesis or from simple to complex, GA generates successive hypotheses by repeatedly mutating and recombining parts of the best currently known hypotheses. The GA algorithm operates by iteratively updating a poll of hypotheses (population). One each iteration, old members of the population are evaluated according to a fitness function. A new generation is then generated by probabilistically selecting the fittest individuals from the current population. Some of these selected individuals are carried forward into the next-generation population, and others are used as bases for creating new offspring individuals by applying genetic operations such as crossover and mutation.

12.2.4 Evolutionary Computing

EC is an approach to the design of learning algorithms that is structured along the lines of the theory of evolution. A collection of potential solutions for a problem compete with each other. The best solutions are selected and combined with each other according to a kind of "survival of the fittest" strategy. Gas are a well-known variant of evolutionary computation [17].

12.2.5 DNA Computing

DNA computing is essential computation that uses biological molecules rather than traditional silicon chips. In recent years, DNA computing has been a research tool for solving complex problems. Despite this, it is still not easy to understand. The main idea behind DNA computing is to adopt a biological (wet) technique as an efficient computing vehicle, where data are represented using strands of DNA. Even though a DNA reaction is much slower than the cycle time of a silicon-based computer, the inherently parallel processing offered by the DNA process plays an important role. This massive parallelism of DNA processing is of particular interest to solving NP-complete or NP-hard problems [18, 19].

It is not uncommon to encounter molecular biological experiments that involve 6 × 1016/ml of DNA molecules. This means that we can effectively realize 60,000 terabytes of memory, assuming that each string of a DNA molecule expresses one character. The total execution speed of a DNA computer can outshine that of a conventional electronic computer, even though the execution time of a single DNA molecule reaction is relatively slow. A DNA computer is thus suitable for problems such as the analysis of genome information, and the functional design of molecules (where molecules constitute the input data) [20].

DNA computing will solve that problem and serve as an alternative technology. It is also known as molecular computing. This computing uses the processing power of molecular information instead of the conventional digital components. It is one of the non-silicon-based computing approaches. DNA has been shown to have massive processing capabilities that could allow a DNA-based computer to solve complex problems in a reasonable amount of time. DNA computing was proposed by Leonard Adleman, who demonstrated in 1994 that DNA could be applied in computations [21, 22].

12.2.6 Analogical Computing

AC is based on the case-based reasoning (CBR) paradigm. CBR is an analogical reasoning method that provides both a methodology for problem solving and a cognitive model of people [23, 24]. CBR means reasoning from experiences or "old cases" in an effort to solve problems, critique solutions, and explain anomalous situations. The case is a list of features that lead to a particular outcome, for example, the information on a patient history and the associated diagnosis. We feel more comfortable with older doctors because they have seen and treated more patients who have had illnesses similar to ours. CBR is a preferred method of reasoning in dynamically changing situations and other situations where solutions are not clear-cut. [25]. The most commonly used application of CBR is in developing expert systems technology. In CBR expert systems, the system can reason from analogy from the past cases. This system contains "case memory" which contains the knowledge in the form of old cases (experiences). CBR solves new problems by adapting solutions that were used for previous and similar problems. The methodology of CBR directly addresses the problems found in rule-based technology, namely, knowledge acquisition, performance, adaptive solution, and maintenance (Figure 12.2).

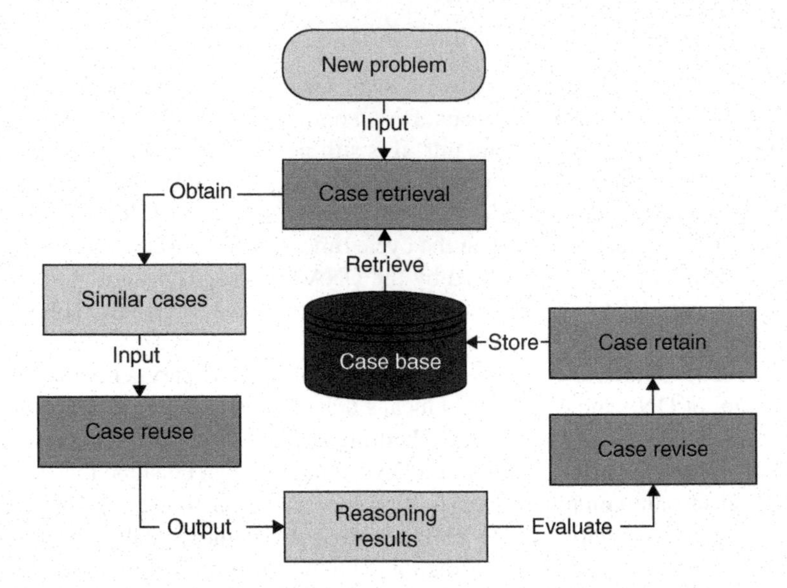

FIGURE 12.2 Case-based reasoning methodology.

According to Kolonder [24], from the computational perspective CBR refers to a number of concepts and techniques (e.g., data structures and intelligent algorithms) that can be used to perform the following operations:

- Record and index cases
- Search cases to identify the ones that might be useful in solving new cases when they are presented
- Modify earlier cases to better match new cases
- Synthesize new cases when they are needed.

12.2.7 Rough Sets Computing

Rough set theory was proposed as a new approach to vague concept description from incomplete data. The rough set theory is one of the most useful techniques in many real-life applications, such as medicine, pharmacology, engineering, banking, and market analysis [26]. This theory provides a powerful foundation to reveal and discover important structures in data and to classify complex objects. In the following, we can summarize the benefits and advantages of rough set theory:

- Deals with vagueness data and uncertainty.
- Deals with reasoning from imprecise data.
- Used to develop a method for discovering relationships in data.
- Provides a powerful foundation to reveal and discover important structures in data and to classify complex objects.
- Does not need any preliminary or additional information about data.
- Concerned with three basics: granularity of knowledge, approximation of sets, and data mining

12.2.8 Fuzzy Logic Computing

In the rich history of rule-based reasoning in AI, the inference engines almost without exception were based on Boolean or binary logic. However, in the same way that NNs have enriched the AI landscape by providing an alternative to symbol-processing techniques, fuzzy logic has provided an alternative to Boolean logic-based systems [27]. Unlike the Boolean logic, which has only two states, true or false, fuzzy logic deals with truth values that range continuously from 0 to 1. Thus, something could be half true (0.5) or very likely true (0.9) or probably not true (0.1). The use of fuzzy logic in reasoning systems impacts not only the inference engine but also the knowledge representation itself [28]. For, instead of making arbitrary distinctions between variables and states, as is required with Boolean logic systems, fuzzy logic allows one to express knowledge in a rule format that is close to a natural language expression.

The difference between this fuzzy rule and the Boolean logic rules we used in our forward- and backward chaining examples is that the clauses "temperature is hot" and "humidity is sticky" are not strictly true or false. Clauses in fuzzy rules are real-valued functions called membership functions that map the fuzzy set "hot" onto the domain of the fuzzy variable "temperature" and produce a truth value that ranges from 0.0 to 1.0 (a continuous output value, much like the NNs).

Reasoning with fuzzy rule systems is a forward-chaining procedure. The initial numeric data values are fuzzified, that is, turned into fuzzy values using the membership functions. Instead of a match and conflict resolution phase where we select a triggered rule to fire, in fuzzy systems, all rules are evaluated, because all fuzzy rules can be true to some degree (ranging from 0.0 to 1.0). The antecedent clause truth values are combined using fuzzy logic operators (a fuzzy conjunction or/and operation takes the minimum value of the two fuzzy clauses). Next, the fuzzy sets specified in the consequent clauses of all rules are combined, using the rule truth values as scaling factors. The result is a single fuzzy set, which is then defuzzified to return a crisp output value. More technical details and applications can be found in the recent book of Voskoglou [29].

12.2.9 Deep Learning

Deep learning is a branch of AI covering a spectrum of current exciting research and industrial innovation that provides more efficient algorithms to deal with large-scale data in healthcare, recommender systems, learning theory, robotics, games, neurosciences, computer vision, speech recognition, language processing, human–computer interaction, drug discovery, biomedical informatics etc. [30, 31]. In the last decade, with the development of ANN, many researchers have tried to develop further studies using deep learning methods [32].

12.2.10 Pervasive Computing Systems

Pervasive networking has recently emerged as a new research topic in the area of communication network systems. It mainly involves methods, algorithms, and protocols that enable devices to autonomously self-organize in network structures and use those infrastructures to facilitate the exchange of information and delivery of services [32]. These systems typically communicate via low-cost and energy-efficient ambient wireless technologies so as to enable seamless interaction and service provisioning. The objective of this thematic series is to capture recent developments and publish ongoing research activities in the area of pervasive computing systems.

12.3 MATERIALS AND METHODS

Figure 12.3 presents the proposed research methodology of this work. It consist of four stages: preprocessing, feature extraction, dimensionality reduction, and classification.

Stage 1: Preprocessing – X-ray images diagnosed with COVID-19 have been collected and remove the noise after that segmentation has been applied.

Stage 2: Feature extraction – In medical image processing extracting the features from the X-ray image, it is not possible to extract the feature from a single pixel; it interacts with the neighbors also. Feature extractor is used to extract the feature from chest X-ray images, especially lungs of COVID-19 patients.

Stage 3: Dimensionality reduction process – After extracting the feature from HOG, the PCA will be applied for the dimension reduction of the features.

Stage 4: Classification process – Classify normal and healthy people without lung disease and X-ray images diagnosed with COVID-19 through classifiers such as KNN and SVM.

12.3.1 Data Set

Two data sets were used in this study: COVID-19 (–) taken from Kaggle repository (www.kaggle.com [Accessed March 16, 2020]) [7] and COVID-19(+) collected from the Open-i repository (https://openi.nlm.nih.gov [Accessed March 16, 2020]) [[8, 9]) as shown in Figure 12.4 and Table 12.1.

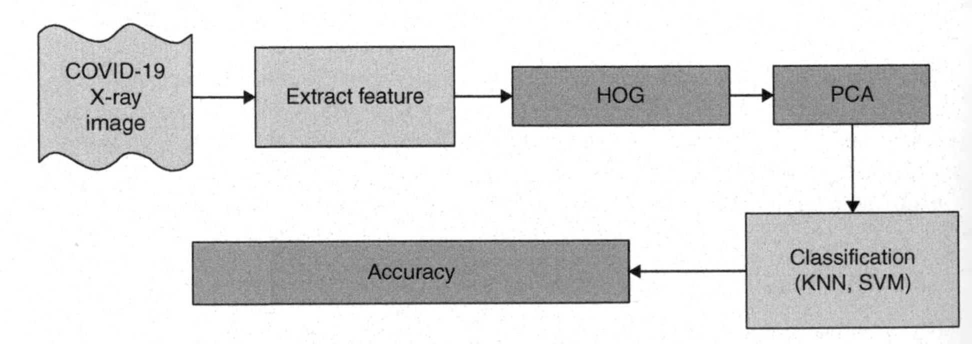

FIGURE 12.3 Flow chart of the proposed work.

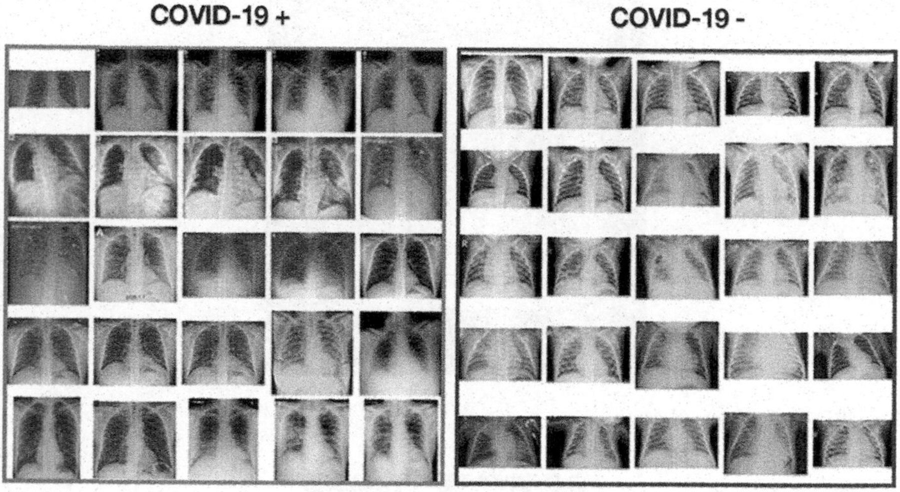

COVID-19 + COVID-19 -

FIGURE 12.4 X-ray of COVID-19(+) and COVID-19(–).

TABLE 12.1
Details of Data Set

Sample	Number	Repository
COVID-19+ without MERS, SARS,ARDS	30	GitHub (Dr. Joseph Cohen)
COVID-19-	30	Kaggle (X-ray images of Pneumonia)

12.3.2 Feature Extraction

12.3.2.1 Histogram of Gradients

HOG depends on the division of the medical image (X-ray image) into small areas called cells [10]. To calculate the edge gradients if 4×4 pixel size cell was selected by default and block size is 8×8, then each of the local cells' (8) orientations are calculated and forms the histogram, of cell then normalize it and normalize the blocks also. A small change is done in the position of window in order to not see the descriptor changing heavily and to get the lesser impact far from center gradients of the descriptors. For each pixel in order to assign a magnitude weight, one half of the width of the descriptor known as sigma is assigned HOG steps in (Matlab) (Figure 12.5).

Implementation **Step1:** Input X-ray medical image (Figure 12.6)

Step 2: Normalize the X-ray image or gamma that is the square root of X-ray image intensity depends on what kind of the X-ray image.

Step 3: Calculate the orientation of gradient and its magnitude.

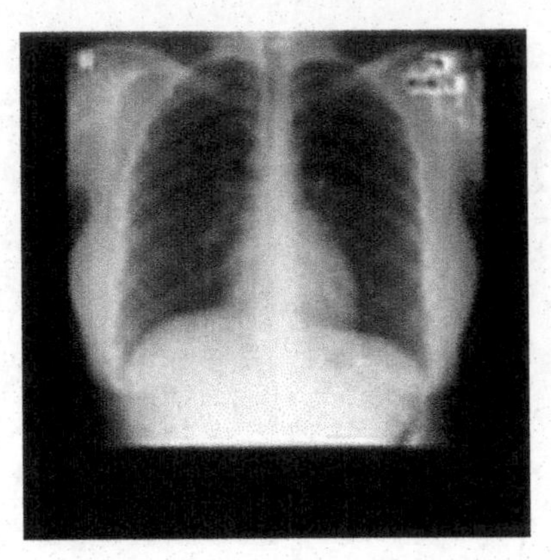

FIGURE 12.5 Input X-ray image.

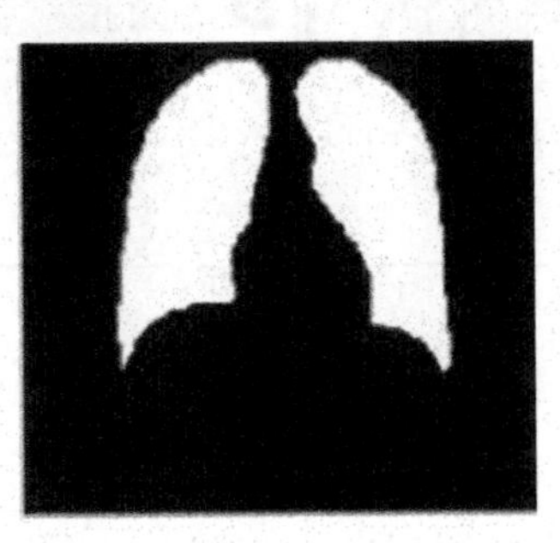

FIGURE 12.6 Gradient computed X-ray image.

Equation 12.1 represents the gradient magnitude while Equation 12.2 represents the gradient direction.

$$(\mathrm{GM}) \| \nabla f(x,y) \| = \sqrt{f_x^2 + f_x^2} \quad (12.1)$$

$$(\mathrm{GD})\, \theta = \tan^{-1} \frac{f_x}{f_y} \quad (12.2)$$

where:

f_x is the derivative with respect to (w.r.t.) x (gradient in the x-direction), f_y is the derivative w.r.t. x (gradient in the y-direction)

Step 4: Create and split the window into cells and each cell represents the pixels and make the histogram of orientation gradient.
Step 5:- Group the cells together into a large one and then normalize it.
Step6:- After extracting data process from HOG, apply the machine learning algorithms or classification process.

12.3.2.2 Principal Component Analysis

After extracting features from the HOG, PCA was applied to reduce the dimensionality of the data set and to reduce the number of dimensions. It utilizes less space. PCA usually helps in the classification of large data set as it takes less time. After reducing the feature space, some noise and redundancies in the features are removed while reducing the dimensionality [11].

12.3.3 Classification Approach

Classification techniques are used to detect the type of disease diagnosis. Classification deals with associating a given input pattern with one of the distinct classes. In this stage, two types of classifier were used in this study: KNN and SVM.

12.3.3.1 K-Nearest Neighbor

KNN is a supervised learning algorithm. It is usually used in machine learning approaches. The best way to classify the feature vectors is to use the closest training as the basis. Being an easy and efficient method that depends on the known samples, it is an important nonparametric, classification approach according to the approximate k-nearest neighbors which classify and specify a class label for unknown samples [12]. If k-nearest = 1, then the object is assigned only to the class of its neighbors, and it can reduce the effect of noise on the major value classification of k-nearest, but can separate the boundaries between the classes.

KNN is classified into testing and training phases.

Training phase:

1. Select the X-ray medical images for the training phase.
2. After that training X-ray medical images will read.
3. Preprocess and resize each X-ray image.
4. Use the preprocessed X-ray medical image to extract the features (through HOG) in order to form a vector of features of X-ray medical image that are local to the image.
5. By the local features, feature vector is constructed of the X-ray medical image as rows in a matrix.
6. Repeat steps 2–5 for all the training X-ray medical images.
7. Train the KNN method for the phase of testing.

Testing phase:

1. Read the images for test.
2. After applying the KNN first, identify the nearest neighbors using the function of Euclidean distance by the training information.
3. If the K neighbors have all the same labels, the image is labeled and exit; otherwise compute pairwise distances between the k-neighbors and construct the distance matrix.

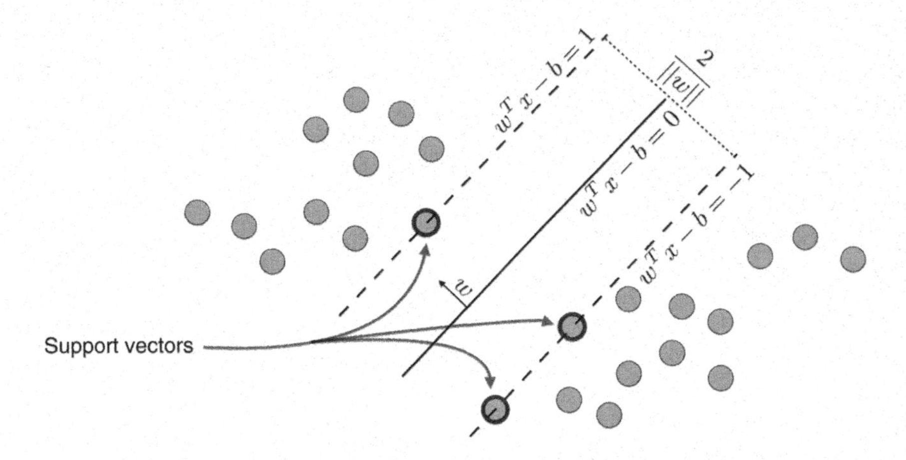

FIGURE 12.7 Support vector machine approach.

12.3.3.2 Support Vector Machine

SVM refers to a binary classifier that uses a hyperplane called the decision boundary between two classes. This hyperplane tries to divide one class containing the target training vector, which is labeled as (+1), and the other class containing the training vectors, which is labeled as (−1). Using these labeled training vectors, the SVM optimizer finds a hyperplane that will then maximize the margin of separation among the two classes [13, 14] (see Figure 12.7).

12.4 RESULT AND ANALYSIS

In this study, we prepared two sets of data sets. The first data set contained 30 number of COVID-19+ and 30 number of COVID-19(−) X-ray medical images. The COVID-19 (+) X-ray medical images were collected from the GitHub repository shared by Dr. Joseph Cohen, a postdoctoral fellow at the University of Montreal [7]. The COVID-19 (−) data sets were the X-ray images of pneumonia collected from Kaggle repository [8]. The COVID-19+ excludes the MERS, SARS, and ARDS. The second data set contains 133 X-ray images of COVID-19 (+) including MERS, SARS, and ARDS. In addition, 133 chest X-ray images were collected from the Open-i repository [9] as COVID-19 (−). The two data sets were examined separately in the proposed models. Two data sets were used for feature extraction based on HOG and PCA. While the SVM was applied to classify the infected lungs from noninfected ones, the experimental studies were implemented using the MATLAB 2015b machine learning toolbox.

In this study, we used a tenfold random cross-validation to evaluate the proposed model and calculated the accuracy of two machine learning algorithms through comparison. Equation 12.3 shows the formula of accuracy. Table 12.2 presents the accuracy between the two classifiers when using the tenfold cross-validation, as shown in Figure 12.8.

TABLE 12.2
The Accuracy of Mortality Prediction in Patients with COVID-19 Using Tenfold Cross-Validation

Classifier	Cross Validation	Accuracy (%)
SVM	Tenfold	89.63
KNN	Tenfold	81.31

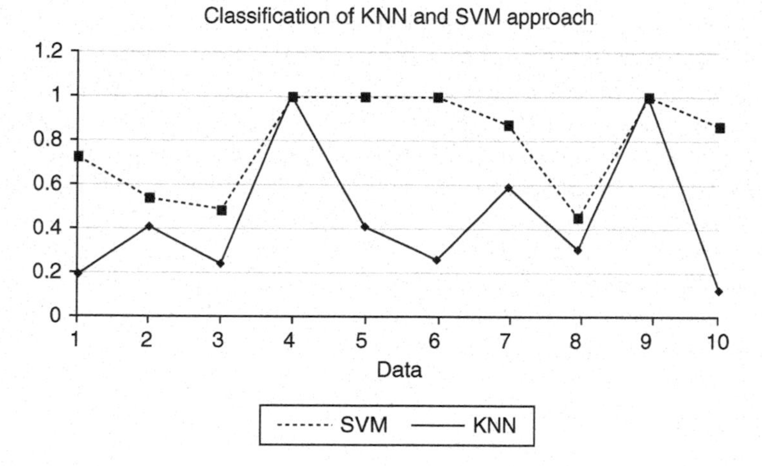

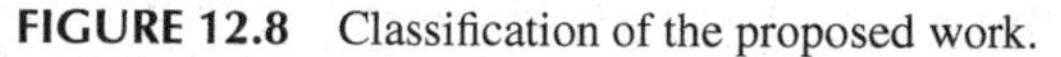

FIGURE 12.8 Classification of the proposed work.

$$\text{Accuracy} = \frac{\text{TP} + \text{TN}}{\text{TP} + \text{TN} + \text{FP} + \text{FN}} \tag{12.3}$$

In addition to analyzing the performance of our proposed system approach, it measures different parameters such as false positive (FP) and false negative (FN) by using equations 12.4 and 12.5, respectively. Table 12.3 shows the results of FP and FN.

$$\text{False Positive} = \frac{\text{FP}}{\text{TP} + \text{TN} + \text{FP} + \text{FN}} \tag{12.4}$$

$$\text{False Negative} = \frac{\text{FN}}{\text{TP} + \text{TN} + \text{FP} + \text{FN}} \tag{12.5}$$

where true positive (TP) is the number of COVID-19 patients that are properly classified, FP is the number of COVID-19 patients that are wrongly classified, true negative (TN) is the number of Flu patients that are properly classified, and FN is the number of Flu patients that are wrongly classified as COVID-19.

TABLE 12.3
Performance Analysis of the Proposed System According to (FP,FN)

Classifier	False Positive	False Negative
SVM	5	7
KNN	6	8

12.5 CONCLUSIONS

AI has the potential to be a tool in the fight against COVID-19 disease and similar pandemics. However, AI systems are still at a preliminary stage to solve COVID-19 problems. In this case of the use of AI within this research, a database must be provided, which would comprise medical images for image analysis and disease diagnosis. For this purpose, two types of data were used. The first type represents people with COVID-19 (infected people), while the second type of data set is for uninfected people. Furthermore, two techniques were used in this study: SVM and KNN. FP and FN were calculated to analyze the proposed work model. Finally, the outcomes are encouraging. The accuracy of detection of COVID-19 with the KNN and SVM is 81.31% and 89.63%, respectively. Through this study, the results showed that the SVM approach is a more reliable method than the KNN.

REFERENCES

1. Lisa Lockerd Maragakis, Johns Hopkins Medicine, "What Is Coronavirus (COVID-19)?", https://www.youtube.com/watch?v=sHP0UIdZyI4&feature=emb_logo [Accessed: 16th March 2020]
2. Shaymaa Adnan Abdulrahman, Abdel-Badeeh M., "A efficient deep belief network for detection of corona virus disease COVID-19" , Vol. 02, No. 01, pp. 05–13, 2020, DOI: 10.5281/zenodo.3931877.
3. Tulin Ozturk, Muhammed Talo, Eylul Azra Yildirim, Ulas Baran Baloglu, Ozal Yildirim, U. Rajendra Acharya, "Automated detection of COVID-19 cases using deep neural networks with X-ray images", *Computers in Biology and Medicine*, 2020, https://doi.org/10.1016/j.compbiomed.2020.103792.
4. Mohamed Amine Ferrag, Leandros Maglaras, Sotiris Moschoyiannis, Helge Janicke, "Deep learning for cyber security intrusion detection: Approaches, datasets, and comparative study", *Journal of Information Security and Applications*, Vol. 50, 2020.
5. L. J. Muhammad Md, Milon Islam, Sani Sharif Usman, Safial Islam Ayon, "Predictive data mining models for novel coronavirus (COVID-19) infected patients' recovery", *SN Computer Science*, 2020.
6. Shuai Wang, Bo Kang, Jinlu Ma, Xianjun Zeng, Mingming Xiao, Jia Guo, Mengjiao Cai, Jingyi Yang, Yaodong Li, Xiangfei Meng, Bo Xu, "A deep learning algorithm using CT images to screen for corona virus disease (COVID-19)", 2020.
7. www.kaggle.com [Accessed:16th March 2020]
8. www.github.com [Accessed: 16th March 2020]
9. https://openi.nlm.nih.gov [Accessed:16th March 2020]
10. Vijay Chandrasekhar, Gabriel Takacs, David M. Chen, Sam S. Tsai, Yuriy Reznik, Radek Grzeszczuk, Bernd Girod, "Compressed histogram of gradients: A low-bitrate descriptor", *International Journal of Computer Vision,* Vol. 96, No. 3, pp 348–399, 2012.

11. Shaymaa Adnan Abdulrahman, Wael Khalifa, Mohamed Roushdy, Abdel-Badeeh M. Salem, "Comparative study for 8 computational intelligence algorithms for human identification", *Journal of Computer Science Review*, Vol. 36, 2020, https://doi.org/10.1016/j.cosrev.2020.100237.
12. Tauno Metsalu, Jaak Vilo, "ClustVis: A web tool for visualizing clustering of multivariate data using principal component analysis and heatmap", *Nucleic Acids Research*, Vol. 43, pp W566–W570, 2015.
13. Shaymaa Adnan Abdulrahman, Mohamed Roushdy, Abdel-Badeeh M. Salem, "Support vector machine approach for human identification based on EEG signals", *Journal of Mechanics of Continua and Mathematical Sciences*, Vol. 15, No. 2, pp. 270–280, February 2020, https://doi.org/10.26782/jmcms.2020.02.00023.
14. Shaymaa Adnan Abdulrahman, Mohamed Roushdy, Abdel-Badeeh M., "Using k-nearest neighbors and support vector machine classifiers in personal identification based on EEG signals", International Journal of Computer Science and Information Security, Vol. 18, No. 5, pp. 29–37, May 2020, https://sites.google.com/site/ijcsis/.
15. S. Simon, Neural Networks and Learning Machines, 3rd Edition, originally published 1993, http://dai.fmph.uniba.sk/courses/NN/haykin.neural-networks.3ed.2009.pdf.
16. C. Cortes, V. Vapnik, "Support vector networks", Machine Learning, Vol. 20, pp. 273–297, 1995.
17. Abdel-Badeeh M. Salem, Abeer M. Mahmoud, "A hybrid genetic algorithm-decision tree classifier", *Proceedings of the 3rd International Conference on New Trends in Intelligent Information Processing and Web Mining*, Zakopane, Poland, pp. 221–232, June 2–5, 2003.
18. L.M. Adleman, "Computing with DNA", *Science*, Vol. 279, pp. 54–61, August 1998.
19. G.H. Paun, G. Rozenberg, A. Salomaa, *DNA Computing: New Computing Paradigms*, Yokomori T (Translated Ed.), Springer, 1999.
20. A. Regalado, "DNA computing", Technology Review, pp. 80–84, May/June 2000.
21. G. Steele, V. Stojkovic, "Agent-oriented approach to DNA computing", *Proceedings of Computational Systems Bioinformatics Conference*, pp. 546–551, 2004.
22. Y. Huang, L. He, "DNA computing research progress and application", *The 6th International Conference on Computer Science & Education*, pp. 232–235, 2011.
23. J.L. Kolodner, "Improving human decision making through case based decision aiding", *AI Magazine*, pp. 52–69, 1991.
24. J. Kolonder, *Case-Based Reasoning*, Morgan Kaufmann, 1993.
25. B. Lopez, E. Plaza, "Case-based planning for medical diagnosis", 1993.
26. Z. Pawlak, *Rough Sets: Theoretical Aspects of Reasoning about Data*, Dordrecht: Kluwer Academic Publishers, 1991.
27. G.J. Klir, T.A. Folger, *Fuzzy Sets, Uncertainty and Information*, London: Prentice Hall International, 1988.
28. T. Mitchell, *Machine Learning*, New York: McGraw-Hill, 1997.
29. Michael Voskoglou, *Special Issue Fuzzy Sets, Fuzzy Logic and Their Applications* (published in Mathematics), 2020, https://doi.org/10.3390/books978-3-03928-521-1.
30. Riccardo Miotto et al., "Deep learning for healthcare: Review, opportunities and challenges", *Briefings in Bioinformatics*, Vol. 19, No. 6, pp. 1236–1246, 2017.
31. Alvin Rajkomar et al., "Scalable and accurate deep learning with electronic health records", *NPJ Digital Medicine*, Vol. 1, No. 1, pp. 18, 2018.
32. Gloria Hyun-Jung Kwak, Pan Hui, "DeepHealth: Deep learning for health informatics reviews, challenges, and opportunities on medical imaging, electronic health records".

Index

Note: Page numbers in *italic* refer to figures, page numbers in **bold** refer to tables.